# PERSPECTIVES ON INDIVIDUAL DIFFERENCES AFFECTING THERAPEUTIC CHANGE IN COMMUNICATION DISORDERS

# PERSPECTIVES ON INDIVIDUAL DIFFERENCES AFFECTING THERAPEUTIC CHANGE IN COMMUNICATION DISORDERS

New Directions in Communication Disorders Research

Edited by **Amy L. Weiss**

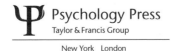

Psychology Press
Taylor & Francis Group

New York   London

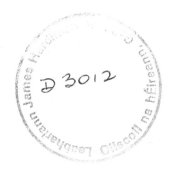

Psychology Press  
Taylor & Francis Group  
270 Madison Avenue  
New York, NY 10016

Psychology Press  
Taylor & Francis Group  
27 Church Road  
Hove, East Sussex BN3 2FA

© 2010 by Taylor and Francis Group, LLC  
Psychology Press is an imprint of Taylor & Francis Group, an Informa business

Printed in the United States of America on acid-free paper  
10 9 8 7 6 5 4 3 2 1

International Standard Book Number: 978-1-84872-887-5 (Hardback)

---

**Library of Congress Cataloging-in-Publication Data**

---

Perspectives on individual differences affecting therapeutic change in communication disorders / editor, Amy L. Weiss.
    p. cm.
    Includes bibliographical references and index.
    ISBN 978-1-84872-887-5 (hbk. : alk. paper)
    1. Communicative disorders--Treatment. 2. Speech therapy. 3. Speech therapist and patient. I. Weiss, Amy L.

RC423.P45 2010
616.85'5--dc22
                         2009042462

---

**Visit the Taylor & Francis Web site at**  
**http://www.taylorandfrancis.com**

**and the Psychology Press Web site at**  
**http://www.psypress.com**

*In memory of my cousin, Pvt. Bernard Bisgeier*
*17th Infantry Battalion*
*12th Armored Division*
*United States Army*
*Harvard University, Class of 1946*
*b. October 7, 1925 (Buffalo, NY)*
*d. December 8, 1944 (French–German border)*

# Contents

# Foreword

We are pleased to present this new volume in our series *New Directions in Research on Communication Disorders: Integrative Approaches.* The purpose of this series is to provide researchers and professionals in the areas of communication development, disability, and related fields with works that supply state-of-the-art information compiled by scientists and practitioners whose goal is to invite collaboration and integrate knowledge on a broad range of emerging issues that pertain to the understanding of human communication and its disorders.

In the present volume, Amy L. Weiss has tackled the difficult question of the role of individual differences in response to intervention for communication disorders. Like so much of the best work in the field, this effort grew out of her clinical experience of trying to understand the differing reactions of clients to her own intervention efforts. From this beginning in creative curiosity, she has assembled a wide-ranging set of not answers but extended discussions that address this crucial issue: What does the client contribute to the outcome of a therapeutic enterprise?

It will surprise no one that the responses to this question by the authors in this volume have a wide range. Some address the issue from the point of view of a particular disorder, such as specific language impairment (Vander Woude, Chapter 5), autism spectrum disorders (Hewitt, Chapter 7), speech sound disorders (Weiss, Chapter 8), cleft lip and palate (Chapman and Hardin-Jones, Chapter 9), dysfluency (Stewart and Leahy, Chapter 10; Hayhow and Shenker, Chapter 11), hearing impairment (Teagle and Eskridge, Chapter 12), and reading disorder (Larrivee and Maloney, Chapter 6). Others come at the question from other angles, such as Brinton and Fujiki's focus on social skill differences (Chapter 2); Capone and Sheng's examination of a particular domain of development, word learning (Chapter 3); and Hammer and Rodríguez's consideration of the role of bilingualism (Chapter 4). Embracing contributions from around the English-speaking world, this compendium of thinking on the subject of individual differences provides one of very few venues for extended consideration of this intriguing but little-studied area.

Although Professor Weiss has focused the discussion here on the client's contribution to the outcome of intervention for disorders of communication, the issues raised will resonate with practitioners from a variety of disciplines that attempt to change human behavior. The capacities clients bring to intervention settings extend beyond parochial concerns of speech therapy to the broader problem of increasing awareness of the ways in which therapists of all stripes come to understand, acknowledge, and build on the skills, interests, and propensities of the complex beings with whom they work. This volume reminds all who attempt to ameliorate behavioral difficulties that these difficulties exist not in isolation or independently but in the context of a person, like any other, with complicated and often conflicting feelings, attitudes, aptitudes, and desires. Only by attempting to understand how this symphony of forces can impact interactions with an equally complicated therapist can we begin to harness these forces in order to maximize clients' achievements of their own goals.

As Professor Weiss so aptly points out, therapy is not only about what the therapist does; it is also about what the client brings to the endeavor and the relationship. Although this term in the equation that predicts therapy outcomes is bafflingly hard to quantify and thus to study systematically, this volume serves as a crucial first step in bringing the issue to the place it belongs, in the forefront of the thinking of any clinician or scholar who seeks to understand how therapy changes behavior. Readers will no doubt be grateful for the guidance on this first leg of what promises to be a long and fascinating journey toward understanding.

**Rhea Paul**

# Contributors

**Bonnie Brinton**, PhD, is professor of communication disorders at Brigham Young University (BYU), Provo, Utah. Her work focuses on language impairment and social communication. Dr. Brinton has been an associate professor at the University of Nevada and BYU, an associate dean in the School of Education at BYU, Dean of Graduate Studies at BYU, and a research scientist at the Parsons Research Center, University of Kansas. She has served as an associate editor for the journal *Language, Speech, and Hearing Services in Schools* and has chaired the American Speech-Language-Hearing Association (ASHA) committee on Language Learning Disabilities. Dr. Brinton is a fellow of the ASHA.

**Nina Capone**, PhD, is an associate professor in the Department of Speech-Language Pathology at Seton Hall University. She earned a BA from Boston University and her MA and PhD from Northwestern University. She has held clinical positions at the Children's Seashore House—Children's Hospital of Philadelphia, Children's Memorial Hospital (Chicago), Bright Futures Early Intervention Clinic (Evanston, IL), and the Westchester Institute for Human Development (Valhalla, NY). In her research, Dr. Capone investigates word learning in young children and the relationship between gesture and language development. She has published in the *Journal of Speech, Language, and Hearing Research* and the *Journal of Child Language*. Dr. Capone presents at national and international conferences (e.g., the American Speech-Language-Hearing Association, the International Association for the Study of Child Language, the Symposium for Research in Child Language Disorders, and the Society for Research in Child Development).Dr. Capone was recently awarded the New Investigators Research grant by the ASHA Foundation.

**Kathy L. Chapman**, PhD, received her doctorate in child language development and disorders from Purdue University. She began her academic career at the University of Montana and then moved to Case Western Reserve University, where she also served as department chair. Dr. Chapman is currently a professor in the Department of Communication Sciences and Disorders at the University of Utah. She has taught courses in language and phonological disorders in young children, cleft palate, and research methods. Her early research focused on children with specific language impairment and more recently on language and phonological development of young children with cleft palate. She is especially interested in the impact of clefting on the developing speech sound system. Dr. Chapman has published numerous data-based articles and given many presentations related to these areas of study. She has served as a reviewer for numerous journals and was associate editor for the *American Journal of Speech-Language Pathology*.

**Hannah Eskridge**, MSP, CCC-SLP, LSLS Cert AVT, is the director of the Center for the Acquisition of Spoken Language Through Listening Enrichment at the University of North Carolina at Chapel Hill (UNC). She directs the professional training program, including presenting on cochlear implantation and auditory habilitation topics and auditory verbal modules. She is also an adjunct professor at UNC. She currently serves as the president-elect on the board of directors for the NC chapter of AG Bell.

**Martin Fujiki**, PhD, is professor of communication disorders at BYU. His work focuses on social competence in children with language impairments. Dr. Fujiki has been an associate professor at the University of Nevada and BYU and a research scientist at the Parsons Research Center, University of Kansas. He has served as an associate editor for the *American Journal of Speech Language Pathology* and the *Journal of Speech, Language, and Hearing Research*. Dr. Fujiki has also served on the ASHA ad hoc committee on social communication. He is a fellow of the ASHA.

**Carol Scheffner Hammer**, PhD, CCC-SLP, received her doctorate in speech pathology from the University of Iowa. She is currently a professor in the Department of Communication Sciences and Disorders at Temple University. Her research focuses on bilingual children's language and literacy development; environmental and cultural influences on children's development; parental beliefs about child rearing and children's language and literacy development; and school readiness interventions. Her work has been funded by the National Institutes of Health, National Institute of Child Health and Human Development; the U.S. Department of Education, Institute of Education Sciences; and the Administration of Children and Families.

**Mary A. Hardin-Jones**, PhD, is a professor in the Division of Communication Disorders at the University of Wyoming. She has been actively involved in the assessment and treatment of children with cleft lip and palate for over 25 years. She is particularly interested in early speech development and treatment outcomes for these children and has numerous presentations and publications pertaining to these topics. She coauthored the fourth edition of *Cleft Palate Speech* in 2009 as well as *The Clinician's Guide to Treating Cleft Palate Speech* in 2006.

**Rosemarie Hayhow**, PhD, has worked in various settings with people who stammer for over 30 years and lectured on disorders of fluency in both under- and postgraduate courses. In the last 10 years she has combined research with clinical work with adults and children who stammer in a local National Health Service Trust in the United Kingdom. She is an advisor for the Royal College of Speech and Language Therapists and the British Stammering Association and a regular contributor to continuing professional development events at the national and local levels. Dr. Hayhow is a member of the Lidcombe Program Trainers' Consortium (LPTC), which trains clinicians in the United Kingdom and in Europe. She has contributed to books, peer review publications, and conferences in areas related to both her research and clinical work. In 2008 Dr. Hayhow completed her doctoral studies, which explored parents' experiences with the Lidcombe Program. She is interested in using qualitative methods to explore children's responsiveness to the Lidcombe Program.

**Lynne E. Hewitt**, PhD, CCC-SLP, is an associate professor in the Department of Communication Disorders at Bowling Green State University, where she has served as graduate coordinator and currently serves as department chair. She writes and researches on the topics of autism, intervention for developmental language disorders, pragmatics, and assessment. She is an associate editor of the journal *Language, Speech, and Hearing Services in the Schools* and is division coordinator for Special Interest Division 1 of the American Speech-Language-Hearing Association, Language Learning and Education. In 2008, she was an Erskine fellow at the University of Canterbury, New Zealand. She frequently presents at national and international meetings on topics related to her research and clinical interests.

**Linda S. Larrivee**, PhD, CCC-SLP, is a professor and department chair in the Department of Communication Sciences and Disorders, Worcester State College (WSC), Worcester, MA. Prior to joining the faculty at WSC, she served as a school-based clinician for several years and held a faculty position in the Department of Communication Science and Disorders at the University of Missouri—Columbia. She has written and presented extensively both nationally and internationally on issues related to phonological awareness, emergent literacy, language impairments and reading disabilities in school-aged children, and psychometric issues associated with assessment, including limitations of age-equivalent scores. Her current research examines English language acquisition in international adoptees.

**Margaret M. Leahy**, MSc, MLitt, MA was formerly head of the Department of Clinical Speech & Language Studies at Trinity College, Dublin, Ireland, and president of the International Fluency Association (IFA). She continues to be a committee member of the International Association of Logopedics and Phoniatrics. As a clinician and academic, she has conducted clinical research and published in the area of stuttering and in the education of speech and language pathologists. She has led research into clinical discourse in the area of stuttering therapy and is involved in normative studies in phonology development in Ireland.

**Emily S. Maloney**, MS, CCC-SLP, is a speech-language pathologist working with preschool and elementary school children in Ellington Public Schools in Connecticut. She has conducted and published research on the limitations of age equivalent scores. In addition, she has presented on how to report performance on standardized tests to Individualized Education Program team members. Her areas of interests include language disorders in young children and the relationship between language and literacy development.

**Barbara L. Rodríguez**, PhD, CCC-SLP, received her doctorate in speech-language pathology from the University of Washington. She is currently an associate professor in the Department of Speech and Hearing Sciences at the University of New Mexico, where she teaches courses in multicultural issues, language intervention and assessment, and bilingual language development and disorders. Her research interests include bilingual language development, literacy development in Spanish-speaking children, and Latino parents' beliefs and practices. She conducted longitudinal research in collaboration with Drs. Carol Scheffner Hammer and Adele W. Miccio on the language and literacy development of bilingual children attending Head Start and on the development of a bilingual phonological assessment tool.

**Li Sheng**, PhD, is assistant professor of communication sciences and disorders at the University of Texas at Austin, where she teaches courses in child language development and disorders and cognitive development. Dr. Sheng received her doctorate from Northwestern University. Her research interests are in the areas of school-age language disorders, lexical-semantic processing and organization, specific language impairment, and semantic development in bilingual speakers of Mandarin-English and Spanish-English. Her publications have appeared in the *Journal of Speech, Language, and Hearing Research*, *Clinical Linguistics and Phonetics*, *Journal of Child Language*, and *Language, Speech, and Hearing Services in Schools*. She serves as editorial consultant for the *Journal of Speech, Language, and Hearing Research*, *Journal of Child Language*, and *Language, Speech, and Hearing Services in Schools*. She has presented her research at numerous national and international conferences.

**Rosalee C. Shenker**, PhD, founder and executive director of the Montreal Fluency Centre, has specialized in fluency disorders for over 30 years. She is also adjunct professor at McGill University, School of Communication Sciences and Disorders, and research associate at the University of Sydney, Australian Stuttering Research Centre. As a charter member of the Lidcombe Program Training Consortium, she coordinates clinical training in North America and has provided presentations and workshops to more than 2000 clinicians. Dr. Shenker has published in peer-reviewed journals and contributed chapters on stuttering to various textbooks. Her interests include long-term follow-up of maintenance of fluency in children and school-age children treated with the Lidcombe Program for early stuttering and evaluation of individual variables influencing treatment outcome including bilingualism.

**Trudy Stewart**, PhD, is currently a consultant speech and language therapist with more than 30 years of clinical experience. She has written numerous journal articles on a number of areas, including psychological issues, client experience, group therapy, and acquired stammering and is the author of several books on stammering. She has been involved in the clinical training of speech therapists at the undergraduate and postgraduate levels in the United Kingdom, the United

States, and Sri Lanka. Dr. Stewart is a specialist advisor for the Royal College of Speech & Language Therapists and the British Stammering Association. She is a committee member of the IFA and on the editorial board for the *Journal of Fluency Disorders*.

**Holly F. B. Teagle**, AuD, is an assistant clinical professor and director of the Carolina Children's Communicative Disorders Program at the University of North Carolina at Chapel Hill. Her career in audiology started at the University of Iowa, where she provided patient care and participated in various aspects of clinical studies related to cochlear implantation in adults and children. She has written and presented on pediatric cochlear implantation and teaches at UNC and through the AG Bell First Years Distance Learning Program. Her research interests include outcomes among special populations of cochlear implant users, including those with auditory neuropathy, cochlear malformations, and bilateral/bimodal assistive devices.

**Judith Vander Woude**, PhD, is a professor and the program director of the Speech Pathology and Audiology Program at Calvin College in Grand Rapids, Michigan. She teaches courses on phonological and language disorders and conducts research on child language disorders. She has authored several articles and book chapters on language and literacy development in addition to a book on planning speech-language pathology treatment. Dr. Vander Woude is currently the associate coordinator of the American Speech-Language-Hearing Association's Special Interest Division 1: Language Learning and Education and the vice president of professional development for the Council of Academic Programs in Communication Sciences and Disorders.

**Amy L. Weiss**, PhD, CCC-SLP, is a professor in the Department of Communicative Disorders at the University of Rhode Island, where she teaches courses in language disorders of young children and school-age children, phonological disorders, fluency disorders, and multicultural issues. A National Institutes of Health grant recipient, Dr. Weiss is also a Board Recognized Specialist in Child Language (ASHA) and the author of one text, *Resource Guide on Preschool Language Disorders*; several book chapters; and more than 30 journal articles. She is currently the chairperson of the Board of Division Coordinators for ASHA's Special Interest Division program and serves as the secretary of the International Fluency Association. Her career experiences in the clinic have included directing a language-based preschool classroom, providing hospital-based services, and the clinical training of hundreds of graduate students at Purdue University, the University of Colorado, and the University of Iowa, prior to her employment at the University of Rhode Island. Dr. Weiss is an ASHA fellow.

# 1 Perspectives on Individual Differences Affecting Therapeutic Change in Communication Disorders

## *Prologue*

*Amy L. Weiss*

As my career as a provider of clinical services to persons with communication disorders has evolved over more than 30 years, I have been struck by several aspects of treatment delivery that were not obvious to me when I was a novice. To begin with, I continue to be overwhelmed by the proliferation of new information that has been made available to speech-language pathologists (SLPs) and audiologists through the efforts of creative and hardworking colleagues focusing first on what was known as treatment efficacy research and more recently on investigations aimed at amassing evidence-based practice data (Dollaghan, 2007). It is nearly impossible to open a scholarly journal that focuses on communication disorders today without finding at least one article with the term "evidence-based practice" in its title. Certainly this trend serves as a response to the ongoing call for accountability in the services we provide, not only to the people we serve but also where reimbursement by third-party payers is concerned.

It is clear to almost anyone invested in selecting the most appropriate intervention approaches for individuals with communication disorders that evidence-based practice has taken center stage with its three decision-making components: (a) What does carefully designed research tell us works? (b) What does our clinical experience suggest will work? and (c) What are the preferences of the particular clients we serve (and their families, of course)? Although several authors have tackled the issue of how professionals can balance these three perspectives in the field of communication disorders (Dollaghan, 2007; Gillam & Gillam, 2006), many professional SLPs and audiologists continue to express concern over how to most appropriately weigh these factors in therapy decision making (E. Strand, personal communication, April 18, 2008).

Second, I recognize that we cannot be cavalier about the heterogeneity of the populations of individuals with communication disorders that we serve and the obvious impact that has on determining best practices. Instead, we have to take the individual differences of our clients into account in both data collection and clinical decision making. Let's take a fairly transparent example to illustrate this point. Not every child with a hearing loss has had the same auditory experiences or the same benefits from auditory input as the standard textbook case, even if that hearing loss looks ostensibly identical when mapped on an audiogram. It can be hypothesized that each child brings to the therapy setting a different history of identification and amplification, even children with a supposedly identical hearing loss, that may contribute a different and more appropriate interface with a particular treatment regimen (see Teagle & Eskridge, Chapter 12, for more information on the particular variables taken into account by professionals serving children with hearing impairments).

Investigators focusing on the efficacy of intervention approaches appear to deal with the issue of heterogeneity in one of two ways, either by utilizing single-subject designs to carefully capture the essential differences inherent in individual clients (see Gierut, 1998) or by attempting to mitigate the presence of individual differences through larger-scale studies (Rvachew & Nowak, 2001; Rvachew, Rafaat, & Martin, 1999). Each approach brings its own set of problems to the interpretation of findings. In the first case, the statistical design allows for a participant to serve as his or her own control. Individual differences between subjects are assumed, and that is one reason why multiple single-subject cases are often reported simultaneously in one article. In the second case, where larger numbers of participants are incorporated into a treatment study, it is assumed that the individual differences presented by these participants will cancel each other out, minimizing the variability in participants' performance.

In a perfect world, professional service providers are able to make inferences about the usefulness of particular interventions when the participants described in treatment studies are similar to clients/patients on their own caseloads. Making such inferences from a single-subject design experiment is more valid if the researcher has provided the reader with a finely tuned description of the participants, taking care to include details that potentially have an impact on the outcome (e.g., age of identification of hearing loss, age at which amplification was supplied, etc.). What is lost in single-subject designs, however, is the ability to make a statistically powerful statement about the inferences of the findings, either positive or negative. Large-scale studies with random assignment of subjects to treatment conditions are more attractive to many consumers of research because findings reflect less of the individual variance that may affect outcomes. Unfortunately, as researchers in communication disorders are well aware, finding large numbers of persons representing low-incidence disorders can be a difficult or impossible task. To that end, selection criteria may be broadened to ensure that a sufficiently large subject population is recruited. Adopting that solution greatly reduces the ability to infer that clients from an individual SLP's caseload will respond the same way that participants in a study responded *on average* to therapeutic regimens. My purpose here is not to support one approach to accruing evidence-based practice data to the exclusion of the other approach. The reality is that our subject populations are inherently more likely to range from 1 to 40 than in the thousands or tens of thousands, as they may for carefully controlled studies comparing drug regimens, for example.

Third, my naïve view of intervention as a new SLP more than 30 years ago posited that successful therapy was mostly about me, my performance as a clinician, and the type of intervention activities I selected. However, over the course of those years as an SLP, I have become interested in exploring the integral role played by the client in determining the success or failure of intervention. Specifically, what does an individual client bring to the therapeutic table?

The topic of the interface between individual differences and therapy progress was discussed in more detail in an earlier article (Weiss, 2004) with a recounting of a clinical experience I had had many years ago as a graduate student assigned to a young, highly unintelligible preschooler. This child made it evident to me that clients I work with likely differ in terms of their motivation, as well as their ability to change. In brief, the child made several explicit comments concerning his recognition that he was talking like a much younger child (e.g., "You think I talk like a baby"). It was not long after these comments were made that the child demonstrated an exponential, positive increase in his intelligibility. This was not a controlled study and so there is no way to make any useful generalization about the relationship between the two occurrences, the comments reflecting self-awareness and rapid improvement in speech intelligibility. This anecdote has stuck with me, however, and although I do not design objectives to elicit comments from preschoolers about the self-perception of their lack of intelligibility, you can be sure that I listen carefully for them. For this particular child, there was a correlation between the two occurrences. Note that I have taken care not to say anything about causality.

It also interests me that within the field of communication disorders, the topic of the client's share of the therapeutic relationship is considered to a greater or lesser extent depending on the particular disorder. For example, in the area of stuttering, it is not unusual for most SLPs to discuss at some point what the impact of a client's stuttering is on his or her activities of daily living (ADL). Please note that I am aware that for those who follow a fluency-shaping approach and favor operant techniques to reduce stuttering, there is often no reference to stuttering except as an isolated behavior, and therefore, the impact of stuttering on ADL is of relatively minimal concern. However, the degree to which a communication disorder impacts on a client's ADL provides the clinician with some perspective on the client's probable motivation to make changes in his or her typical communication behaviors. Again, note that I am not suggesting that for our clients who stutter, the elimination of stuttering is necessarily the only viable outcome. That is my acknowledged bias as an SLP. Changing speech behaviors to foster more successful communication is a worthwhile goal and will probably be defined by the client along with collaboration from relevant family members and a clinician.

Consider a different setting and a different population of individuals with communication disorders. It is much less likely that as a matter of course, SLPs in the schools will provide their clients with questionnaires to determine their level of motivation for change. More often it appears that the SLP forms an opinion about the client's investment in therapy in an indirect manner. When homework is not completed, when the client is not willing to work at the upper limits of his or her capacity, or when the client consistently shows up for therapy sessions several minutes late, the message of low motivation is conveyed. Furthermore, it may not just be about clients and their abilities. Kwiatkowski and Shriberg (1993) referred to a client's contribution to therapy as the intersection of capability and focus. The partnership formed between the client and clinician to some extent dictates the level of success in therapy in many cases. We may already be calling this interaction *rapport*—the working relationship that is built between the clinician and the client. However, the measurement of rapport may entail more than the likelihood that a young client will remain seated during therapy or a somewhat older one will show up on time with homework in hand. Rapport may be enhanced by the degree to which the client buys into the therapy plan developed by the clinician. This is a side benefit to creating goals and selecting targets that are meaningful to a particular client. That is, if I am a client who can understand why learning a certain technique will be useful to me, or if I can see that the technique works, I am that much more invested in the outcome. Any SLP who collaborates with classroom teachers to find out the science or history unit being addressed before selecting vocabulary or reading materials for a school-age client with literacy-learning issues is ultimately doing so to make therapy more relevant. With perceived relevance presumably comes more attention and motivation from the client.

A focus on communication disorders affecting language development presents yet another perspective on individual differences and outcome. Much of my clinical career has been spent working with children who had diagnosed language disorders or who were at risk for developing language disorders. When not working directly with young clients, I was investigating (or musing about) how the language development patterns I observed reflected both general trends and individual differences (Goldfield & Snow, 2009, p. 285). In the area of child language disorders, it has been my experience that SLPs are more likely to consider the level of language competence the child possesses going into therapy and the particular style of language learning exhibited by the child to be two of the most essential factors prescribing the course of therapy and its relative rate of progression toward a favorable outcome, more important than the child's motivation to learn, per se. When Bates, Dale, and Thal (1995) explored the individual differences observed in children's language development, they addressed variability in the rate of development within specific language components (e.g., semantics) and across language components (i.e., comprehension outpaces production for most children), as well as reported differences among children related to language-learning style. These investigators went so far as to conclude that "the Average Child is a fiction, a descriptive convenience like the Average Man or the Average Woman" (Bates et al., 1995, p. 151). This statement throws into disarray the assumptive usefulness of normative data to the exclusion of monitoring evidence of the individual differences represented by our clients.

The purpose of this text was to compile the contributors' responses and reflect on how their perspectives on the relationship between clients' individual differences and therapy outcomes may inform us about practice in the field of communication disorders. To that end, I asked a number of my colleagues who are SLPs and/or audiologists both inside and outside the United States to consider the area of communication disorders they have focused most of their professional attention on and write about their perceptions of how the notion of individual differences fits with therapy outcomes. That is, I asked them not only what the available research says to them that aids in their clinical decision making but also how their own clinical experiences square with the notion that clients treated for communication disorders are not uniform in their ability to benefit from therapy. I purposely gave the authors very little guidance about how to go about that mission because I did not want any template followed that might stifle their clinical problem-solving creativity.

Each contributor agreed that she or he was cognizant of the crucial effect of personal factors on therapy outcomes, and as you will see, the authors differed quite strikingly in how they attacked the questions presented. Some used a case study approach to illustrate different outcomes stemming from individual differences. Others paid close attention to the evidence-based practice model that we have become so very used to in our literature within the last several years. For others, where there was a heartier research base available, you will notice less speculation and more of a review of the research literature. I believe that most of the authors will agree, however, that they were forced to make more speculations than they may have been entirely comfortable with. I include myself in that group.

The topics covered in this text range from an overview of the individual differences in children's acquisition of social language competencies to the very specific topic of the individual client differences that influence changes in stuttering behavior when the Lidcombe Program is implemented. Given the expanded scopes of practice experienced by audiologists and SLPs over the time I have practiced, it would have taken a text at least twice the size of this one to cover every disorder and every context of practice, so it is probably wise to consider the chapters that have been included as a first wave of attack on an intriguing topic. It is our collective hope that you will find the chapters both informative and thought provoking.

## REFERENCES

Bates, E., Dale, P., & Thal, D. (1995). Individual differences and their implications for the theories of language development. In P. Fletcher & B. MacWhinney (Eds.), *Handbook of child language* (pp. 96–115). Oxford, United Kingdom: Basil Blackwell.

Dollaghan, C. (2007). *The handbook for evidence-based practice in communication disorders.* Baltimore: Paul H. Brookes Publishing Co.

Gierut, J. (1998). Treatment efficacy: functional phonological disorders in children. *Journal of Speech, Language, and Hearing Research, 41,* S85–S100.

Gillam, S., & Gillam, R. (2006). Making evidence-based decisions about child-language intervention in schools. *Language, Speech, and Hearing Services in Schools, 37,* 304–315.

Goldfield, B., & Snow, C. (2009). Individual differences: Implications for the study of language acquisition. In J. Berko Gleason & N. Bernstein Ratner (Eds.), *The development of language* (7th ed., pp. 285–314).

Kwiatkowski, J., & Shriberg, L. (1993). Speech normalization in developmental phonological disorders: A retrospective study of capability-focus theory. *Language, Speech, and Hearing Services in Schools, 24,* 10–18.

Rvachew, S., & Nowak, M. (2001). The effect of target-selection strategy on phonological learning. *Journal of Speech, Language, and Hearing Research, 44,* 610–623.

Rvachew, S., Rafaat, S., & Martin, M. (1999). Stimulability, speech perception skills, and the treatment of phonological disorders. *American Journal of Speech-Language Pathology, 8,* 33–43.

Weiss, A. (2004). The child as agent for change in therapy for phonological disorders. *Child Language Teaching and Therapy, 20,* 221–244.

# 2 "The Social Stuff Is Everything"

*How Social Differences in Development Impact Treatment for Children With Language Impairment*

*Bonnie Brinton and Martin Fujiki*

## INTRODUCTION

A number of years ago, we conducted a study looking at the social competence of elementary school-age children with language impairment (LI) (Brinton, Fujiki, Montague, & Hanton, 2000). This work involved detailed observations of the children in a variety of contexts, including cooperative work and playground interactions. Each of the children then participated in a social communication intervention study that was followed by a repeat of the detailed observations conducted before the study began. As a group, these children performed more poorly than their typical peers on almost every measure of social competence we employed. They were less well accepted by peers, had fewer friends, and were rated by teachers as being more withdrawn and less sociable than their typical classmates. As individuals, however, some notable differences were evident. Six of the children were in the same first-grade classroom. Despite the generally poor social performance of the group, one child with LI was one of the most popular children in the class. Conversely, another child was singled out by peers as being the most disliked and feared student in the classroom. Although the children with LI, as a group, were not more aggressive than expected, this particular child was highly aggressive.

As noted, the children diagnosed with LI participated in cooperative work groups that involved two typical peers. In these interactions we found something we did not expect, although in retrospect it now seems rather obvious. The children's ability to interact effectively in these groups was influenced not only by their language skills but also by their social abilities. The child who showed high levels of aggressive behavior had difficulty working effectively with peers. Over the course of four cooperative learning group sessions, she took materials from the other children, criticized her peers, told them to "shut up," pushed them out of the way to get materials, and on one occasion hit another child. Needless to say, her interactions during the cooperative learning group were less than satisfying to her peers. Two other children were rated as highly withdrawn. Their levels of interaction often depended on the behavior of the other children in the group. If their partners sought to include them, they participated effectively, albeit somewhat passively. If the partners did not include them, they were isolated, and the cooperative nature of the group broke down. The two children with the strongest social functioning also had the most successful cooperative learning sessions. Both spent a relatively high percentage of their time in interactions that were collaborative and cooperative. Not only were these interactions more positive socially, they were also more conducive to learning (Brinton, Fujiki, Montague, & Hanton, 2000). Although it was not evident to us when we started, it became more and more clear as we worked with these children that it was of primary importance to address their social functioning as we planned our interventions as speech-language pathologists (SLPs).

## THE SOCIAL NATURE OF LANGUAGE INTERVENTION

Language acquisition and language intervention are inherently social in nature. In essence, we facilitate children's ability to produce and understand language by having them talk, listen, read, and write. In a school context, these are generally social acts. The language behaviors that we target in intervention have potential social impact, and we conclude that those behaviors have generalized when we see them put to competent social use.

In designing language treatment for any child with LI, we know it is essential to evaluate the abilities and challenges the child brings to the treatment context. Traditional assessment procedures tend to concentrate on what a child knows about language comprehension and production, as well as his or her ability to attend to and process information. The child's social functioning has sometimes been an afterthought, however, considered only to the extent that it might predict how easily the child's behavior could be managed within clinical tasks.

Each child brings a unique personality to the intervention context. We use the term *social profile* to refer to patterns of an individual's social behavior in interactional contexts. Describing a social profile helps us consider the child's social strengths and limitations across a range of behavioral realms or domains. These domains include, but are not limited to, aggressive, withdrawn, sociable, victimizing, and impulsive behaviors. It is important to note that each of these general domains may be further broken into subtypes of behavior. For example, not all types of aggressive behavior are similar. Aggressive behavior displayed in response to the aggressive behaviors of others may be viewed differently than aggressive actions initiated without provocation. Describing a child's social profile not only requires consideration of types of behavior and levels of competence across behavioral domains and contexts, it also requires consideration of the meaning and impact of a child's behavior on that child's social world.

The child's social profile is critical in determining how well that child can form and maintain relationships with others. The primary reason to consider the social profile in intervention is to facilitate a child's ability to connect with others and have fulfilling relationships with others in his social world. This should be our primary focus. We would also contend, however, that the social profile is an extremely important parameter influencing how a child responds to treatment, acquires new behaviors, and generalizes new skills. Understanding the social profile is particularly central in judging how a child will respond to various learning contexts, such as dyadic interactions or group work. As in the example provided at the beginning of the chapter, social profile can determine a child's access to important learning contexts, such as reading groups, problem-solving discussions, and joint class assignments. In addition, a child's social profile may also influence learning in individual work tasks and other academic endeavors that are not designed to be particularly social in nature. For example, an anxious, reticent child and an outgoing, confident child may approach such tasks very differently.

## CATEGORIES OR CONTINUA OF IMPAIRMENT

SLPs have long been aware that a diagnostic label provides only a general indication of a child's communication strengths and limitations, since individuals within a diagnostic category may vary so markedly (Paul, 2001). Similarly, a child's social profile will depend upon behaviors the child demonstrates rather than the diagnostic category used to identify the child. Diagnostic labels provide a general indication of what to expect, but this expectation may not be realized for an individual child. Illustrative of this, children diagnosed with autism spectrum disorder (ASD) by definition have pragmatic problems that complicate their social interactions. In contrast, children with LI are sometimes thought to have difficulty with vocabulary and grammar in the face of relatively intact pragmatic skills. It has been documented, however, that some of the pragmatic difficulties commonly associated with ASD have also been observed in children with LI (Bishop, 2000). This overlap can be puzzling, particularly when attempting to identify a child within a diagnostic category. For instance, a child with LI may show a nonresponsive conversational pattern reminiscent of a child with Asperger syndrome. However, the child may also have a history of language formulation problems consistent with a primary diagnosis of LI.

The overlap between LI and ASD has been described as representing a continuum between the two categories (Bishop, 2003). It is important to keep in mind that the term *continuum*, as applied here, does not imply gradual and consistent movement from mild to severe impairment in the same way that a color continuum might move from pink to red. Rather, it is a general way of characterizing the overlap between diagnostic categories and the fact that at times, the borders of these disorders can be particularly fuzzy. Recognizing that social behaviors may vary within a category as well as between categories, and that a child's social profile must be determined on an individual basis, will be helpful concepts in sorting out the social behaviors of individual children.

## SOCIAL PROBLEMS OF CHILDREN WITH LI: GROUP RESULTS

To provide background for our discussion of how social profile may impact intervention, we begin by reviewing what we know about the social problems that children with language problems may experience. First, we discuss the results of group studies. We later present several case studies, illustrating how the generalizations made from the findings of group studies reflect what we see in individual children. In discussing the results of group studies, we focus on three related lines of research. First, we consider studies examining the socioemotional difficulties of children with language problems. We then focus on research considering the ability of these children to perform specific social tasks. Finally, we consider specific social outcomes, such as whether children with LI have friends or are well accepted by peers.

### SOCIOEMOTIONAL DIFFICULTIES IN CHILDREN WITH LI

There is a considerable amount of research documenting the socioemotional problems of children with LI, so much that a comprehensive review is well beyond the scope of this chapter. Also complicating a summary of this work is the fact that studies often vary markedly in the methods used and the populations sampled (e.g., who exactly is considered to have LI). Despite these differences, it may generally be said that children with LI are at a notably higher risk for socioemotional difficulties than are typically developing children. These problems may appear early in development, with difficulties reported in late talkers near age 2 (Irwin, Carter, & Briggs-Gowan, 2002; Paul, Looney, & Dahm, 1991). In older children, a variety of problems have been documented, including high rates of withdrawal (Fujiki, Brinton, Morgan, & Hart, 1999; Fujiki, Spackman, Brinton & Hall, 2004; Hart, Fujiki, Brinton, & Hart, 2004; Redmond & Rice, 1998), internalizing disorders (Coster, Goorhuis-Brouwer, Nakken, & Lutje Spelberg, 1999), attention difficulties (Snowling, Bishop, Stothard, Chipchase, & Kaplan, 2006), and behavior problems in general (Benasich, Curtiss, & Tallal, 1993). Although internalizing problems appear to be more common, externalizing disorders have also been observed (Horowitz, Jansson, Ljungbeg, & Hedenbro, 2005; Tomblin, Zhang, Buckwalter, & Catts, 2000). Of particular interest are longitudinal studies that document high rates of anxiety and social phobia in adolescence (Beitchman et al., 2001) and increased risk for serious psychiatric difficulties in young adults with LI (Clegg, Hollis, Mawhood, & Rutter, 2005).

Of the behaviors discussed above, withdrawal merits elaboration because it illustrates how individual children with a particular behavioral label may still be very different from one another. As noted, children with LI tend to be more withdrawn than their typical peers. It is important to recognize, however, that there are different types of withdrawal, and that simply preferring to be alone may not necessarily be negative (Rubin & Asendorpf, 1993). In recognition of this fact, social psychologists have identified different subtypes of withdrawal, each having specific social consequences (Coplan & Rubin, 1998; Coplan, Rubin, Fox, Calkins, & Stewart, 1994; Harrist, Zaia, Bates, Dodge, & Pettit, 1997; Nelson, Hart, & Evans, 2008).

One subtype of withdrawal has been labeled solitary-passive withdrawal (Coplan & Rubin, 1998) and is characterized by playing or working alone in constructive activities. Thus, a child sitting alone reading a book would be exhibiting solitary-passive withdrawal. Teachers and parents are generally not concerned by this type of behavior, although in early and middle childhood it may be viewed negatively by peers (Younger & Daniels, 1992).

A second subtype, solitary-active withdrawal, is "characterized by repeated sensorimotor action with or without objects and/or … solitary dramatizing" (Coplan et al., 1994, p. 130). For example, a group of children might be pretending to be on a space ship traveling to Mars. One child is physically sitting with these children, and also playing like he is on a space ship, but is not playing with the other children. Thus, as the other children are enacting a pretend landing sequence, this child is engaged in a high-speed chase of an alien space ship. Although relatively rare, when solitary-active withdrawal does occur in free play it is highly noticeable and invites peer rejection (Coplan et al., 1994). Recent work has suggested that solitary-active withdrawal may more accurately be divided into two unrelated constructs, solitary-pretend play (solitary dramatizing) and solitary-functional play (repeated sensorimotor action), each with its own negative social outcomes (Nelson et al., 2008).

A third type of withdrawal, reticence (Coplan & Rubin, 1998), is seen in children who would like to interact with others but are afraid of doing so. These children may spend a good deal of time on the outside of interactions, watching other children play. They may also spend time wandering about doing nothing (Rubin & Asendorpf, 1993).

In a series of studies referred to previously, we asked elementary teachers to rate the social behaviors of children with and without LI in their classrooms. Although all three types of withdrawal were observed, children with LI were most consistently rated as significantly more reticent than typical peers (Fujiki, Brinton, Morgan, et al. 1999; Fujiki et al., 2004). Teachers indicated that children with LI spent a good deal of time hovering on the edge of interactions, apparently wanting to interact but not being able to do so. Children with LI were also characterized as avoiding or failing to respond to the overtures of other children. Finally, teachers indicated that these children spent time in class doing nothing when they had plenty of work to do, another characteristic of reticence. These findings were confirmed by observational data in which children with LI were videotaped during interactions on the playground. As in the studies involving teacher ratings, children with LI were more reticent than their typical peers (Fujiki, Brinton, Isaacson, & Summers, 2001).

In considering these and other findings documenting the social difficulties of children with LI, it is notable that in some of the studies cited, children with LI performed below their typical peers, but still not poorly enough to fall into the clinical range on the measures used (e.g., Redmond & Rice, 1998). It should be kept in mind, however, that as socioemotional problems become more serious, children are no longer considered to have LI but are likely to be identified in other categories of impairment, such as behavior disorder or ASD. The fact that group differences exist, despite this "ceiling," is indicative of both the pervasiveness and the seriousness of these problems.

## THE ABILITY OF CHILDREN WITH LI TO PERFORM SOCIAL TASKS

There has been a considerable amount of research looking at the ability of children with LI to perform social tasks such as accessing ongoing group interactions or participating in cooperative work groups. Before discussing these tasks, however, it is useful to consider sociable behaviors in general. Positive behaviors such as offering help, sharing, providing comfort, and cooperating are often grouped under the behavioral dimension of sociability, or sociable behavior (Hart, Robinson, McNeilly-Choque, Nelson, & Olsen, 1995; Ladd & Price, 1993). These behaviors are often critical to effective participation in social tasks. In addition, the negative influence of some forms of withdrawal (e.g., solitary-passive withdrawal) might be moderated by strong sociable skills. A person who is quiet by nature might do quite well if he or she can interact effectively when the need arises. Thus, it is important to consider sociable skills at the same time one considers withdrawal. We first briefly consider general ratings of the sociable behaviors of children with LI and then focus on their performance on specific social tasks.

Teachers have consistently rated children with LI as being less sociable than typically developing children (Fujiki, Brinton, Morgan, et al. 1999; Fujiki et al., 2004). Furthermore, there is evidence that level of LI severity is related to a child's proficiency in displaying sociable behavior. This makes good sense in that many sociable behaviors are heavily dependent upon spoken language (Hart et al., 2004). Children who have difficulty producing and understanding language are likely to have problems effectively performing sociable tasks such as comforting others or demonstrating empathy.

A number of investigations have considered how children with LI perform on specific social communication tasks. One important social task is accessing, or entering, ongoing social interactions. This task is particularly difficult for children with LI, and it has repeatedly been demonstrated that they have more trouble than typical children in joining ongoing activities (Brinton, Fujiki, Spencer, & Robinson, 1997; Craig & Washington, 1993; Liiva & Cleave, 2005). Children with LI also have difficulty negotiating with peers and are limited not only by their poor structural language skills but also by the fact that they use less effective negotiation strategies (Brinton, Fujiki, & McKee, 1998). Children with LI have also been found to be less effective participants in cooperative work groups, a common context employed in school (Brinton, Fujiki, & Higbee, 1998; Brinton et al., 2000).

Even in situations in which children with LI are specifically placed in groups with others to facilitate their interactions, they may still end up isolated. For example, as noted above, we examined whether children with LI could enter an ongoing interaction consisting of two typically developing peers (Brinton et al., 1997). Of the six children with LI observed, three successfully accessed the interaction. Even for the children who were able to join the group, however, the triad frequently evolved into a dyadic conversation involving the two children with typical language competencies.

Difficulty with basic social communication tasks is likely to impact the social outcomes that children with LI experience. Acceptance, friendship, and victimization are considered in the following section.

## Peer Acceptance, Friendship, and Victimization

Social psychologists often separate peer acceptance and friendship when considering peer relationships in childhood (Rubin, Bukowski, & Parker, 1998). Peer acceptance is a reflection of group popularity, which is often measured by asking peers how much they enjoy playing or spending time with a specific child. Friendship, on the other hand, is a reciprocal relationship—it exists only when two children recognize each other as friends. To cite an oft quoted bit of parental wisdom, "to have a friend you have to be a friend." If either of the children pulls out, the friendship is dissolved (Asher, Parker, & Walker, 1996). Although both acceptance and friendship are important, lack of friendship makes the larger contribution to loneliness, particularly in a school context. Even among well-accepted children, those without close friends are more lonely at school than those with friends (Parker & Asher, 1993).

As a group, children with LI are less well accepted and have fewer friends than their typical peers. Children with LI as young as preschoolers are viewed as less desirable playmates than typical peers in social tasks, such as dramatic play (Gertner, Rice, & Hadley, 1994). In our own work, we studied peer acceptance and friendship in 8 elementary school children with LI. Although there were some notable exceptions that we will discuss later, as a group these children were both less well accepted and had fewer friends than their typical peers (Fujiki, Brinton, Hart, & Fitzgerald, 1999).

More recently, Durkin and Conti-Ramsden (2007) examined friendship quality in a group of 120 adolescents with a history of specific language impairment (SLI). As a group, these individuals indicated that they had significantly poorer quality friendships than typical peers. It is notable that there was relatively little variability in the typical group, with almost all of the individuals reporting good quality friendships (over 90%). The adolescents with SLI showed considerably more variability, with an overall mean of about 60% reporting good quality friendships. Social strengths and weaknesses played an important predictive role in friendship outcomes, as did language ability.

Tomblin (2007) described the social status of a large group of 10th-grade students originally diagnosed with SLI at age 6. For measurement at the older age level, the individuals with SLI were divided into two groups, those who still could be considered as having an SLI and those with more general LI, defined by nonverbal IQ scores below the typical cut off of 85 but above 75 (to eliminate intellectual disability). On a self-report composite measure of social activity and friendship, individuals in both these groups rated themselves significantly lower than did typical peers. The results of scales completed by parents produced similar findings.

Given their poor showing on measures of friendship and acceptance, it would be expected that children with LI would experience high levels of loneliness. This expectation has been supported by two studies (Fujiki, Brinton, & Todd, 1996; Tomblin, 2007). Fujiki et al. (1996) administered the Williams and Asher lone-liness questionnaire to elementary school-age children. Children with LI rated themselves as being significantly more lonely than did typical peers. Tomblin used a different questionnaire, the UCLA Loneliness Scale. He reported that adolescents with more general LI reported greater levels of loneliness than either persons with SLI or the typical group on this scale. Adolescents with SLI did not differ from their typical peers, however.

Finally, we consider whether children with LI are frequently targeted by bullies. Despite the great interest in victimization with typical children, there has been surprisingly little study of this behavior in children with LI. In one of the few available studies, Conti-Ramsden and Botting (2004) presented self-report data indicating that 11-year-old children with SLI were three times as likely to be victimized at school than were their typically developing peers.

## SUMMARY

Children with LI are more likely to have socioemotional difficulties than typical children. They are also more likely to experience problems with basic social tasks, such as joining ongoing interactions or negotiating with peers. Children with LI are also more lonely, more likely to be rejected by peers, and more likely to be bullied. Despite all of these negatives, it is important to keep in mind that not all children with LI have social difficulties. For example, Fujiki, Brinton, Morgan, et al. (1999) found that as a group, children with LI were rated by teachers as being significantly more withdrawn and less sociable than typical children. Despite overall group performance, 8 of the children with LI (representing 20% of the sample) were rated as not having problems in any of the social areas studied. Durkin and Conti-Ramsden (2007) found that adolescents with LI reported significantly more problems with friendship than typical adolescents. Still, 60% of the individuals with LI reported that they had good friendships.

The point of highlighting the fact that not all children with LI have social challenges is not to minimize the seriousness of these problems. Rather, we wish to emphasize that even in the face of strong evidence that these children have social difficulties, there are individual exceptions to the group experience. In the following section we highlight the experience of several children, illustrating how these individuals both conform to and vary from group expectations. In each of these cases, it was important to understand how the social profile of the individual children impacted their response to intervention and generalization of communicative treatment targets.

## SOCIAL PROFILES OF INDIVIDUAL CHILDREN

### AMY—ATTACK AND RETREAT: AGGRESSIVE AND WITHDRAWN BEHAVIOR COMBINED

Amy, age 6 years 6 months, came from a large, middle-class, Tongan-American family. English was spoken in the home. She was the youngest of 13 children. By the time she was in the first grade, Amy was identified with LI. She attended a regular classroom and was followed for speech and language services on a pull-out basis. Formal test measures yielded scores more than 1.5 standard deviations below the mean on expressive and receptive subtests. Her nonverbal IQ score was within normal limits. Results of hearing and vision screening measures revealed no concerns. In terms of her social profile, Amy reflected results of group research in many ways. She was the least accepted child in her first-grade classroom. She had no reciprocal friends in her class; when she was asked to name her best friends, she named children who reported they did not like to play with her. Amy indicated that she was lonely at school.

As might be predicted by the literature, Amy frequently demonstrated the withdrawn behaviors observed in children with SLI in school setting. Sometimes she played or worked alone (solitary-passive withdrawal), and other times she played at group activities around other children, but not with them (solitary-pretend play). At recess, she often wandered from group to group without really joining in the play (reticence). However, Amy's profile was not limited to withdrawal. She demonstrated much more aggression that we would have expected considering the literature. As with withdrawal, subtypes of aggression have also been described (Crick & Dodge, 1996). Although a review of these subtypes is beyond the scope of this discussion, it may suffice to say that Amy displayed various types of aggressive behavior. For example, in play and work situations she tended to place herself too close to her classmates, and she often hit, pushed, or otherwise annoyed them.

Amy's sociable behaviors were limited. When she tried to enter playgroups, she often burst into the middle of play. She was frequently unresponsive to peers and at times totally ignored the interactional bids of others. She seemed unaware of the needs of others and rarely tried to help or comfort other children. Rather, she tended to "run over" her peers at play. Classmates were afraid of Amy and often marginalized and sometimes taunted her—from a safe distance.

Amy illustrated the fact that withdrawal and aggression can be found in the same child, with serious social consequences. Her response to treatment was highly influenced by this challenging social profile. At times, she could not participate effectively in intervention tasks because of the various types of withdrawal she exhibited. At other times, she dominated and intimidated other children. She needed intervention approaches that would help her gear up to participate in interaction with others and, at the same time, teach her to regulate her emotions and behavior to respond appropriately to others.

## MARIE—ON THE OUTSKIRTS: RETICENCE AND POOR SOCIABLE SKILLS

Marie, 6 years 3 months old, was a Caucasian child living with her middle-class parents, her older sister, and younger twin brothers. She was identified with LI and attended a regular first grade. She was followed by the school SLP for language intervention on a pull-out basis. Marie scored more than 1.5 standard deviations below the mean on both receptive and expressive subtests on standardized language measures. Marie's IQ score was also more than 1.5 standard deviations below the mean, but she was tested using a measure that relied heavily on language skills. The school psychologist was confident in ruling out general intellectual delay. Results of hearing and vision screening yielded no concerns. Socially, Marie was moderately well accepted in her classroom. Although she had two reciprocal friends within the class, one of whom was also identified with LI, Marie reported that she felt lonely at school.

Marie's social profile reflected the group trends reported in the literature. She was highly withdrawn at school, and in comparison with her classmates, she worked and played alone much of the time. She sometimes performed the same activity as other children, but she did it alongside them, not with them (solitary-pretend play). She also showed reticent behavior such as doing nothing when there were lots of things to do, or hovering around groups without joining in. At recess, she often played alone or wandered from group to group. She reported feeling isolated at school. Marie's teacher did not observe much aggressive behavior.

Marie's sociable behaviors were also problematic. She had difficulty entering group interactions, and when she did enter, she seldom participated or collaborated with peers. She was often unresponsive to peers, and she rarely reached out to others to empathize or provide comfort. Even though she had two friends, these friendships proved to be rather fragile, and Marie seemed to exist on the periphery of the classroom.

Marie's response to treatment was also highly influenced by her social profile. Although generally cooperative and compliant, she was hesitant to interact with others or to try new things. She needed support to extend herself to participate with others and to try new tasks and behaviors.

## CASEY—A MIXED BAG: ANXIETY, WITHDRAWAL, AND POOR SOCIABLE SKILLS

Casey, a 7-year-old male, lived with his middle-class, Caucasian parents and three older brothers and younger sister. Another brother joined the family when Casey was 8. Casey was enrolled in a regular first-grade class and received language intervention services delivered within his classroom. Casey was identified with LI and scored 1.5 standard deviations below the mean on receptive and expressive subtests of standardized language measures. His IQ as measured on a nonverbal test of intelligence was within normal limits. Casey was well accepted within his classroom, but he did not have reciprocal friends. He reported loneliness and isolation at school and in his neighborhood.

Casey seemed outgoing and gregarious by nature, and in that respect, he did not seem to fit the profile of the withdrawn children with LI described in the literature. In fact, his outgoing nature belied the fact that he was quite withdrawn at times. He showed anxious or reticent behavior and sometimes seemed immobilized when there was plenty to do. On rare occasions, Casey became frustrated and had brief episodes of aggressive behavior toward peers. He sometimes had difficulty in group interactions if the group did not act on his suggestions and ideas.

Although Casey was not nearly as aggressive as Amy, he still demonstrated a mix of internalizing and externalizing behaviors. Casey willingly joined group play at recess if he understood the activity (e.g., simple sociodramatic play). At other times, he was unable to enter and was excluded from group work or play. He was often unresponsive to peers, and he tended to monopolize the conversational floor. He talked on and on even after his listener had clearly lost interest. He had trouble in situations where he needed to problem-solve or negotiate with peers. Casey was anxious to befriend others, but he seemed unable to anticipate or appreciate their needs in conversation.

Like that of Amy and Marie, Casey's response to treatment was highly influenced by his social profile. He needed intervention designed to facilitate his integration into interactions with others. At the same time, he needed a great deal of support to learn to gear his contributions to the needs of his conversational partners.

## SUMMARY

Amy, Marie, and Casey had a number of things in common. Each had deficits in language comprehension and language production. Each was frequently reticent, and none had strong prosocial skills. It followed that each child had negative social outcomes, including problems interacting with peers, loneliness at school, and difficulty making friends. However, each child presented a distinctive social profile. Amy was sometimes unresponsive and at other times highly aggressive. Marie was isolated, withdrawn, and lonely. Casey was outgoing but sometimes withdrawn. As much as he wanted to make friends, he could not adjust his behavior to meet the needs of his listeners. Certainly, each child had social challenges that needed to be addressed. Their social development and ability to use social language were primary considerations. In addition, each child had social tendencies that impacted their performance in language intervention, regardless of what specific treatment target might be adopted. Amy, Marie, and Casey illustrate the need to consider how both general and specific aspects of a child's social profile figure into the treatment process.

## DESCRIBING THE SOCIAL PROFILE: GENERAL CONSIDERATIONS

There are several aspects of a child's history that influence the child's social profile, as well as the way the child approaches learning contexts. These aspects may be intertwined and include the child's cultural background, family environment, social experience, and social goals.

## CULTURAL BACKGROUND

All social learning takes place in a cultural context that influences beliefs and behaviors. A child's educational background, religious beliefs, gender roles, and various other factors all contribute to this context and play an important role in determining what is viewed as appropriate or inappropriate behavior (Kalyanpur & Harry, 1999). It follows, then, that a child's social behavior must be considered in terms of the culture in which he or she has been reared. If an individual interacts with peers, teachers, and other individuals who have differing cultural expectations of appropriate behavior, there is the potential for misinterpretation and miscommunication. Both the verbal and nonverbal aspects of interaction are important. For example, in a classroom context, knowing how to answer when called upon, how to address the teacher and classmates, and what topics are appropriate for conversation will communicate social competence. Students who do not know these culturally dictated standards may communicate ignorance, apathy, or disrespect in their responses. Similarly, subtle differences in eye contact, proximity (how close one stands to another), physical contact, and body movement may all communicate unintended messages. One illustration of this point can be found by considering reticent withdrawal. As noted, this type of withdrawal is problematic for middle-class American children (Coplan & Rubin, 1998). For a child growing up in some cultures, however, interacting in a reserved manner, particularly when talking with an adult, may be appropriate (Cheng, 1987). Thus, consideration of the child's cultural background would be key to determining whether reserved behavior represented reticent withdrawal or a self-determined style of interaction appropriate within a cultural context.

The influence of culture on social behavior is a broad topic that can only briefly be addressed in the context of this chapter. For additional information see Lynch and Hanson (2004) and Johnson and Johnson (2002).

## FAMILY ENVIRONMENT

Within the greater cultural context, the family structure provides a miniature culture in which a child learns which social behaviors are appropriate and which are ineffective or unacceptable. We can expect a child to be highly influenced by the way parents view, model, and teach social behavior. Therefore, it is important to understand, to the extent possible, the social behaviors that are valued within a child's family. For example, we once worked with a 6-year-old boy diagnosed with LI who showed frequent aggression in reaction to the actions of others. This behavior was problematic in and of itself, and it also affected the way he functioned in group learning contexts. His teachers noted that he sometimes fought unusually violently with his brother when they interacted with each other at school. In considering how best to approach this child, it was important to communicate with the parents to determine how they viewed their sons' combative behavior. If the parents were unhappy with the fighting but felt unable to handle it effectively, a team approach assisting them to manage the boys' interaction within the home would seem warranted. If, on the other hand, the parents viewed their boys' aggression toward each other as a typical developmental pattern, we would have our work cut out for us. It would be necessary to emphasize to the child, as well as to the parents, that physical fighting interferes with learning in a school context.

In addition to considering the social behaviors valued within a child's family, it is also important to understand that specific parenting styles may influence the child's social behavior. The research on parenting style is far too extensive to do justice to it in the context of this chapter. It should be emphasized, however, that parenting style is likely to interact with a child's temperament with an important impact on child behavior. For further information the reader is referred to Hart, Newell, and Olsen (2003).

## PRIOR SOCIAL EXPERIENCE

A child's social history will influence how that child approaches others. It is well accepted that children with histories of abuse bring a number of complicating issues to the treatment process. Even children who have nurturing and supportive families, however, may have histories of unsatisfactory experiences with peers. As indicated earlier, children with LI may have experienced difficult interactions in work and play and may even have been victimized by peers. Children with LI may have low expectations for peer interaction and may avoid it.

A child with negative experience interacting with adults or peers may bring a particular set of challenges to the therapeutic process. For example, Marie experienced considerable isolation at school, seemed wary or anxious about communicative tasks, and was less than enthusiastic when attempting new behaviors within those contexts. Her prior experience may have taught her that avoiding interaction through withdrawal was the safest course of action. Amy seemed fearless around peers, but she had very little experience with supportive peer relationships. Her experience may have reinforced the idea that she should either avoid interaction or "shoot first and ask questions later." Casey was eager to interact with peers, but he was frequently frustrated when things did not go as he planned. His experience seemed to bolster the notion that peer interaction was a source of anxiety. For Marie, Amy, and Casey, prior social experience may have contributed to their difficulties in interaction and encouraged the adoption of negative social goals (see Redmond & Rice, 1998).

## SOCIAL GOALS

An individual usually approaches an interaction with one or more personal social goals. For example, a child may approach a game with peers with any of several possible social goals. The child might have goals such as having fun with peers, helping others have fun, or making friends. On the other hand, a child may have less friendly social goals, such as protecting himself or herself from embarrassment, dominating others, or exacting revenge for past losses. The social goals a child adopts are directly related to how that child behaves in social situations (Erdley & Asher, 1999). Therefore, we can expect a child's social goals to influence the way that child interacts in treatment. Many children with LI seem to have social goals that are self-protective. These children may be hesitant to try new tasks and may avoid interaction altogether. This bodes ill for the acquisition of new behaviors. Children who have aggressive social goals may look for opportunities to control the interaction or act out against others. This, too, can limit a child's ability to learn. In short, negative social goals can seriously sabotage a child's response to treatment, especially if group work or collaboration is involved.

## CONSIDERING SOCIAL PROFILE IN INTERVENTION

As we have discussed earlier, the social difficulties that many children with LI experience have negative consequences in terms of their ability to establish and maintain positive relationships with others. In this respect, social problems can seriously undermine a child's quality of life. In addition, aspects of a child's social profile can influence the way that child learns in very important ways. The social profile can help shape, and sometimes restrict a child's readiness and availability to learn as well as the style in which a child most successfully learns. Even in effectively designed classrooms, social difficulties can sabotage a child's learning in many activities.

In considering social profile in language intervention, it is important to take into account not only the child's social behaviors but also the factors that may motivate those behaviors. To illustrate this point, we first discuss the impact of a child's social goals. We then examine three general types of behavior: aggression, withdrawal, and sociability. In focusing our discussion, we acknowledge that these parameters may overlap in complex ways and will certainly vary from child to child. We also recognize that there are additional motivating factors and social behaviors that could be discussed if space allowed.

### Social Goals

As already discussed, social goals motivate social behavior. Social goals may also be intertwined with a child's perception of his or her ability to learn or sense of self-efficacy. For example, a child who seeks to avoid interacting in a reading group may not feel that he or she has much of value to contribute to that group. Thus, that child's self-perception is likely to be self-fulfilling.

As important as social goals are, they cannot be "remediated" directly (Taylor & Asher, 1984). It is not possible to impose a social goal on another individual. A child whose parents told him to "go in there and make friends" when they dropped him off at preschool is unlikely to adopt making friends as a social goal just because he has been told to do so. Still, it may be possible to foster the adoption of desirable social goals implicitly. For example, Amy wanted to interact with other children, but she approached most interactions with self-protective social goals. She either avoided interaction altogether or dominated others. Part of her intervention involved helping her view felicitous interaction with other children as enjoyable and worth pursuing. We often commented, "It's fun to play with other kids," or pointed out, "Look at those kids. They're working together. That looks like fun." We called her attention to times when she had fun interacting with her peers. We also videotaped her interacting with others and reviewed the best part of the interaction with her, drawing her attention to the smiles and laughter that had communicated friendly interaction. Amy gradually began to approach other children in a more prosocial way. Her teacher observed that she first did this by initiating interaction at recess with children in a self-contained class for lower functioning students. Perhaps she viewed these children as less threatening than some of her own classmates.

Like Amy, Marie needed to understand that playing and working cooperatively with peers was worth the effort involved to participate. Casey needed to internalize more other-oriented social goals in order to motivate increased responsiveness to his conversational partners' needs. The adoption of positive and cooperative social goals was important to all three children in order to enhance their social functioning and to facilitate their inclusion in important learning activities within the school setting. It was also important to help them view themselves as capable members of the learning community.

The following subsections focus on three types of behavior, or behavioral styles, that may impact the child's ability to participate in the therapeutic process: aggression, withdrawal, and sociability.

## Aggression

There are many types of aggressive behavior, and they can all interfere with learning in various ways. As mentioned previously, when children with LI are considered as a group, aggression may appear neither prevalent nor obvious. There are exceptions, however, in that externalizing behaviors have been reported (Tomblin et al., 2000), and these externalizing behaviors tend to be aggressive in nature. In our own work, we have not found significant levels of aggressive behaviors in children with LI when compared with their typically developing peers. It has been the case, however, that aggressive behaviors have been an issue for individual children. For example, children like Casey may be noncombative for long periods of time, but on rare occasions, when experiencing high stress or anxiety, they may suddenly boil over and show physical aggression.

Amy, on the other hand, often pushed, hit, called others names, or otherwise annoyed peers (proactive aggression) and also tended to react quickly to any perceived aggression from peers (reactive aggression). Amy's case illustrates that although aggressive behavior is not typical, individual children with LI may be aggressive. We have not observed much relational aggression (excluding peers from play, trying to break up friendships of others, gossiping, etc.) in young children with LI, possibly because this type of behavior often requires sophisticated emotion understanding and language (e.g., knowing what will hurt someone's feelings and how best to phrase what one wants to say to achieve that outcome).

Aggressive behavior, whether it is rare or frequent, interferes with learning in a dramatic way. For one thing, aggressive behavior disrupts educational contexts and tasks. For another, when children are angry, frustrated, or in an otherwise high emotional state, they are not in a position to learn. It can be hard for them to calm themselves sufficiently to participate constructively in learning groups or to complete individual tasks. Accordingly, aggressive behavior is difficult to manage in the moment that it is occurring. Telling a child who is throwing things at his classmate to calm down and consider his actions is usually an exercise in futility. It is far more helpful to prevent aggressive behaviors when possible.

For children like Casey, it is important to look for events and circumstances that precipitate acting out. Once these are identified, it may be possible to help the child avoid these situations. Since not all tense situations can be avoided, it is also important to help a child anticipate and plan strategies to deal with frustration and anger in difficult conditions. For example, Casey gradually learned several strategies to calm himself when he became frustrated. These included physical relaxation, determining where to go for help, and problem solving. These strategies were effective but not totally failsafe. Amy needed more comprehensive intervention to help her improve her impulse control and regulate the negative emotions that motivated her aggression. One particularly helpful strategy was to help her put appropriate space between herself and her peers. When she did not stand or sit too close to them she had fewer opportunities and less motivation to push or hit them. Amy also needed help to anticipate difficult situations and strategies to regulate her emotions and actions when they arose.

It is particularly important in supporting children like Amy and Casey to team with teachers, special service providers, parents, and others in planning and carrying out intervention strategies. Treatment techniques will be effective only if they are consistently applied across a wide variety of contexts.

## WITHDRAWAL

As indicated earlier, there are different types of behavior that are described under the umbrella term *withdrawal*. Each of these types of withdrawal can interfere with learning in various ways. Even the most benign type, solitary-passive withdrawal (i.e., playing or working constructively alone), may lead to peer rejection as children grow older (Younger & Daniels, 1992). An isolated child may be more vulnerable to teasing, victimization, and exclusion. Children who often play or work alone may miss out on opportunities to learn from and with other children. This may be particularly problematic for children with LI who can benefit from cooperative learning contexts and from interacting with peers who provide good communication models. It is important to draw withdrawn children into peer interactions, but it must be done with care so that the work or play experience is productive and positive. For example, when we put Marie into a small group, she was usually excluded. She needed specific intervention and support to integrate her into interactions and to prepare her to take advantage of peer interaction in learning contexts.

Solitary-pretend play and solitary-functional play are more noticeable and disruptive than solitary passive withdrawal. These types of withdrawal may look unusual or bizarre to peers and almost certainly will call negative attention to a child. Both types contribute to peer rejection. From a clinical viewpoint, these types of withdrawal are concerning because they can block access to positive peer interactions. Like solitary-passive withdrawal, these forms of withdrawal can also sabotage learning in cooperative groups. It is difficult (but important) to draw a child who is demonstrating these types of withdrawal into the mainstream of group activity. This can be a challenging proposition because a child who engages in solitary-pretend play or solitary-functional play may not understand what it means to cooperate with a group and may also have contrary social goals.

Reticence is the most commonly observed type of withdrawal in children with LI. It can be particularly worrisome in a classroom for the very reason that it calls so little attention to itself. A reticent child may not immediately elicit teacher concern and may easily fall into the cracks. Amy, Marie, and Casey were all reticent at times, but it was most problematic for Marie. Like many reticent children, she seemed to exist on the outskirts of her classroom's culture. Her spontaneous participation in classroom work and play activities was minimal, and thus her inclusion in the learning community was compromised.

Reticent withdrawal is not only concerning because it isolates children from learning contexts. Just as aggressive children may have trouble calming themselves down, reticent children may be unable to gear themselves up to try a new task or participate in a group. They may be fearful and anxious about attempting new behaviors. These children need consistent support from adults or classmates trained to serve as confederates to assist them to attempt new behaviors and to enter and become integrated in group interaction. Special consideration may also need to be given to the procedures used to generalize learning from clinical to more real-world settings.

## SOCIABILITY

The impact of withdrawal may be tempered by the positive social behaviors a child demonstrates. In essence, sociable behaviors allow a child to reach out to others in a positive way. Children who tend to work or play alone much of the time may do well if they employ strong sociable behaviors when they do interact. Some people are obviously more reserved than others by nature, but they may be well accepted if they are responsive when they do interact. The problem is, as Amy, Marie, and Casey illustrate, most children with LI who are withdrawn do not show strong sociable behaviors. Withdrawal and poor sociability make a poor combination in terms of a child's social functioning and successful response to intervention. Withdrawn children with limited sociable skills may not participate in treatment activities with other children, and they are likely to be excluded from the classroom culture.

In working with Amy, Casey, and Marie, we found it helpful to focus language therapy on targeting specific sociable skills in conversation, such as entering ongoing interactions, making cooperative and responsive comments in conversation, making positive comments to others, negotiating, and problem solving. Each child made marked progress in producing more sociable behaviors in interaction, and in turn this facilitated a range of educational activities and tasks designed to support language and academic learning. In addition, as Amy, Casey, and Marie acquired more positive sociable behaviors, the effects of their withdrawn behavior were less serious, and their interaction with their peers improved as well. In fact, we have found that facilitating prosocial behaviors is the most effective way to handle withdrawal.

## CONCLUSIONS

We can generally say that children with LI have social difficulties, but they will exhibit a good deal of individual variation in their social profiles. As Amy, Casey, and Marie illustrate, children with LI may exhibit various combinations of withdrawn, sociable, and aggressive behavior. These social difficulties limit a child's ability to form and maintain positive relationships with others, and thus they impact quality of life. Social difficulties also interfere with the learning process in significant ways and impede the child's access to instruction and knowledge. In approaching treatment, it is important for SLPs to consider the nature of an individual child's social profile and how that profile affects both the child's social functioning and the child's learning in specific contexts and activities. This is true not only in cases where we focus on interactional or social language targets, but also in cases in which intervention involves structural aspects of language. In rare cases, children with LI may have relative social strengths that can be capitalized on to enhance therapeutic contexts. Far more often, however, children with LI require ongoing intervention to enhance their social functioning. In any event, children with LI are best served when consideration of the social profile is an integral aspect of our treatment approach. The mother of a young man who had grown up with LI recently emphasized this point. In reflecting on more than 15 years of her son's intervention and development, she concluded, "The social stuff is everything."

## REFERENCES

Asher, S. R., Parker, J. G., & Walker, D. L. (1996). Distinguishing friendship from acceptance: Implications for intervention and assessment. In W. M. Bukowski, A. F. Newcomb, & W. W. Hartup (Eds.), *The company they keep: Friendship in childhood and adolescence* (pp. 366–405). New York: Cambridge University Press.

Beitchman, J. H., Wilson, B., Johnson, C. J., Atkinson, L., Young, A., Adlaf, E., et al. (2001). Fourteen-year follow-up of speech/language-impaired and control children: Psychiatric outcome. *Journal of the American Academy of Child and Adolescent Psychiatry, 40*, 75–82.

Benasich, A., Curtiss, S., & Tallal, P. (1993). Language, learning and behavioral disturbances in childhood: A longitudinal perspective. *Journal of the American Academy of Child and Adolescent Psychiatry, 32*, 585–594.

Bishop, D. V. M. (2000). Pragmatic language impairment: A correlate of SLI, a distinct subgroup, or part of the autistic continuum? In D. V. M. Bishop & L. B. Leonard (Eds.), *Speech and language impairments in children: Causes, characteristics, intervention, and outcome* (pp. 99–113). Philadelphia: Taylor and Francis.

Bishop, D. V. M. (2003). Autism and specific language impairment: Categorical distinction or continuum? *Novartis Foundation Symposium, 251*, 213–234.

Brinton, B., Fujiki, M., & Higbee, L. (1998). Participation in cooperative learning activities by children with specific language impairment. *Journal of Speech, Language, and Hearing Research, 41*, 1193–1206.

Brinton, B., Fujiki, M., & McKee, L. (1998). The negotiation skills of children with specific language impairment. *Journal of Speech, Language, and Hearing Research, 41*, 927–940.

Brinton, B., Fujiki, M., Montague, E. C., & Hanton, J. L. (2000). Children with language impairment in cooperative work groups: A pilot study. *Language, Speech, and Hearing Services in Schools, 31*, 252–264.

Brinton, B., Fujiki, M., Spencer, J. C., & Robinson, L. A. (1997). The ability of children with specific language impairment to access and participate in an ongoing interaction. *Journal of Speech, Language, and Hearing Research, 40*, 1011–1025.

Cheng, L. (1987). *Assessing Asian language performance: Guidelines for evaluating limited-English-proficient students.* Rockville, MD: Aspen.

Clegg, J., Hollis, C., Mawhood, L., & Rutter, M. (2005). Developmental language disorders—A follow-up in later adult life. Cognitive, language and psychosocial outcomes. *Journal of Child Psychology and Psychiatry, 46*, 128–149.

Conti-Ramsden, G., & Botting, N. (2004). Social difficulties and victimization in children with SLI at 11 years of age. *Journal of Speech, Language, and Hearing Research, 47*, 145–161.

Coplan, R. J., & Rubin, K. H. (1998). Exploring and assessing nonsocial play in preschool: The development and validation of the preschool play behavior scale. *Social Development, 7*, 72–91.

Coplan, R. J., Rubin, K. H., Fox, N. A., Calkins, S. D., & Stewart, S. L. (1994). Being alone, playing alone, and acting alone: Distinguishing among reticence, and passive and active-solitude in young children. *Child Development, 65*, 129–137.

Coster, F. W., Goorhuis-Brouwer, S. M., Nakken, H., & Lutje Spelberg, H. C. (1999). Specific language impairments and behavioural problems. *Folia Phoniatrica et Logopaedica, 51*, 99–107.

Craig, H. K., & Washington, J. A. (1993). The access behaviors of children with specific language impairment. *Journal of Speech and Hearing Research, 36*, 322–336.

Crick, N. R., & Dodge, K. A. (1996). Social information-processing mechanisms in reactive and proactive aggression. *Child Development, 67*, 993–1002.

Durkin, K., & Conti-Ramsden, G. (2007). Language, social behavior, and the quality of friendships in adolescents with and without a history of specific language impairment. *Child Development, 78*, 1441–1457.

Erdley, C. A., & Asher, S. (1999). A social goals perspective on children's social competence. *Journal of Emotional and Behavioral Disorders, 7*, 156–168.

Fujiki, M., Brinton, B., & Todd, C. M. (1996). Social skills of children with specific language impairment. *Language, Speech, and Hearing Services in Schools, 27*, 195–202.

Fujiki, M., Brinton, B., Hart, C. H., & Fitzgerald, A. (1999). Peer acceptance and friendship in children with specific language impairment. *Topics in Language Disorders, 19*(2), 34–48.

Fujiki, M., Brinton, B., Morgan, M., & Hart, C. (1999). Withdrawn and sociable behavior of children with specific language impairment. *Language, Speech, and Hearing Services in Schools, 30*, 183–195.

Fujiki, M., Brinton, B., Isaacson, T., & Summers, C. (2001). Social behaviors of children with language impairment on the playground: A pilot study. *Language, Speech and Hearing Services in Schools, 32*, 101–113.

Fujiki, M., Spackman, M. P., Brinton, B., & Hall, A. (2004). The relationship of language and emotion regulation skills to reticence in children with specific language impairment. *Journal of Speech Language and Hearing Research, 47*, 637–646.

Gertner, B. L., Rice, M. L., & Hadley, P. A. (1994). Influence of communicative competence on peer preferences in a preschool classroom. *Journal of Speech and Hearing Research, 37*, 913–923.

Harrist, A. W., Zaia, A. F., Bates, J. E., Dodge, K. A., & Pettit, G. S. (1997). Subtypes of social withdrawal in early childhood: Sociometric status and social-cognitive differences across four years. *Child Development, 68*, 278–294.

Hart, C. H., Newell, L. D., & Olsen, S. F. (2003). Parenting skills and social/communicative competence in childhood. In J. O. Greene & B. R. Burleson (Eds.), *Handbook of communication and social interaction skills* (pp. 753–800). Mahwah, NJ: Lawrence Erlbaum Associates.

Hart, C. H., Robinson, C. C., McNeilly-Choque, M. K., Nelson, L., & Olsen, S. (1995, April). *Multiple sources of data on preschooler's playground behavior.* Paper presented at the meeting of the American Educational Research Association, San Francisco, CA.

Hart, K. I., Fujiki, M., Brinton, B., & Hart, C. H. (2004). The relationship between social behavior and severity of language impairment. *Journal of Speech Language and Hearing Research, 47*, 647–662.

Horowitz, L., Jansson, L., Ljungberg, T., & Hedenbro, M. (2006). Interaction prior to conflict and conflict resolution in preschool boys with language impairment. *International Journal of Language and Communication Disorders, 41*, 441–466.

Irwin, J. R., Carter, A. S., & Briggs-Gowan, M. J. (2002). The social-emotional development of "late-talking" toddlers. *Journal of the American Academy of Child & Adolescent Psychiatry, 41*, 1324–1332.

Johnson, D. W., & Johnson, R. T. (2002). *Multicultural education and human relations: Valuing diversity.* Boston: Allyn & Bacon.

Kalyanpur, M., & Harry, B. (1999). *Culture in special education: building reciprocal family-professional relationships.* Baltimore: P. H. Brookes.

Ladd, G. W., & Price, J. M. (1993). Play styles of peer-accepted and peer-rejected children on the playground. In C. H. Hart (Ed.), *Children on playgrounds: Research perspectives and applications* (pp. 130–161). New York: State University of New York Press.

Liiva, C. A., & Cleave, P. L. (2005). Roles of initiation and responsiveness in access and participation for children with specific language impairment. *Journal of Speech, Language, and Hearing Research, 48*, 868–883.

Lynch, E. W., & Hanson, M. J. (2004). *Developing cross-cultural competence* (3rd ed.). Baltimore: Paul H. Brookes.

Nelson, J. R., Hart, C. H., & Evans, C. A. (2008). Solitary-functional play and solitary-pretend play: Another look at the construct of solitary-active behavior using playground observations. *Social Development, 17*, 812–831.

Parker, J. G., & Asher, S. R. (1993). Beyond group acceptance: Friendship adjustment and friendship quality as distinct dimensions of children's peer adjustment. In D. Perlman & W. H. Jones (Eds.), *Advances in personal relationships* (Vol. 4, pp. 261–294). London: Kingsley.

Paul, R. (2001). *Language disorders: From infancy through adolescence* (2nd ed.). St. Louis, MO: Mosby.

Paul, R., Looney, S. S., & Dahm, P. S. (1991). Communication and socialization skills at ages 2 and 3 in "late-talking" young children. *Journal of Speech and Hearing Research, 34*, 858–865.

Redmond, S. M., & Rice, M. L. (1998). The socioemotional behaviors of children with SLI: Social adaptation or social deviance? *Journal of Speech, Language, and Hearing Research, 41*, 688–700.

Rubin, K. H., & Asendorpf, J. B. (1993). Social withdrawal, inhibition, and shyness in childhood: Conceptual and definitional issues. In K. H. Rubin & J. B. Asendorpf (Eds.), *Social withdrawal, inhibition, and shyness in childhood* (pp. 291–314). Hillsdale, NJ: Lawrence Erlbaum Associates.

Rubin, K. H., Bukowski, W. J., & Parker, J. G. (1998). Peer interactions, relationships, and groups. In W. Damon & N. Eisenberg (Eds.), *Handbook of child psychology* (5th ed., Vol. 3, pp. 619–700). New York: Wiley.

Snowling, M. J., Bishop, D. V. M., Stothard, S. E., Chipchase, B., & Kaplan, C. (2006). Psychosocial outcomes at 15 years of children with a preschool history of speech-language impairment. *Journal of Child Psychology and Psychiatry, 47*, 759–765.

Taylor, A. R., & Asher, S. (1984). Children's goals in social competence: Individual differences in a game playing context. In T. Field, J. L. Roopnarine & M. Segal (Eds.), *Friendship in normal and handicapped children* (pp. 53–78). Norwood, NJ: Ablex.

Tomblin, J. B. (2007). *Validating diagnostic standards for SLI using adolescent outcomes.* Unpublished manuscript.

Tomblin, J. B., Zhang, Z., Buckwalter, P., & Catts, H. (2000). The association of reading disability, behavioral disorders, and language impairment among second-grade children. *Journal of Child Psychology and Psychiatry, 41*, 473–482.

Younger, A. J., & Daniels, T. M. (1992). Children's reasons for nominating their peers as withdrawn: Passive withdrawal versus active isolation. *Developmental Psychology, 28*, 955–960.

# 3 Individual Differences in Word Learning
## *Implications for Clinical Practice*

*Nina Capone and Li Sheng*

## INTRODUCTION

This chapter discusses the individual differences that children bring to the task of word learning. Although development of language form (phonology, syntax, morphology) is largely completed by 8 years of age, word learning is a prolonged and continuous process that evolves across the life span. Also, grammatical and phonological rules for the most part do not vary among contexts, one subtle exception being dialectical variations. Vocabulary, though, can be specific to academic areas of study (science, math, computer science), social contexts (religious ceremony, extracurricular activity), and work or career environments (medicine, business, theater, politics); each context has its own relevant lexicon. Consider the following examples. Two 10-year-old boys share a math lexicon because they are in the same grade, yet the math lexicon of a 6-year-old is different from that of a 10-year-old by virtue of exposure to taught concepts. Furthermore, each 10-year-old child will have a different extracurricular lexicon. One may have a football lexicon (e.g., *uprights, spear, stunt, onside*), whereas the other may have a music lexicon (e.g., *treble clef, refrain, crescendo, al coda*). A 10-year-old Jewish boy may know the meaning of words such as *Bar Mitzvah, shiva,* and *bima,* whereas his Native American peer can compare and contrast *tepee, chickee, wigwam,* and *igloo* with great detail. As adults we add a career-specific lexicon to our repertoire. Also, vocabulary is continually added to a language as a cultural phenomenon. This can yield individual differences between generations. For example, new vocabulary tends to be associated with a casual youth culture (e.g., *groovy, phat*) or advances in technology that may be used more by younger people (e.g., *blogging, e-mail, texting*).

As these examples illustrate, one of the most influential factors of the individual differences observed in word learning and use is having had experience with a word (Bjorklund, 1987; Bjorklund & Schneider, 1996). The quality of experience and the quantity (i.e., frequency) of experience with a word can vary greatly between words and between individuals for particular words. The result is a continuum of word knowledge across words in the lexicon. Some words are newly learned or infrequently encountered and as such are weakly represented in the lexicon. We do not know much about a word we have only recently or rarely experienced. Other words are more frequently encountered, such that they are more richly stored in memory. The richness of word learning affects word use, and accurate word use has a functional impact on communication. Specifically, when a word is richly represented it is more likely to be recalled, whereas children tend to produce word retrieval errors when words are weakly represented (e.g., McGregor, Friedman, Reilly, & Newman, 2002; McGregor, Newman, Reilly, & Capone, 2002).

This chapter provides a discussion of several factors that contribute to the individual differences observed in word learning, including age, gender, phonological repertoire, phonological loop capacity, bilingualism, and language impairment. However, we focus primarily on an individual's experience as a contributing factor to individual differences because experience can supersede even age and IQ effects on memory (Bjorklund, 1987). Experience with words changes how the brain processes words. Neural processing in infancy is diffuse between the two hemispheres, but by toddlerhood, left-hemisphere specialization for word processing has evolved (e.g., Mills, Coffey-Corina, & Neville, 1997). There is evidence that this neural organization is related to vocabulary size (i.e., experience with word learning) and not brain maturation that comes with age. Also, it has been shown that neural processing for an individual object strengthens as a child has more experience with it (Mills, Plunkett, Prat, & Schafer, 2005).

From an associative learning model of language learning, the child brings an innate learning mechanism to the task of word learning. This mechanism is the ability to compute statistical probabilities from the language they hear (Plunkett, 1997). Children extract regularities from the ambient language (e.g., regularities in syntax) as well as nonverbal cues (e.g., gesture) that help them become more efficient with subsequent word learning (Hollich et al., 2000). Therefore, experience with individual words enriches those words in memory; also, the more experience children have with the process of word learning, the more efficient word learners they become.

If experience is an important component of word learning, then clinicians are fortunate. Intervention provides an enriched quality of experience and an increased frequency of word encounters when session objectives are well planned. As such, intervention should be tailored to the individual child's word learning needs. Target vocabulary should take into account specific words that each child needs for social, cultural, and academic success.

## A WORD ABOUT EXTERNAL FACTORS

Much of the scientific literature focuses, and rightly so, on factors that are external to the child to explain the variations in vocabulary development. Factors such as birth order, family size, socioeconomic status, and caregiver input (e.g., child-directed speech) exert an influence on the child's vocabulary development

(Hart & Risley, 1995). Recently, phonotactic probability has been the focus of some important research (e.g., Storkel, 2004c). Phonotactic probability refers to the frequency with which a sound sequence is heard in the ambient language. Common phonotactic probability words comprise more frequent sound sequences heard in the child's language, whereas uncommon phonotactic probability words comprise less frequent sound sequences.

Storkel (2001) found that preschoolers learn words composed of common sound sequences more quickly than uncommon sequences. Children with language impairment represent an individual difference in word learning. In Storkel (2004b), preschoolers with phonological disorders showed the reverse pattern, with more uncommon than common sequences learned. Storkel suggested that children with phonological disorders may have more difficulty with common sound sequences because they present competition or interference in memory among words that share them. Uncommon sequences may be more distinct from each other in memory and as such provide less competition among words that share them. We return to the issue of lexical (i.e., word) competition later in the chapter.

## MILESTONES OF WORD LEARNING

Individual differences must be considered within the timeline that most children meet vocabulary milestones. These milestones are age ranges at which the typical child meets certain expectations of vocabulary development. For example, between 11 and 13 months of age, typically developing infants speak their first words (Bates, Bretherton, & Snyder, 1988). Expressive word learning is relatively slow between 12 and 18 months of age as the child accumulates a small, stable lexicon. Some time during the second half of the 2nd year, usually between 18 and 24 months, the child will have accumulated approximately 50–100 words in his or her expressive vocabulary. It is at this time that the child will begin learning words at an exponential rate. This rapid onset of word learning is referred to as the *word spurt* (Gershkoff-Stowe & Smith, 1997).

During the word spurt, the toddler begins mapping many new words into memory. Gershkoff-Stowe and Smith (1997) found that during this shift to rapid word learning, toddlers had a parallel increase in naming errors, even errors on words that, before the word spurt, the toddlers had retrieved without difficulty. Toddlers' naming errors during the word spurt period were predominantly semantically related to the target word, such as saying *pig* for *cow,* but perseverative errors were also prevalent. A perseverative error is a repetition of a recently said word. Phonological errors, such as saying *kitchen* for *chicken,* were less common.

Perseverative errors reflect a general fragility in the process of retrieving words because children are still relatively new at the word-learning process (Gershkoff-Stowe & Smith, 1997). After the initial spurt in word learning, the retrieval process itself stabilized and perseverative errors declined. However, semantic errors persisted as the primary error type. Word retrieval errors in older children continue to be predominantly semantic in nature, even though other types of errors can occur (e.g., phonological, visual misperception; McGregor, 1997).

Another milestone tied to the word spurt is the appearance of two-word combinations. Although this aspect of semantics is outside the scope of this chapter, suffice it to say that word combinations express relationships between words, and they are an important aspect of semantic development in their own right.

Even though changes in vocabulary size occur with age, vocabulary development varies widely even between same-age peers. For example, the MacArthur-Bates Communicative Development Inventory (CDI; Fenson et al., 2007) provides normative data separately for boys and girls at ages 9–16 months (infant form) and at ages 16–30 months (toddler form). A lexicon of 276 words places a 24-month-old boy at the 50th percentile for his age. Vocabulary size at this age has a range, however, of 48 (5th percentile) to 630 (99th percentile) words. As a comparison, a 24-month-old girl has a vocabulary size of 370 words at the 50th percentile but a range of 70 (5th percentile) to 647 (99th percentile) words. Here we see that at an early stage of word learning, gender can also be an individual difference that affects vocabulary size in particular.

For most children, the early lexicon is largely composed of nouns even though there are some other word classes represented (e.g., classes including words such as *hi* or *gimmie*). Bates et al. (1988) described children with a dominant object vocabulary (i.e., more nouns than other word classes) as *referential children*. A smaller group of children are referred to as *expressive children*. These children demonstrate a learning difference characterized by a larger number of social phrases and other nonproductive or unanalyzed phrases. Several additional differences in language development are observed between referential and expressive children. Specifically, referential children show advantages in language learning in general that include larger vocabularies overall, more timely meeting of semantic and morphological milestones, and more flexible word use. Expressive children show slower vocabulary development, a less robust to absent word spurt, and later productive use of close-classed words.

Verb acquisition becomes more evident during the word spurt. Verb learning is important for the acquisition of verb-related morphology and some aspects of syntax that are verb-dependent, such as argument structure and subcategorization frames. Argument structure refers to the number of "players" needed for a grammatical sentence, and subcategorization frame refers to the linguistic phrases allowed in a sentence to maintain grammaticality (for review of relevant linguistic theory, see Shapiro, 1997).

The toddler and preschooler expand the types of word classes they are acquiring to include locative terms (e.g., *in*, *on*, *under*), temporal terms (e.g., *first*, *after*), determiners (e.g., *a*, *the*), conjunctions (e.g., *and*, *because*), adjectives (e.g., *big*), and *wh-* words (e.g., *how*, *what*, *where*, *when*, *that*, etc.), among others (Owens, 2008). By 6 years of age, the average child has a vocabulary of 14,000 words (Templin, 1957). Acquisition of polysemous terms also emerges in preschool (Nippold, 2007). Children learn the concrete meaning of these multiple meaning words first, and later they map the more abstract meaning. For example, the preschooler initially understands that *cold* refers to temperature but later he begins to understand the psychological meaning (i.e., personality trait).

Vocabulary learning has a new source for school-age children. Children continue to learn many words through oral communication, but the transition to reading offers the child more novel word experiences through written text. The child who presents difficulty with reading has an individual difference that may affect *breadth* and *depth* of word learning. Breadth refers to the number of words learned; depth refers to the richness of word knowledge. Children with language impairments have difficulty with both aspects of word learning, breadth and depth.

School-age children and adolescents acquire increasingly abstract vocabulary, as well as a new lexical form, idioms (Nippold, 2007). Idioms are metaphorical phrases that function as a single vocabulary item. They convey a meaning that is not necessarily discernable from the individual words that make up the phrase (e.g., *it's raining cats and dogs*, *long in the tooth*, or *beat around the bush*). Many of the same factors that influence single-word learning also play a role in children's development of idioms, experience with idioms being one of the most important factors. Exposure to idioms provides a context for the child to make inferences about their figurative meanings.

By the time students graduate from high school, they have an estimated vocabulary of 40,000 words. This number is doubled when proper nouns and idiomatic phrases are added, and quadrupled when all the morphological variations of the word roots are included (Miller & Gildea, 1987; Nagy & Herman, 1987).

## WORD LEARNING

It is also important to place individual differences in the context of what it means to learn a word. Word learning can grossly be thought of as learning a word label (lexical representation), its meaning (semantic representation), and the connection between them, as well as other grammatical specifications (e.g., word class, syntactic environments). The richness of each aspect of word learning is related to experience. Carey (1978) described word learning as consisting of two phases, *fast mapping* and *slow mapping*. Fast mapping is the initial phase of word learning. When children first hear a word, they must link it to the referent (i.e., its meaning). Children come equipped with several innate biases to help them constrain the possible referents of the heard word. For example, children assume that when they hear a word it refers to an object that they do not already have a name for (*novel-name-nameless category bias*; Markman, 1989). A word is said to be fast mapped when the link between lexeme and referent has been established. The fast-mapped word is weakly represented in memory because the child does not know much about a newly heard word.

Slow mapping refers to the extended period of experiences that the child has with a word after it has been fast mapped. It is through the slow-mapping process that children enrich the lexical representation, the semantic representation, and the connections within the system. Individual words will vary in terms of slow-mapping experience because some words are encountered more frequently than others. Remember the example of the 10-year-old who plays football and does not play music; this child will have greater experience hearing and using a football lexicon than a music lexicon. Therefore, his football lexicon will be richly represented, whereas his music lexicon will be comparatively quite weak. Frequently encountered words provide the child greater opportunity to enrich the lexical-semantic representations of those words. Infrequently encountered words maintain weaker representations because no new information is integrated with existing information. Take the following as a personal example. One of this chapter's authors was discussing her profession with a new acquaintance. The acquaintance remarked "ah, you can tell me what a *fricative* is." To the author's surprise this acquaintance knew the word *fricative*, a lexical item specific to language specialists. When the author asked how the acquaintance knew the word, the friend replied that she had taken a speech class in college. She remembered the word but not its meaning. In this example, one can see that even for adults, brief exposure to a word is insufficient to fully enrich its meaning. Also, of all the novel words she was exposed to in the class (e.g., fricative, nasals, affricates, glides, and many more), the acquaintance remembered only one, *fricative*, 20 years later. In other words, without repeated exposure to enrich the lexical-semantic representations of these words, the lexemes remained weak and largely forgotten.

Variations in experience affect word learning and word use. These variations include *frequency of exposure* (Dell, 1990; McGregor, Sheng, & Ball, 2007), *practice* in saying words (Gershkoff-Stowe, 2002), *neighborhood density* surrounding the lexeme (Luce & Pisoni, 1998; Sheng, 2007), and richness of *semantic representation* (Capone, 2008; Capone & McGregor, 2005; Sheng & McGregor, in press). The influence of frequency (representational richness), as well as neighborhood density, on word learning and word use can be understood within an associative learning model of the lexical-semantic system. Before discussing these factors, we first provide a general description of the associative learning model in the next section.

## LEXICAL-SEMANTIC REPRESENTATIONS ARE DISTRIBUTED WITHIN A NEURAL NETWORK

Lexical and semantic information are connected within a distributed network in the brain (Bjorklund & Schneider, 1996; Plunkett, Karmiloff-Smith, Bates, Elman, & Johnson, 1997; for review of neural imaging evidence, see Nobre & Plunkett, 1997). Semantic representations are derived from multimodal experiences (Barsalou, 2008). The child maps visual, auditory, olfactory, gustatory, tactile, and proprioceptive information that is experienced when encountering a word and its referent. Multimodal information is part of a referent's meaning. The concept of *bone*, for example, comprises visual information (shape, color), thematic associates (dogs chew bones), actions (chewing), the proprioceptive-tactile experience of feeling its weight and rough texture, and its lexeme (/bon/). Lexemes are divisible into phonemes (/b/, /o/, and /n/) and stress and syllable structure. Each of these can be conceptualized as a *node* of information (semantic, phonological, lexical) in the network. Individual nodes of information are linked or connected as a distributed neural network throughout the brain. Therefore, a rich representation can be distinct, consisting of many and unique nodes of information, and it can be richly connected between nodes.

By contrast, a weak representation will have few nodes and connections and may overlap with other weak representations in memory or be missing defining information. For example, one of this chapter's authors learns her graduate students' names by calling students by name at the beginning of the term. She referred to one student, Kimberly, as Jacqueline for two class periods. Here, we illustrate a weak lexical representation in which the stress and syllable structure were mapped, and perhaps the salience of the dorso-velar /k/ phoneme, but the full phonological sequence was clearly missing. Only through repeated exposure (which included humorous feedback for the professor) did the student's name become committed to memory.

Nodes and connections carry electrical activation. When one node is activated, electrical activity travels to other nodes in the network via the connections between them. That is, when a bone is visualized, the shape node activates, but through connections in the network there is activation of the other nodes as well, including the lexeme *bone*. A richer semantic representation is distinct, with unique information represented, and is well connected. This richer representation provides more neural activation at an intended target lexeme than a weak semantic representation. The target lexeme of a rich semantic representation will more likely be retrieved for production because greater neural activation is sent to it. When a threshold of activation is met, the lexeme is recalled. A weak semantic representation may not support word retrieval for production of a target. The result is that a semantic neighbor may be activated instead.

Remember that weak representations are most likely the result of being newly fast-mapped or infrequently encountered words. Not much is known about a word after a brief or rare exposure to it. Weak representations are not distinct from other weakly represented words because they may share some features. For example, upon seeing an image of a *pig,* a child may activate several lexical-semantic representations that are weak if he or she has little experience with farm animals. These representations perhaps all have two ears, four legs, and a tail. There are several possible lexemes to name this weak representation—*pig, horse, cow.* The child is just as likely to say any one of them. As the child acquires a richer knowledge of pigs, horses, and cows, only the relevant lexeme will be activated because the distinct semantic features for one will send greater activation to it. Nodes and connections are enriched and strengthened through experience. Because quantity and quality of word experience differs, we can think of lexical-semantic representations within the network as existing along a continuum of representational strength, from weak to richer. That is, richness is dependent upon experience with a particular word, experience being of varying quantity and quality (Capone & McGregor, 2005).

In addition to semantic nodes and lexical nodes, there is a distinction made between lexical nodes and phoneme nodes (Dell, 1986, 1988; Dell, Schwartz,

Martin, Saffran, & Gagnon, 1997). Lexeme and phoneme nodes are connected bidirectionally such that activation spreads from higher level units (e.g., lexemes) to lower level units (e.g., phonemes) and back to the higher level units. Accordingly, activation spreads from a target to its neighbors and back to the target via their shared phonemes. For example, when /bon/ is activated, /bot/ will receive spreading collateral activation from the /b/ and /o/ phoneme activity. As a result, a large number of similar-sounding neighbors may increase activation of the phonemes that make up the target words (Dell & O'Seaghdha, 1992; Storkel, 2004a; Vitevitch & Sommers, 2003). Of importance to the clinician is the understanding that strengthening storage of individual words with enriched quality and quantity of experiences may reduce the competition effects of other lexical neighbors. Distinct and enriched lexical and semantic representations will set the target lexeme apart from its competitors.

## NEIGHBORHOOD DENSITY AND PRACTICE WITH WORDS: LEXICAL REPRESENTATIONS

Neighborhood density refers to the number of words that are phonologically similar to a target word. More specifically, density is determined by the number of words that can be created from a target word when a single phoneme is added, deleted, or changed (Luce & Pisoni, 1998; Storkel, 2004c). Density is described as sparse (e.g., *vogue*), with few neighbors (e.g., *rogue, vague, vole, vote*) surrounding the representation in memory, or dense (e.g., *pan*), a word with many neighbors (e.g., *pad, pack, pal, pass, pat, man, ran, tan, van, span, pant, pen, an*, among others).

Neighborhood density influences word identification, word production, and word learning. For children, words from sparser neighborhoods are identified more accurately and more quickly. As for word production, there is some conflicting evidence. On the one hand, Newman and German (2002) found an advantage of sparse neighborhoods over dense neighborhoods in naming for typically developing children as well as children with word-finding difficulties. On the other hand, Sheng (2007) found an advantage of dense neighborhoods for naming in children with and without specific language impairment (SLI). German and Newman (2004) also found a dense neighborhood advantage in the naming performance of children with word-finding difficulties. Finally, with regard to word learning, denser neighborhoods appear to give the child an advantage in learning new words (for review, see Storkel, 2004c). It is of importance to the clinician that the words that children learn and use are affected by their existing (i.e., already learned) vocabulary. In this instance, the denseness or sparseness of a neighborhood will affect the child's new word learning and use.

Another experiential factor of word learning and use is practice in saying a word. With increased frequency of exposure to a word comes the opportunity for the child to practice saying it more often. Gershkoff-Stowe (2002) found that when toddlers had more practice saying words, they retrieved them more often than words they had little practice producing. Specifically, in one condition toddlers had practice naming pictures from a picture book, but in a second condition toddlers had extra practice naming the same pictures from a book and picture cards. Toddlers in the extra-practice condition produced fewer naming errors than toddlers in the low-practice condition. Children also had an opportunity to map more semantic information about words because they saw pictures of the referents more often. The additional opportunity to see pictured referents may have also enriched their semantic representations.

## SEMANTIC REPRESENTATION AND LEXEME RETRIEVAL

The influence of semantic representation on lexeme retrieval has been studied in typically developing children and children with SLI (Capone, 2008; Capone & McGregor, 2005; McGregor & Appel, 2002; McGregor, Friedman, et al., 2002; McGregor, Newman, et al., 2002; Sheng & McGregor, in press). McGregor (1997) showed that children with SLI make the same types of naming errors that typically developing children make. The difference is that children with SLI make more errors than their typically developing peers (see also Lahey & Edwards, 1999). Naming errors by both groups of children tend to be semantically related to the target word (e.g., saying *glass* for *cup*) more often than other error types, including phonological errors (e.g., saying *miracleride* for *merry-go-round*). A semantic error suggests that the breakdown in the retrieval process occurred at the level of semantic representation or at the link between semantic and lexical representation. Indeed, research shows that semantic richness is one important aspect of word learning and word use.

McGregor, Friedman et al. (2002) examined typically developing 5–8-year-old children's accuracy in naming a set of target words. Children then defined and drew pictures of target words as two pieces of converging evidence of semantic knowledge. Words that were named accurately were associated with (a) definitions that contained more information units and (b) more semantically specific drawings (rich semantic representations) than words named in error. When target words resulted in a naming error, they were (a) defined with fewer information units and (b) rendered as less semantically specific drawings (weak semantic representations). McGregor, Friedman et al. used a set of target words that were drawn from the children's established vocabulary; therefore, frequency of exposure could not be controlled. Also, an association between semantic richness and word retrieval was found, but the study could not establish a cause–effect relationship. Capone and McGregor (2005) conducted a word learning experiment that trained novel word–referent pairs. This experiment controlled frequency of experience but varied semantic enrichment. The study established a causal link of semantic enrichment, semantic learning, and lexeme retrieval.

Capone and McGregor (2005) examined the influence of enriched quality of semantic learning for its effect on word retrieval in typically developing toddlers. These were children who were post-word spurt, ages 27–31 months. Children heard objects labeled a total of nine times across three separate learning sessions.

The quality of experience varied among three conditions of semantic enrichment: shape, function, and control. Object shape (shape condition) and object function (function condition) were enriched in their respective conditions via gestures; no semantic enrichment was provided in the control condition. At the test, toddlers named more objects when those words were learned with semantic enrichment (i.e., gestures that highlighted shape or function) than when words were learned without it. In addition, semantic learning was assessed. Toddlers knew more about the objects in the shape and function conditions than in the control condition. Therefore, semantic enrichment via gesture strengthened semantic learning and retrieval of trained lexemes. For the same participants, Capone (2007) discovered that semantic knowledge was sometimes expressed in gestural communication even though it was not expressed via spoken language. Children's gestures are hypothesized to express knowledge that is not rich enough to support the demands of spoken expression (for review, see Capone & McGregor, 2004). As such, Capone (2007) argued that for some objects, semantic representations were weakly represented, but the objects were not altogether missing representations.

Capone (2008) replicated and extended the evidence that semantic enrichment influences lexeme retrieval by again comparing word learning among three conditions: shape, function, and point. Here, the test of lexeme retrieval was in the more challenging context of lexeme extension. *Lexeme extension* refers to the application of a known word to a novel exemplar of its referent category (principle of extendability; Markman, 1989). This is an important aspect of word use because each instance of a word–referent pair need not be taught explicitly. Indeed word learning would be quite laborious without it! Also, words reach symbolic status when they are extended to name multiple exemplars, and symbolic status is required for functional communication.

Lexeme extension is a challenging test of the relationship between semantic enrichment and word retrieval. When children extend a lexeme, they must first make an inference about the untrained object's semantic category. Children make such inferences on the basis of shared semantic features between the novel exemplar and the trained referent. In the case of objects, inferences are made on the basis of shared shape and/or function (Landau, Smith, & Jones, 1988; Kemler Nelson, 1999). For example, after children learn that the thing one drinks from is labeled *cup*, they will start naming other objects that look like it *cup* because they share shape and function with the original cup. By contrast, objects that share the same material are not named *cup* (e.g., plastic objects).

Capone (2008) found that typically developing toddlers, ages 27–42 months, extended lexemes to name three untrained exemplars when they learned lexemes with shape enrichment (via gesture) over simply pointing to an object in teaching lexemes; naming performance under the function condition fell between the shape and point conditions. Performance across word-learning conditions illustrated the gradient continuum of word learning, with the strongest learning achieved when lexemes were enriched with shape cues. Capone & McGregor (2005) and

Capone (2008) provided converging evidence that semantic enrichment positively influences lexeme learning and use by young children.

## SEMANTIC REPRESENTATIONS IN CHILDREN WITH SLI

Children with SLI demonstrate the same relationship between semantic richness and naming performance as their typically developing peers. McGregor, Newman et al. (2002) recruited children with SLI and replicated the results of McGregor, Friedman, et al. (2002). Specifically, children with SLI produced more information units and drew more semantically specific drawings for words that they named accurately than for those that resulted in an error. The difference between children with SLI and typically developing children was that children with SLI made more errors. Sheng and McGregor (in press) then studied the effect of SLI on children's semantic network development. A word association task was used to tap semantic networks around test stimuli. Children were asked to retrieve three words that were semantically associated with each target word. Associates that are semantically related to a target (e.g., *dog—pet*, *bark*, *furry*) reflected activation of the semantic network surrounding the target word in memory. Children with SLI produced fewer semantic associations than their typically developing peers. Also, children with SLI produced more errors (i.e., words that do not bear a relationship to the target such as *dog—lamp*) than age-matched peers and younger children who were matched for expressive vocabulary. These and other studies show that children with SLI are less adept at developing rich semantic representations and develop less richly connected semantic networks (Alt & Plante, 2006; Alt, Plante, & Creusere, 2004; Gray, 2005; Nash & Donaldson, 2005). If semantic richness influences word retrieval, and if children with SLI are poor semantic learners, then children with SLI need increased frequency and quality of word exposure to map semantic information (as well as lexical information) for word use. In particular, it is important to remember that intervention goals should include increasing vocabulary size (i.e., breadth) as well as vocabulary knowledge (i.e., depth of semantic and lexical knowledge). We will return to this discussion in the clinical implications section below.

Gray (2005) examined the effect of phonological and semantic cues on word learning in preschoolers with SLI. Preschoolers participated in several word-learning sessions that provided word models and prompts for the child to repeat words. These procedures provided children increased practice with saying new words. The children were also provided feedback from the experimenter on accuracy of responses. In addition, children were provided either a phonological enrichment cue or a semantic enrichment cue. Semantic cues included superordinate category, physical characteristics, function, or associations with the target object. Phonological cues highlighted initial sound or syllable, or a rhyming cue. For example, the experimenter said "This is a *fogut*. Say *fogut*." Children were then provided a semantic cue—"It's made of plastic"—or a phonological cue—"It starts with /f/" (Gray, 2005, p. 1457). When learning was assessed, Gray found that semantic cues appeared to strengthen children's ability to comprehend trained words, whereas phonological cues appeared to strengthen their production of them. Wing (1990) also compared phonologically and semantically based enrichment cues and found an advantage for phonologically based cues in naming.

One caveat is worth considering. If children with SLI have difficulty processing and learning verbal symbols as in language learning, then perhaps the clinician should consider implementation of nonverbal enrichment cues, such as gesture cues to semantic information, and other multimodal experiences. For example, Capone & McGregor (2004) provided a review of the positive effects gesture cues have on verbal learning. It is also possible that children benefit from different types of cues at different points in development. For example, McGregor & Capone (2004) provided gesture + word labels to a set of quadruplets who were at risk for language impairment. These were infants who were followed longitudinally from the prelinguistic period through toddlerhood. McGregor and Capone found that words paired with gestures emerged in each child's expressive vocabulary (i.e., to name) before other words. Research is still needed to examine the individual differences between factors that could influence intervention, such as modality and developmental age.

## PHONOLOGICAL REPERTOIRE AS AN INDIVIDUAL DIFFERENCE IN WORD LEARNING

For very young children at the start of word learning, the size and composition of their *phonological repertoire* can exert influence on word learning. McCune & Vihman (2001) suggested that the size of children's consonant inventory at the earliest stage of language development is predictive of children's later vocabulary growth. In the babbling period, the proportion of vocalizations that include consonants grows over time. Consonant production in prelinguistic vocalizations is the most useful predictor of speech onset, long-term phonological development, and children's transition to using referential vocabulary.

McCune and Vihman (2001) followed a group of 20 children from the time they were 9 months old until they reached 16 months. Monthly free-play sessions of mother–child dyads were recorded for each participant. These researchers inventoried each child's consonant repertoire. A consonant was included in the child's repertoire if it was produced at least 10 times in each of three or more monthly half-hour sessions. Consonants that met this criterion were characterized as a *vocal motor scheme*. Vocal motor schemes are defined as a productive sound sequence that is consistent and generalized to other contexts, much like real words. Among the consonants that met the criterion for vocal motor scheme, /t, d/ were produced by 17 children, /p, b/ by 10 children, and /k, g/ by 7 children. The remaining consonants that appeared, /s/, /m/, /n/, and /l/, were produced by fewer than 5 children.

The researchers then tallied words that occurred across at least two different contexts and/or in relation to at least two different objects (e.g., *baby* to refer to the child herself and to a doll). The third dependent measure was the age at which children made a transition to referential word use. This transition was operationally defined as the time when children (a) produced two or more referential words in a session and (b) exhibited those or other referential words in subsequent sessions. Three findings are pertinent to the close interaction between phonological and lexical learning. First, the transition to using referential vocabulary varied between individual children. Children who made the transition early (by 13–14 months) had a larger number of vocal motor schemes in their repertoire than those who made the transition later (by 15–16 months). This latter group, in turn, had more vocal motor schemes than those who never made the transition during the study period.

Second, the number of vocal motor schemes turned out to be a strong predictor of the number of different referential word types produced by age 16 months, accounting for 43% of the variance between children. Third, the researchers examined the consonants in words occurring at both 15 and 16 months and found that the vocal motor schemes accounted for the consonants in 91% of these words. In other words, these vocal motor schemes were privileged production routines, and children relied on these routines when producing their first words. Taken together, infant consonant production is a strong predictor of early lexical milestones and may act as a gauge for children's readiness to say words.

The McCune and Vihman (2001) study has at least two important implications. First, the size of children's sound inventories shared a positive relationship with the same children's ability to learn words. Second, individual children may show selectivity when incorporating new words in their lexicon by relying on their individual repertoire of well-practiced consonants. This second finding is consistent with a number of earlier studies that investigated the composition of children's sound inventories in relation to their early word productions (Ferguson & Farwell, 1975; Leonard, Newhoff, & Mesalam, 1980).

Lexical selection that is based on the child's established phonological repertoire is referred to as *phonological selectivity and avoidance* (Ferguson & Farwell, 1975). As a case example, Ferguson and Farwell documented a rather rare case of phonological selectivity. One of the children they studied favored words with sibilant fricatives and affricates, producing words such as *ice*, *eyes*, *shoes*, and *juice* at an earlier age than is typical. The two remaining children had few to no words containing these sounds. Leonard et al. (1980) studied the word-initial sounds attempted and produced by 10 children early in word learning development. Words with initial /m/, /b/, and /d/ were attempted by all children, words with initial /k/ were attempted by 9 children, and words with initial /h/, /w/, /n/, /g/, and /p/ were also attempted by 5 or more children. In contrast, none of the children attempted words with initial /v/, /θ/, /z/, /l/, or /r/, and fewer than half of the children attempted words beginning with other consonants. These results showed some general consistency in children's selectivity patterns overall but some individual differences as well.

Experimental studies have examined the effect of individual phonological repertoire on young children's word learning. Specifically, studies compared learning of *in phonology* (IN) versus *out of phonology* (OUT) novel words

(Leonard, Schwartz, Morris, & Chapman, 1981; Leonard et al., 1982; Schwartz & Leonard, 1982). IN words contained consonants or structures that were observed in the child's productive phonological repertoire. OUT words were those that contained consonants or syllable structures not inventoried as part of the child's phonological repertoire In these studies, children at the early stage of word learning (vocabulary size ranged from 5 to 75 words) were exposed to nonsense words (e.g., *bobo, meb*) paired with novel referents over an extended period of time. For each child, half of the words were IN words and half were OUT words.

In a review of this literature, Schwartz (1988) concluded that a significant IN word advantage emerged for the number of words learned and the rate of learning. A higher number of IN words were acquired than OUT words, and the IN words were acquired more rapidly than the OUT words. One of these investigations (Leonard et al., 1982) included children with SLI. Children with SLI were compared with younger children who were matched for expressive vocabulary size. Children with SLI also showed an advantage for learning IN words over OUT words. Therefore, children abide by the constraints of their productive phonology when it comes to expressive word learning, regardless of their language learning abilities (but see Storkel, 2004b, as described above).

To summarize, the size of an infant's consonant inventory signals the child's readiness to learn words and make the transition to referential word use. Furthermore, the ease of acquiring words is affected by a child's existing pho-nology, with words containing IN sounds acquired more rapidly than words containing OUT sounds. Although these constraints will eventually become less durable with development, a close examination of the infant-toddlers' current sound inventory can provide clinicians with valuable information for therapy planning and target selection.

## PHONOLOGICAL LOOP CAPACITY INFLUENCES WORD LEARNING

The capacity children have to process words in working memory is another important individual difference observed in children's word learning. Working memory refers to the memory involved in active, online processing of information. We first review, generally, the working memory model of Baddeley and Hitch (1974; Baddeley, 2000). Within this model of working memory there are several components—*central executor, phonological loop, visual-spatial sketchpad,* and *episodic buffer*—each of which has a separate function. The visual-spatial sketchpad and the phonological loop are work spaces in the model. The visual-spatial sketchpad is the work space for nonverbal information (e.g., visual recognition, stimuli orientation). The phonological loop is the work space for processing speech-based information (i.e., encoding and rehearsing sound sequences). The central executor is the component of working memory that is responsible for directing attention and delegating neural resources between the two workspaces. The central executor is also responsible for retrieving information from long-term memory. Processing novel information in the context of known information (long-term memory) places new information in a meaningful context. The newest component of the model to be described is the episodic buffer. The episodic buffer integrates multimodal information—visual and verbal—into something meaningful before it is stored in long-term memory.

Neural resources for processing information in working memory are limited in capacity. The central executor is responsible for maximizing these limited neural resources by efficiently directing attention and distributing resources between the visual-spatial sketchpad and the phonological loop. In this section we focus our discussion on the phonological loop. To date, the phonological loop is a well-studied component of the model because of its relationship with word learning. Specifically, early vocabulary development is linked to the integrity of the phonological loop, and children bring individual differences in phonological loop capacity to the task of word learning.

Two common measures of phonological loop capacity are digit span repetition and nonword repetition. Digits and nonwords are used because they do not have visual referents or previous exposure associated with them. Therefore, they are believed to be processed exclusively by the phonological loop without the support of information from long-term memory and without the demand of visual spatial processing. Consider that all new words a child encounters are essentially nonwords upon first encounter. The nonword repetition task is often used with children to measure capacity of the phonological loop. They are asked to imitate phoneme sequences from their native language that are not real words (e.g., "say *ballop*"). These are also nonwords of increasing length, one to four syllables (e.g., *ballop, blonterstaping*).

Research dating back to the 1980s and continuing to the present day supports a relationship between nonword repetition performance and receptive vocabulary size in children as young as 22 months of age, and for children with and without language impairments (e.g., Gathercole & Baddeley, 1989, 1990; Hoff, Core, & Bridges, 2008; Jarrold & Baddeley, 1997). Gathercole and Baddeley (1989) found that 4- and 5-year-old children with larger vocabularies were better at nonword repetition than children with smaller vocabularies. Phonological memory at 4 years of age also predicted vocabulary size at 5 years, even after nonverbal IQ and 4-year-old vocabulary size were statistically controlled.

Gathercole, Willis, Emslie, and Baddeley (1992) studied children from 4 to 8 years of age. Again, nonword repetition at age 4 years predicted vocabulary size at age 5 years; vocabulary size at 4 years of age did not predict nonword repetition at 5 years of age. Therefore, the direction of the relationship between nonword repetition and vocabulary development is this: the variance observed between children in processing nonwords is directly related to the individual differences observed in their vocabulary development 1 year later. At 6–8 years of age, however, the direction of that relationship changed. Vocabulary size became a significant predictor of later nonword repetition, but the reverse was no longer true. By 8 years of age, children have accumulated a substantial vocabulary size. This increase in vocabulary knowledge apparently provides the opportunity for the child to scaffold the temporary retention of nonwords in working memory.

As with other aspects of word learning, children with language impairments show the same relationship between nonword repetition and vocabulary size as their unimpaired peers. The exception, of course, is that they are poorer at nonword repetition than their peers, and they have smaller vocabularies. Gathercole and Baddeley (1990) used the nonword repetition task with a group of children with SLI and two groups of control children, one matched on verbal ability, the other matched on nonverbal ability. Children with SLI performed more poorly than both control groups, particularly when words were longer, 3- and 4-syllable nonwords. The difficulty that children with SLI have with nonword repetition has been replicated (Dollaghan & Campbell, 1998; Edwards & Lahey, 1998; Ellis Weismer et al., 2000; Montgomery, 1995). Of particular importance for the clinician is that there is consensus that poor nonword repetition performance is a clinical marker for SLI (Conti-Ramsden & Hesketh, 2003; Dollaghan & Campbell, 1998; Ellis Weismer et al., 2000; Graf Estes, Evans, & Else-Quest, 2007). In fact, Campbell, Dollaghan, Needleman, and Janosky (1997) published a standardized diagnostic measure of nonword repetition, the Non-Word Repetition Test, for clinicians to use.

Children with Down syndrome (DS) represent another group of children with language impairment. Children with DS have moderate to severe intellectual disabilities, with verbal ability being more impaired than nonverbal ability. In a longitudinal study, Laws and Gunn (2004) administered tests of language and memory to 30 adolescents and young adults with DS at two sessions that were completed 5 years apart. As with typically developing (but much younger) children, there was a significant correlation between nonword repetition at Time 1 and vocabulary size at Time 2 after controlling for nonverbal ability and early vocabulary knowledge.

Interestingly, when the DS group was divided into two subgroups—vocabulary age equivalent under 5 years of age and vocabulary age equivalent over 5 years of age—there was a significant correlation between receptive vocabulary at Time 1 and nonword repetition performance at Time 2 only for the subgroup whose vocabulary was above the age equivalent of 5 years. This pattern also paralleled the relationship found in typical development that we discussed above. There appears to be a shift in how phonological memory and vocabulary size interact with experience in word learning (i.e., vocabulary size). Having accrued a sufficient number of vocabulary words enables children to draw on their extant vocabulary knowledge to scaffold maintaining novel sound sequences in working memory.

The relationship between nonword repetition (i.e., the measure of phonological loop capacity) and new word learning is unclear. For example, Alt and Plante (2006) found that nonword repetition scores were positively correlated with the fast mapping of novel words. Alternatively, Gray (2006) failed to find a relationship between nonword repetition and fast mapping of novel words. Furthermore, the durability of the fast-mapped representation into the slow mapping period has not yet been tested for its relationship with nonword repetition. Horst and Samuelson (2008) have suggested that fast and slow mapping may represent distinct processes. In fact, it is likely that nonword repetition, fast mapping, and slow mapping all represent distinct processes. Whereas the relationship between nonword repetition and existing vocabulary (a measure of slow mapping) is well documented, the relationship between nonword repetition and the gradual process of slow mapping of new words for children remains a fruitful area of research.

## THE CASE OF BILINGUALISM

A discussion of individual differences in lexical learning is not complete without consideration of children who are bilingual. Although the general patterns of language learning are believed to be similar between monolingual and bilingual individuals, vocabulary development is the exception. Individual differences can manifest themselves in bilingual children in the proportion of time spent using each language, the context in which they use each language, and the conversational partners they have for each language. A detailed discussion of how each of these factors affects word learning can be found in Patterson and Pearson (2004), Peña and Kester (2004), and Hammer and Rodríguez (Chapter 4). Here we highlight important issues for assessing and treating the bilingual lexicon.

The first issue concerns how to calculate vocabulary size in bilingual people. In our foregoing discussion of word learning, we bolstered the view that word learning consists of learning the lexeme, the meaning, and the link between the two (Gupta, 2005). In the bilingual child, word learning has an added layer of complexity because each meaning unit needs to be linked with two language-specific lexemes (i.e., one from each language). To further complicate matters, even translation equivalents may not have the same referent for the child. For example, a child may use *dog* to refer to the family pet but *perro* to refer to dogs in general.

Several alternative scoring methods should be used to calculate a bilingual child's vocabulary. The clinician can calculate a *total vocabulary* score by summing all lexemes across both languages. This method is likely to yield a vocabulary size that is equal to or higher than that of the monolingual child. This approach may be appropriate for assessing infants and toddlers because it recognizes each sound-meaning pairing as an achievement. A second scoring method tallies the bilingual child's *conceptual vocabulary* (Pearson, Fernández, & Oller, 1993). Here, the clinician tallies all lexemes, including translation equivalents, only once. For example, *dog* and *perro* are tallied as one item for the child who is bilingual Spanish–English. This method tends to yield a vocabulary size that is comparable to that of the monolingual child. This method is recommended when assessing older children in particular. Sheng, McGregor, and Marian (2006) adapted this method to assess depth of semantic knowledge as well. Here, the experimenters administered the repeated word association task to 5–8-year-old children who were bilingual in Mandarin–English. Children generated three associations to each word, and the proportion of categorical associations (e.g., dog: pet, cat, golden retriever) was compared between the bilingual Mandarin–English and the monolingual English-speaking children. However, the performance entered in the comparison for the bilingual child was the best language performance.

To determine the child's best language performance, Sheng et al. compared the bilingual child's performance in Mandarin and in English and took scores from the high-scoring language to represent the child's performance. This best performance score is derived from the idea of conceptual scoring and reflects the highest level of development attained by the bilingual children instead of the level reflected in one language only. In Sheng et al., English contributed to the best performance score 53% of the time and Mandarin 47% of the time. Performance on the word association task was fairly comparable between bilingual and monolingual participants using this method. However, bilingual children showed a slight advantage over monolingual children in categorical (*cold–hot*) responding. The interpretation of the result was that bilingual children showed an advantage in the development of semantic networks in memory.

Finally, the clinician may opt to calculate vocabulary score in a single language. This approach can identify critical gaps in language-specific contexts (e.g., academic success versus social context). Caution is needed with this method because this score is likely to be lower than that of the monolingual child. Because a single language score will *not* be a comprehensive reflection of the child's semantic knowledge across languages, it is critical that clinicians use a variety of scoring methods to accurately characterize semantic development of the bilingual child.

Another assessment issue for bilingual lexical acquisition pertains to the amount of overlap in a bilingual child's two lexicons. Pearson, Fernández, and Oller (1995) suggested that the degree of overlap or translation equivalents in each lexicon of a bilingual toddler is similar to the degree of overlap between the lexicons of two monolingual children. In other words, knowing a word in one language does not necessarily facilitate learning the translation equivalents in the other language. Bilingual children do not appear to privilege learning two names for the same concept. This may be a reflection of bilingual children's experience, because bilingual children may use one language exclusively at school and the other language only in the home context. For example, Peña, Bedore, and Zlatic-Giunta (2002) examined the responses produced by 4–7-year-old bilingual children who spoke Spanish and English in a category generation task (e.g., "Name all the animals you can think of in one minute"). Comparisons between the two languages revealed that a considerable proportion (68.4%) of the responses were unique to either language. Also using the category generation task, Ward, Chu, Vaid, and Heredia (2005) found that the percentage of unique items ranged from 42% to 69% across the 10 categories sampled in the Mandarin–English bilingual adults.

Young bilingual children may learn different vocabulary words in each of their languages because of differences in experience. These differences in vocabulary learning persist during development such that older children (and adults) who are bilingual show considerable between-language variations in their semantic representations. There is a degree of independence between word learning in the two languages of the bilingual individual. Transfer from one language to the other may be limited for this domain of language (Ordóñez, Carlo, Snow, & McLaughlin, 2002; Patterson & Pearson, 2004).

## LATE TALKERS

Late-talking children are generally identified between their 2nd and 3rd birthdays. *Late talkers* warrant a special section in our chapter because their initial delay is characterized by difficulty learning words. Specifically, late talkers present with a small vocabulary, too few object words, and a less diverse verb lexicon than their peers (Hadley, 1998; Paul, 1996; Rescorla, Mirak, & Singh, 2000). An expressive vocabulary score below the 10th percentile on the CDI is one measure that reflects a child at risk for persistent language impairment (Tsybina & Eriks-Brophy, 2007). The reader is reminded that in typical development large object vocabularies are associated with larger vocabularies overall and the more timely achievement of other language milestones. Rescorla et al. (2000) found that late-talking children with larger vocabularies (although smaller vocabularies than those of their typically developing peers) also made greater gains in vocabulary and grammar development compared with those with the smallest vocabularies. Development of the object vocabulary in typically developing children is positively related to the child's bias toward using shared object shape when extending lexemes (Gershkoff-Stowe & Smith, 2004). Jones (2003) showed that late-talking toddlers do not use shape information in extending lexemes to novel exemplars. Therefore, late-talking toddlers may not be taking advantage of the statistical regularity with which an object's shape and its lexeme are correlated for word learning.

Many of the toddlers identified as late talkers will outgrow their early language delay. These children are later referred to as *late bloomers* (Paul, 1996; Thal & Tobias, 1992). Late talkers who persist in having language impairments are later referred to as *specific language impaired* or *language learning disabled* (Paul, 2007). For children with SLI or a language learning disability (LLD), initial delays in vocabulary development transcend the domain of semantics to affect the development of morphosyntax, narratives, and other pragmatic areas. But what puts a late talker at risk for SLI/LLD? Some prognostic indicators have been identified. All late talkers are initially identified by their small expressive vocabularies. However, children who also have an initial delay in receptive language and in play and other gestural schemes are the children who tend to persist with their language delays into the school years (e.g., Thal, Reilly, Seibert, Jeffries, & Fenson, 2004; Thal & Tobias, 1992). By contrast, children who are later recognized as late bloomers tended to fall within normal limits for receptive language and play, and they express communicative intents via gestures early on. Throughout elementary school, late bloomers are reported to perform within a typical range of development on formal tests of language. However, their performance remains significantly below their same-age peers (e.g., Rescorla, 2002, 2005).

## CLINICAL IMPLICATIONS

Attention to individual differences in word learning is particularly important in clinical practice. Individual differences come from several sources, including age, gender, language ability, phonological loop capacity, bilingualism, and experience.

The reader is reminded that children can present with overlapping differences. For example, the child who is bilingual may also present with language impairment. Successful communication, of course, depends on the development of a general lexicon that we all share. However, we must also acquire context-specific lexicons that support individual academic and social areas of communication. The clinician can remember that assessing and training a variety of *core lexicons* can have a broad functional impact on communication. It is also important to remember that intervention goals should increase vocabulary size, as well as the depth or richness of lexical and semantic knowledge.

This chapter has focused on the effect that quality and quantity of experience have on word learning. Intervention provides the child with increased frequency of exposure to important words, as well as richer quality of experience. Quality of experience refers to the clinician's therapeutic scaffolding (e.g., cues, prompts, models, control of linguistic and situational complexity) and experiential activity planning. Our discussion of the associative learning model provides the theoretical foundation for interventions to take place in a variety of contexts and with direct experiential activities. Within this model, we understand how multimodal experience enriches lexical-semantic representations. Enriched representations support retrieval and extension of lexemes. We conclude the chapter with a final discussion of clinically specific issues.

Effective interventions are guided by thorough evaluations. Expressive vocabulary is generally assessed using formal tests (e.g., Expressive Vocabulary Test [EVT]; Williams, 1997) and formal analyses (e.g., type:token ratio, number of different words; for review, see Retherford, 2000). These tests and analyses compare the child's naming performance to same-age peers. The EVT, for example, gives us a sense of a child's expressive vocabulary *size* relative to other children of the same age but not the individual vocabulary items that comprise that child's lexicon. Also, formal tests tend to sample the most typical vocabulary items found in the lexicon at each age level and not the more individually specific items, which can vary across individuals and contexts. By making comparisons of the child's vocabulary size with a normative data set, we remove the rich information that individual differences can provide the clinician regarding (a) the types of words a child does or does not know, (b) words that would impact the child's functional communication for academic and/or social success, and (c) any unique learning strategies that the child may bring to the task of word learning. Therefore, our best clinical practices may be missing important information that could help clinicians plan and execute interventions for individual children.

Formal tests of vocabulary also do not analyze naming errors. An error analysis could help the clinician identify the types of words or word classes that the child with language impairment may have difficulty learning. Furthermore, error analysis could reveal whether the child is having more difficulty with the semantic aspects of word learning (a prevalence of semantic errors), the phonological aspects of word learning (a prevalence of phonological errors), or other weaknesses that are reflected through errors (visual misperception/encoding). Interventions could be customized toward semantic enrichment (i.e., multimodal experiences; Manolson, 1992; see also Gray, 2005) versus phonological enrichment (e.g., sound marking, syllable marking; see, for example, German, 2002; Gray, 2005; McGregor, 1994) depending upon the types of errors children make. More often than not, a combination of semantic and phonologically based enrichment programs will be implemented (Wing, 1990). As we have discussed, children with language impairments tend to have difficulty learning both types of information. However, individual differences that are discerned through error analysis can guide the clinician to weight each of these more effectively. It is also wise to remember that both oral and written language may need to be targeted if children present with reading impairments.

Sampling children's spontaneous language is central to any language evaluation (e.g., Capone, 2010). A tally of the types of words a child is using can be taken from a *spontaneous language sample analysis*. However, we suggest that more than one topic area be used to elicit spontaneous language. For example, two or three short samples can be elicited around an academic topic, an extracurricular topic, and perhaps a topic that relates to religious or cultural ceremony. Once the more general measures are computed (e.g., number of different words), the clinician can examine the individual words used, words not used, and error types. This assessment (and intervention) process should be conducted in collaboration with the child's parent or teacher. The parent and teacher can provide lists of core vocabularies needed for communication success in each context. A second source of core vocabulary targets for intervention can come from academic texts and literature related to the child's social, religious, or cultural interests. A third method of organizing target words for intervention is to have children journal words and idioms that they encounter in their daily academic and social contexts. This may capitalize not only on individual differences in word learning needs but also on the child's motivation to participate in the intervention process. When children journal important words and draw vocabulary from their functional communication contexts, it can give them ownership over the vocabulary learning process. It will also ensure that individual differences in word learning needs are addressed.

For much younger children, parents and other caregivers remain the primary source of relevant and functional vocabulary. However, the CDI is also an excellent source of vocabulary targets for intervention. Not only does the CDI provide the clinician with the most typical words in toddlers' vocabularies, it is also organized by word class (e.g., actions, prepositions, and a variety of nouns—body parts, animals, vehicles, toys, and others). Therefore, the CDI allows the clinician to assess whether vocabulary is limited to certain items within a word class or is spread thinly across word classes. Individual intervention goals can be determined by word class or category. For example, a late talker may have two separate target goals: body parts and action words.

It is prudent to remember that evaluation and intervention are best conducted when tasks, materials, techniques, scaffolds, and goals are developmentally appropriate and with consideration of the child's bilingual status (American Speech-Language-Hearing Association, 2004; Capone, 2010). The child's age is one source of individual difference, but more importantly, the child's language ability and experience with learning language (or more than one language) can exert greater influence. Assessment and intervention need to be developmentally appropriate such that intervention goals are determined on the basis of where the child's current abilities fall along the continuum of milestones discussed above. For example, the 30-month-old child with a lexicon of fewer than 10 words has a vocabulary development placed (grossly) at the 12–18-month-old age level. Therefore, one of this child's vocabulary goals will be to increase his or her lexicon to at least 50 words (a vocabulary milestone for children 18–24 months). Another goal will be to increase this child's noun vocabulary given what is known about the importance and prevalence of nouns in the early vocabulary.

The child's existing sound inventory should also be considered when working with children whose vocabularies are under the 50-word mark. An inventory of the child's individual sound repertoire is necessary when selecting targets in teaching vocabulary. There is ample normative information for individual phoneme production that provides clinicians with an expectation of when sounds are acquired (Smit, Hand, Freilinger, Bernthal, & Bird, 1990). These norms are valuable in identifying generalities in learning. However, observational and experimental studies have confirmed that young children may show individualized preference for words containing certain categories of sounds. The reason for this preference is not entirely clear and may be underlined by factors such as frequency in the input, motor limitations, or perceptual limitations (Schwartz, 1988).

Finally, the results of investigations into the development of the vocabularies of children learning more than one language have indicated that intervention focused on the vocabulary development of the bilingual child requires a variety of methods. When a clinician understands vocabulary development of the bilingual child, she can minimize incorrectly diagnosing a language impairment where a language difference exists. The clinician is reminded that calculating a vocabulary score in a single language may be appropriate *in conjunction with other measures* to identify critical gaps in specific contexts, such as academic success. Where language impairment exists, the clinician can make context-specific decisions regarding which language to use as the basis for treatment and who is most competent to provide that intervention. Please refer to the American Speech-Language-Hearing Association (2004) for preferred practice patterns when assessing and treating bilingual individuals.

## REFERENCES

Alt, M., & Plante, E. (2006). Factors that influence lexical and semantic fast mapping of young children with specific language impairment. *Journal of Speech, Language, and Hearing Research, 49*, 941–954.

Alt, M., Plante, E., & Creusere, M. (2004). Semantic features in fast-mapping: Performance of preschoolers with specific language impairment versus preschoolers with normal language. *Journal of Speech, Language, and Hearing Research, 47*, 407–420.

American Speech-Language-Hearing Association. (2004). *Preferred practice patterns for the profession of speech-language pathology.* Retrieved June 22, 2009, from http://www.asha.org/docs/html/PP2004-00191.html

Baddeley, A. D. (2000). The episodic buffer: A new component of working memory? *Trends in Cognitive Science, 4*(11), 417–423.

Baddeley, A. D., & Hitch, G. J. (1974). *Working memory.* In G. H. Bower (Ed.), The psychology of learning and motivation (Vol. 8, pp. 47–90). New York: Academic Press.

Barsalou, L. W. (2008). Grounded cognition. *Annual Review of Psychology, 59,* 617–645.

Bates, E., Bretherton, I., & Snyder, L. (1988). *From first words to grammar: Individual differences and dissociable mechanisms.* New York: Cambridge University Press.

Bjorklund, D. F. (1987). How age changes in knowledge base contribute to the development of children's memory: An interpretive review. *Developmental Review, 7,* 93–130.

Bjorklund, D. F., & Schneider, W. (1996). The interaction of knowledge, aptitude and strategies in children's memory performance. *Advances in Child Development and Behavior, 26,* 59–89.

Campbell, T., Dollaghan, C., Needleman, H., and Janosky, J. (1997). Reducing bias in language assessment: Processing-dependent measures. *Journal of Speech, Language, and Hearing Research, 40,* 519–525.

Capone, N. (2010). Language assessment and intervention: A developmental approach. In B. S. Shulman & N. C. Capone (Eds.), *Language development, foundations, processes, and clinical applications.* Baltimore: Jones & Bartlett.

Capone, N. C. (2007). Tapping toddlers' evolving semantic representation via gesture. *Journal of Speech, Language, and Hearing Research, 50,* 732–745.

Capone, N. C. (2008, July). *Iconic gesture cues facilitate lexical-semantic learning for naming and extension of object labels.* Poster presented at the meeting of the International Association for the Study of Child Language, Edinburgh, Scotland.

Capone, N. C., & McGregor, K. K. (2004). Gesture development: A review for clinical and research practices. *Journal of Speech, Language, and Hearing Research, 47,* 173–186.

Capone, N. C. & McGregor, K. K. (2005). The effect of semantic representation on toddlers' word retrieval. *Journal of Speech, Language and Hearing Research, 48,* 1468–1480.

Carey, S. (1978). The child as word learner. In M. Halle, J. Bresnan, & C. A. Miller (Eds.), *Linguistic theory and psychological reality* (pp. 264–293). Cambridge, MA: Massachusetts Institute of Technology Press.

Conti-Ramsden, G., & Hesketh, A. (2003). Risk markers for SLI: A study of young language-learning children. *International Journal of Language and Communication Disorders, 38,* 251–263.

Dell, G. S. (1986). A spreading-activation theory of retrieval in sentence production. *Psychological Review, 93,* 283–321.

Dell, G. S. (1988). The retrieval of phonological forms in production: Tests of predictions from a connectionist model. *Journal of Memory and Language, 27,* 124–142.

Dell, G. S. (1990). Effects of frequency and vocabulary type on phonological speech errors. *Language and Cognitive Processes, 5,* 313–349.

Dell, G. S., & O'Seaghdha, P. G. (1992). Stages of lexical access in language production. *Cognition, 42,* 287–314.

Dell, G. S., Schwartz, M. F., Martin, N., Saffran, E. M., & Gagnon, D. A. (1997). Lexical access in aphasic and nonaphasic speakers. *Psychological Review, 104,* 801–838.

Dollaghan, C. & Campbell, T. (1998). Nonword repetition and child language impairment. *Journal of Speech, Language, and Hearing Research, 41,* 1136–1146.

Edwards, J., & Lahey, M. (1998). Nonword repetition of children with specific language impairment: exploration of some explanation for the inaccuracies. *Applied Psycholinguistics, 19,* 279–309.

Ellis Weismer, S., Tomblin, B., Zhang, X., Buckwalter, P., Chynoweth, J., & Jones, M. (2000). Nonword repetition performance in school-age children with and without language impairment. *Journal of Speech, Language, and Hearing Research, 43,* 865–878.

Fenson, L., Marchman, V. A., Thal, D. J., Dale, P. S., Bates, E., & Resnick, J. S. (2007). *MacArthur-Bates communicative development inventories* (2nd ed.). Baltimore: Paul Brookes Publishing.

Ferguson, C., & Farwell, C. (1975). Words and sounds in early language acquisition. *Language, 51,* 419–439.

Gathercole, S. E., & Baddeley, A. D. (1989). Evaluation of the role of phonological STM in the development of vocabulary in children: A longitudinal study. *Journal of Memory and Language, 28,* 200–213.

Gathercole, S. E., & Baddeley, A. D. (1990). Phonological memory deficits in language disordered children: Is there a causal connection? *Journal of Memory and Language, 29,* 336–360.

Gathercole, S., Willis, C. Emslie, H., & Baddeley, A. (1992). Phonological memory and vocabulary development during the early school years: A longitudinal study. *Developmental Psychology, 28,* 887–898.

German, D. J. (2002). A phonologically based strategy to improve word finding abilities in children. *Communication Disorders Quarterly, 23*(4), 177–190.

German, D. J., & Newman, R. S. (2004). The impact of lexical factors on children's word finding errors. *Journal of Speech, Language, and Hearing Research, 47,* 624–636.

Gershkoff-Stowe, L. (2002). Object naming, vocabulary growth, and the development of word retrieval abilities. *Journal of Memory and Language, 46,* 665–687.

Gershkoff-Stowe, L., & Smith, L. B. (1997). A curvilinear trend in naming errors as a function of early vocabulary growth. *Cognitive Psychology, 34,* 37–71.

Gershkoff-Stowe, L., & Smith, L. B. (2004). Shape and the first hundred nouns. *Child Development, 75*(4), 1098–1174.

Graf Estes, K., Evans, J. L., & Else-Quest, N. M. (2007). Differences in the nonword repetition performance of children with and without specific language impairment: A meta-analysis. *Journal of Speech, Language, and Hearing Research, 50,* 177–195.

Gray, S. (2005). Word learning by preschoolers with specific language impairment: Effect of phonological or semantic cues. *Journal of Speech, Language, and Hearing Research, 48,* 1452–1467.

Gray, S. (2006). The relationship between phonological memory, receptive vocabulary, and fast mapping in young children with specific language impairment. *Journal of Speech, Language, and Hearing Research, 49,* 955–969.

Gupta, P. (2005). What's in a word? A functional analysis of word learning. *Perspectives on Language Learning and Education, 12,* 4–8.

Hart, B., & Risley, T. R. (1995). *Meaningful differences in the everyday lives of young American children.* Baltimore: Paul Brookes Publishing.

Hoff, E., Core, C., & Bridges, K. (2008). Non-word repetition assesses phonological memory and is related to vocabulary development in 20- to 24-month-olds. *Journal of Child Language, 35,* 903–916.

Horst, J. S., & Samuelson, L. K. (2008). Fast mapping but poor retention by 24-month-old infants. *Infancy, 13*(2), 128–157.

Hollich, G. J., Hirsh-Pasek, K., Golinkkoff, R. M., Brand, R. M., Brown, E., Chung, H. L., et al. (2000). Breaking the language barrier: An emergentist coalition model for the origins of word learning. *Monographs of the Society for Research in Child Development, 65.*

Jarrold, C., & Baddeley, A. D. (1997). Short-term memory for verbal and visuospatial information in Down's syndrome. *Cognitive Neuropsychiatry, 2*(2), 101–122.

Jones, S. S. (2003). Late talkers show no shape bias in a novel name extension task. *Developmental Science, 6*(5), 477–483.

Kemler Nelson, D. G. (1999). Attention to functional properties in toddlers' naming and problem solving, *Cognitive Development, 14*, 77–100.

Lahey, M., & Edwards, J. (1999). Naming errors of children with specific language impairment. *Journal of Speech, Language, and Hearing Research, 42*, 195–205.

Landau, B., Smith, L. B., & Jones, S. S. (1988). The importance of shape in early lexical learning. *Cognitive Development, 3*, 299–321.

Laws, G., & Gunn, D. (2004). Phonological memory as a predictor of language comprehension in Down syndrome: A five-year follow-up study. *Journal of Child Psychology and Psychiatry, 45*, 326–337.

Leonard, L. B., Newhoff, M., & Mesalam, L. (1980). Individual differences in early child phonology. *Applied Psycholinguistics, 1*, 7–30.

Leonard, L. B., Schwartz, R. G., Chapman, K., Rowan, L., Prelock, P., Terrell, B., Weiss, A., & Messick, C. (1982). Early lexical acquisition in children with specific language impairment. *Journal of Speech and Hearing Research, 25*, 554–564.

Leonard, L. B., Schwartz, R. G., Morris, B., & Chapman, K. (1981). Factors influencing early lexical acquisition: lexical orientation and phonological composition. *Child Development, 52*, 882–887.

Luce, P. A., & Pisoni, D. B. (1998). Recognizing spoken words: The neighborhood activation model. *Ear and Hearing, 19*, 1–36.

Manolson, A. (1992). *It takes two to talk: A parent's guide to helping children communicate.* Toronto, Ontario, Canada: The Hanen Centre.

Markman, E. M. (1989). *Categorization and naming in children: Problems in induction.* Cambridge, MA: Massachusetts Institute of Technology Press.

McCune, L., & Vihman, M. M. (2001). Early phonetic and lexical development: A productivity approach. *Journal of Speech, Language, and Hearing Research, 44*, 670–684.

McGregor, K. K. (1994). Use of phonological information in a word-finding treatment for children. *Journal of Speech and Hearing Research, 37*, 1382–1393.

McGregor, K. K. (1997). The nature of word finding errors of preschoolers with and without word-finding deficits. *Journal of Speech and Hearing Research, 40*, 1232–1244.

McGregor, K. K., & Appel, A. (2002). On the relationship between mental representation and naming in a child with specific language impairment. *Clinical Linguistics and Phonetics, 16*, 1–20.

McGregor, K. K., & Capone, N. C. (2004). Genetic and environmental interactions in determining the early lexicon: Evidence from a set of tri-zygotic quadruplets. *Journal of Child Language, 31*, 311–337.

McGregor, K. K., Friedman, R. M., Reilly, R. M., and Newman, R. M. (2002). Semantic representation and naming in young children. *Journal of Speech, Language, and Hearing Research, 45*, 332–346.

McGregor, K. K., Newman, R. M., Reilly, R. M., and Capone, N. (2002). Semantic representation and naming in children with specific language impairment. *Journal of Speech, Language, and Hearing Research, 45*, 998–1014.

McGregor, K. K., Sheng, L., & Ball, T. (2007). Complexities of expressive word learning over time. *Language, Speech, and Hearing Services in Schools, 38*, 353–364.

Mills, D. L., Coffey-Corina, S., & Neville, H. J. (1997). Language comprehension and cerebral specialization from 13 to 20 months. *Developmental Neuropsychology, 13*, 397–445.

Mills, D. L., Plunkett, K., Prat, C., & Schafer, G. (2005). Watching the infant brain learn words: Effects of vocabulary size and experience. *Cognitive Development, 20*, 19–31.

Miller, G., & Gildea, P. (1987). How children learn words. *Scientific American, 257,* 94–99.

Montgomery, J. W. (1995). Examination of phonological working memory in specifically language impaired children. *Applied Psycholinguistics, 16,* 355–378.

Nagy, W. E., & Herman, P. A. (1987). Breadth and depth of vocabulary knowledge: Implications for acquisition and instruction. In M. G. McKeown & M. E. Curtis (Eds.), *The nature of vocabulary acquisition* (pp. 19–35). Hillsdale, NJ: Erlbaum.

Nash, M., & Donaldson, M. L. (2005). Word learning in children with vocabulary deficits. *Journal of Speech, Language, and Hearing Research, 48,* 439–458.

Newman, R. S., & German, D. J. (2002). Effects of lexical factors on lexical access among typical language-learning children and children with word-finding difficulties. *Language and Speech, 45,* 285–317.

Nippold, M. A. (2007). *Later language development. School-age children, adolescents, and young adults* (3rd ed.). Austin, TX: Pro-Ed.

Nobre, A. C., & Plunkett, K. (1997). The neural system of language: Structure and development. *Current Opinion in Neurobiology, 7,* 262–268.

Ordóñez, C. L., Carlo, M. S., Snow, C. E., & McLaughlin, B. (2002). Depth and breadth of vocabulary in two languages: Which vocabulary skills transfer? *Journal of Educational Psychology, 94,* 719–728.

Owens, R. (1988). *Language development: An introduction.* Boston: Allyn & Bacon.

Paul, R. (1996). Clinical implications of the natural history of slow expressive language development. *American Journal of Speech-Language Pathology, 5,* 5–21.

Paul, R. (2007). *Language disorders from infancy through adolescence: Assessment and intervention* (3rd ed.). St. Louis, Missouri: Mosby.

Patterson, J. L., & Pearson, B. Z. (2004). Bilingual lexical development: Influences, contexts, and processes. In Goldstein, B. A. (Ed.), *Bilingual language development & disorders in Spanish-English speakers* (pp. 77–104). Baltimore: Paul Brookes Publishing.

Pearson, B. Z., Fernández, S. C., & Oller, D. K. (1993). Lexical development in bilingual infants and toddlers: Comparison to monolingual norms. *Language Learning, 43,* 93–120.

Pearson, B. Z., Fernández, S. C., & Oller, D. K. (1995). Cross-language synonyms in the lexicons of bilingual infants: One language or two? *Journal of Child Language, 22,* 345–368.

Peña, E. D., Bedore, L. M., & Zlatic-Giunta, R. (2002). Category-generation performance of bilingual children: The influence of condition, category, and language. *Journal of Speech, Language, and Hearing Research, 45,* 938–947.

Peña, E. D., & Kester, E. S. (2004). Semantic development in Spanish-English bilinguals: Theory, assessment, and intervention. In Goldstein, B. A. (Ed.), *Bilingual language development & disorders in Spanish-English speakers* (pp. 105–128). Baltimore: Paul Brookes Publishing.

Plunkett, K. (1997).Theories of early language acquisition. *Trends in Cognitive Sciences, 1*(4), 146–153.

Plunkett, K., Karmiloff-Smith, A., Bates, E., Elman, J. L., & Johnson, M. (1997). Connectionism and developmental psychology. *Journal of Child Psychology and Psychiatry, 38,* 53–80.

Retherford, K. (2000). *Guide to analysis of language transcripts* (3rd ed.). Eau Claire, WI: Thinking Publications.

Rescorla, L. (2002). Language and reading outcomes to age 9 in late-talking toddlers. *Journal of Speech, Language, and Hearing Research, 45,* 360–371.

Rescorla, L. (2005). Language and reading outcomes of late-talking toddlers at age 13. *Journal of Speech, Language, and Hearing Research, 48*, 1–14.

Rescorla, L., Mirak, J., & Singh, L. (2000). Vocabulary growth in late talkers: Lexical development from 2.0 to 3.0. *Journal of Child Language, 27*, 293–311.

Schwartz, R. G. (1988). Phonological factors in early lexical acquisition. In M. Smith & J. Locke (Eds.), *The emergent lexicon* (pp. 185–222). New York: Academic Press.

Schwartz, R. G., & Leonard, L. B. (1982). Do children pick and choose? Phonological selection and avoidance in early lexical acquisition. *Journal of Child Language, 9*, 319–336.

Shapiro, L. (1997). Tutorial: An introduction to syntax. *Journal of Speech, Language, and Hearing Research, 40*, 254–272.

Sheng, L. (2007). *Lexical access and semantic organization in children with specific language impairment.* Unpublished doctoral dissertation, Northwestern University, Evanston, IL.

Sheng, L., & McGregor, K. K. (in press). Lexical-semantic organization in children with specific language impairment: Evidence from a repeated word association task. *Journal of Speech, Language, and Hearing Research.*

Sheng, L., McGregor, K. K., & Marian, V. (2006). Lexical-semantic organization in bilingual children: Evidence from a repeated word association task. *Journal of Speech, Language, and Hearing Research, 49*, 572–587.

Smit, A. B., Hand, L., Freilinger, J. J., Bernthal, J. E., & Bird, A. (1990). The Iowa articulation norms project and its Nebraska replication. *Journal of Speech and Hearing Disorders, 55*, 779–798.

Storkel, H. L. (2001). Learning new words: Phonotactic probability in language development. *Journal of Speech, Language, and Hearing Research, 44*, 1321–1337.

Storkel, H. L. (2004a). Do children acquire dense neighborhoods? An investigation of similarity neighborhoods in lexical acquisition. *Applied Psycholinguistics, 25*, 201–221.

Storkel, H. L. (2004b). The emerging lexicon of children with phonological delays: Phonotactic constraints and probability in acquisition. *Journal of Speech, Language, and Hearing Research, 47*, 1194–1212.

Storkel, H. L. (2004c). Methods for minimizing the confounding effect of word length in the analysis of phonotactic probability and neighborhood density. *Journal of Speech, Language and Hearing Research, 47*, 1454–1468.

Templin, M. (1957). *Certain language skills in children.* Minneapolis, MN: University of Minnesota Press.

Thal, D. J., & Tobias, S. (1992). Communicative gestures in children with delayed onset of oral expressive language use. *Journal of Speech and Hearing Research, 35*, 1281–1289.

Thal, D. J., Reilly, J., Seibert, L., Jeffries, R., & Fenson, J. (2004). Language development in children at risk for language impairment: Cross-population comparisons. *Brain and Language, 88*, 167–179.

Tsybina, I., & Eriks-Brophy, A. (2007). Issues in research on children with early language delay. *Contemporary Issues in Communication Science and Disorders, 34*, 118–133.

Vitevitch, M. S., & Sommers, M. S. (2003). The facilitative influence of phonological similarity and neighborhood frequency in speech production in younger and older adults. *Memory and Cognition, 31*, 491–504.

Ward, T. B., Chu, Ah., Vaid, J., & Heredia, R. R. (2005). Divergence and overlap in bilingual concept representations. In *Proceedings of the 27th Annual Conference of the Cognitive Science Society* (pp. 2342–2346). Mahwah, NJ: Lawrence Erlbaum.

Williams, K. T. (1997). *Expressive Vocabulary Test*. Circle Pines, MS: American Guidance
     Service.
Wing, C. S. (1990). A preliminary investigation of generalization to untrained words fol-
     lowing two treatments of children's word-finding problems. *Language, Speech, and
     Hearing Services in Schools, 21*, 151–156.

# 4 Individual Differences in Bilingual Children's Language Competencies
## *The Case for Spanish and English*

*Carol Scheffner Hammer and*
*Barbara L. Rodríguez*

The number of children who speak two languages is increasing in the United States. Over a 10-year period from 1995–1996 to 2005–2006, the number of English language learners (ELLs) has grown from 3.2 million to 5.1 million, a 57% increase (Office of English Language Acquisition, 2007). Note that these figures do not include bilingual children who are proficient speakers of English. Of the languages spoken by bilingual children, Spanish is by far the most common. Approximately 80% of ELLs speak Spanish. The languages that are next most commonly spoken by ELLs are Vietnamese, spoken by 2%; Hmong, spoken by 1.5%; and Cantonese, spoken by 1% (United States Department of Education, 2002). Given the large numbers of children in the United States who are learning two languages, it is critical that speech-language pathologists (SLPs) understand bilingual children's language development and the individual differences that are observed in this population. Therefore, the purpose of this chapter is to discuss factors that may lead to individual differences in bilingual children's developing language competencies, specifically the variation that occurs in children's semantic and morphosyntactic development, and considerations for service delivery. Because Spanish–English bilinguals constitute the largest group of children learning two languages in the United States, the focus of the chapter will be on this population.

## FACTORS LEADING TO INDIVIDUAL DIFFERENCES IN LANGUAGE DEVELOPMENT

Although bilingual children acquire first words, produce two-word phrases, and use morphosyntactic structures at the same time as monolingual children, their language development differs from that of children learning one language. As Grosjean (1989) stated nearly 20 years ago, "The bilingual is not the sum of two complete or incomplete monolinguals; rather, he or she has a unique and specific linguistic configuration" (p. 6). This is because bilingual children's language development is affected by a number of factors that can lead to individual differences in their developmental paths. These factors are most often considered to be generational status, length of time in the country, parents' and siblings' language usage, gender, age and amount of exposure to the second language, the larger community, and the dialects of Spanish and English spoken (cf. Arriagada, 2005; Genesee, Paradis, & Crago, 2004; Hammer, Miccio, & Rodríguez, 2004; Hurtado & Vega, 2004; Portes & Rumbaut, 2001; Veltman, 1981). Each of these factors is discussed in the following sections.

## GENERATIONAL STATUS

Bilingual individuals' generational status may impact their proficiency in their first and second languages, as the amount of language usage has been shown to differ among generations (Hurtado & Vega, 2004). Research on language usage in immigrant populations has demonstrated that first-generation immigrants are more likely to use their native language than subsequent generations (Arrigada, 2004). This first generation, however, tends to learn English quickly, using their native language at home and learning English for communication at work (Hurtado & Vega, 2004; Portes & Hao, 2002). In a large-scale study of Latino immigrants' language usage, nearly 7% of adults reported using English as their primary language within 18 months of their arrival in the United States, and another 24% reported using English often. Within 4 years, a large percentage of immigrants spoke English regularly, and the majority used English on a regular basis within 9 years. Ten percent made English their primary language (Veltman, 1988). The greatest changes in language usage are observed in this generation (Veltman, 1981).

Individuals in the second generation are typically proficient speakers of English who tend to prefer communicating in English over their native language (Hurtado & Vega, 2004; Portes & Hao, 1998). Within this generation, knowledge of the native language is more variable, with many individuals losing the native language of their parents (Portes & Hao, 2002; Portes & Rumbaut, 2001).

By the third generation, language usage has completely shifted away from the native language. English typically is the language used by members of this generation. Relatively few individuals have knowledge of their parents' language. In fact, parents of children in this generation typically speak English to their children. Because few children know their parents' native language, native language usage is not observed in subsequent generations (Hurtado & Vega, 2004; Portes & Hao, 2002; Veltman, 1983).

## LENGTH OF TIME IN THE UNITED STATES

In addition to generational status, the length of time individuals have lived in the United States impacts the usage of their native language and the likelihood that they will become fluent bilinguals. Studies have shown that individuals who have spent longer periods of time in the United States are more likely to use English as their primary language (Portes & Shauffler, 1994; Veltman, 1981, 1988) and less likely to become bilingual. Portes and Rumbaut (2001) found that a child's chances of becoming a fluent bilingual decreases by 1% each year he or she lives in the United States.

In addition, the amount of time spent in the United States interacts with the age at the time of immigration, with younger individuals gravitating toward English language usage faster than older immigrants who have lived in the United States for comparable lengths of time (Veltman, 1981). As a result, children who immigrate to the United States use English more commonly than older immigrants and are less likely to become fully bilingual, having never developed proficiency in their native language (Portes & Schauffler, 1994).

## Parents' and Siblings' Language Usage

The language used by parents and siblings also impacts children's language usage. In a study of non-English speakers, Veltman (1981) found that the presence of one parent who speaks English leads children to use English as their primary language, regardless of the language choice of the other parent. The language characteristics of mothers, however, are even more significantly related to whether or not their children become bilingual or English monolinguals. Less than 20% of children with a mother who spoke a non-English language were English monolinguals, whereas 60–70% of children with English bilingual mothers and the vast majority of children with English monolingual mothers were English monolinguals themselves. In other words, children of mothers who spoke a language other than English were more likely to become bilingual and less likely to become monolingual speakers of English. Maternal bilingualism, however, did not necessarily assist children in becoming bilingual. This was true even in households where both parents were bilingual.

The presence of siblings in the household may also lead children toward the usage of English, particularly when one or more siblings are older and attend school. Research has shown that the language used among siblings shifts to English earlier than among the adult population (Hakuta, 1994).

## Gender

Gender also affects children's language proficiencies. In immigrant families, girls are typically more proficient in their native language than boys (Arriagada, 2005; Portes & Hao, 2002; Portes & Schauffler, 1994). For example, Veltman (1981) found that 20% of girls ages 4–17 years were English monolinguals compared with half of the boys in this age group. In addition, girls are more likely to become fluent bilinguals than boys from comparable familial and socioeconomic backgrounds (Portes & Hao, 2002; Portes & Rumbaut, 2001). In fact, Portes and Rumbaut found that gender was the strongest predictor of bilingualism in their study of second-generation immigrants.

These gender differences have been explained by differences in the socialization practices that male and female children experience. For example, in traditional Latino homes, males assume the dominant role of breadwinner and decision maker. The primary role of women is motherhood, with the performance of domestic tasks being a high priority, even if the woman works outside the home (De Von Figueroa, Ramey, Keltner & Lanzi, 2006; Flannagan, Baker-Ward, & Graham, 1995; González, Umana-Taylor, & Bamaca, 2006; Zentella, 1997). Children are socialized into these roles very early in life, which results in different language experiences. For example, in order to learn domestic skills, girls spend more time with their mothers, grandmothers, and other female relatives inside their homes. As a result, girls are exposed to Spanish through the interactions that they are involved in or that they overhear. Boys, on the other hand, are encouraged to be independent and to spend time outside. Therefore, boys are more commonly immersed in English-speaking environments as they play with others outside their family context (Arriagada, 2005; Portes & Rumbaut, 2001; Portes & Schauffler, 1994; Zentella, 1997). Thus, differences between boys and girls in Spanish and English language competencies may result.

## AGE AND AMOUNT OF LANGUAGE EXPOSURE

Individual differences in language acquisition may also occur because the age at which bilingual children are exposed to two languages may vary. Bilingual children have traditionally been described as being simultaneous or sequential language learners. Simultaneous language learners are children who have been exposed to two languages from birth, whereas sequential language learners are children who were exposed to their parents' native language from birth and then were exposed to a second language later in their development. Although a cutoff point has not been agreed upon to distinguish between simultaneous and sequential learners, 3 years of age has traditionally been used as the age that differentiates the two groups (Genesee et al., 2004; McLaughlin, 1984; Meisel, 1994).

More recently, Hammer and colleagues (Hammer, Lawrence, & Miccio, 2007, 2008) have classified bilingual children on the basis of the timing of exposure to school entry. Building on the work of Butler and Hakuta (2004), Genesee (2004), and Oller and Eilers (2002), Hammer et al. (2007, 2008) have argued that the findings of studies of bilingual children developing in nonschool settings may not apply to the development of children who experience a change in language exposure when they enter school. Therefore, the investigators classified Spanish-speaking children into two groups on the basis of whether or not they were exposed to and expected to communicate in English before or after entry into school. Children who were exposed to Spanish and English at home were classified as home English communicators (HECs), and children who were exposed to Spanish at home and not expected to communicate in English until entrance into Head Start were considered school English communicators (SECs).

Differences in the language development of children in the two groups have been found. For example, a longitudinal study of children's receptive vocabulary development during 2 years in Head Start revealed that children in the HEC group had higher English vocabulary scores than children in the SEC group at the beginning of Head Start and that children in the SEC group had higher Spanish vocabulary scores than HEC children. In addition, SEC children's Spanish and English vocabularies grew at a faster rate than those of HEC children. Thus, the age and timing of exposure to English resulted in differences in bilingual children's development of vocabulary competencies. Also, large variations in children's abilities were found in both groups, revealing within-group as well as between-group differences in language development (Hammer et al., 2008).

In addition to the age of exposure, the amount of exposure to the two languages may also impact children's language development. Bilingual children experience differences in the language input they receive not only because the language usage of their parents, relatives, and other significant people varies but because they may attend educational programs that may or may not promote the maintenance of Spanish while the children are learning English. Therefore, some bilingual children may receive relatively equal exposure to the two languages, whereas others may experience differential exposure to the two languages over time (Hammer et al., 2004).

Furthermore, children's development in one of their languages may progress or regress as a result of changes in their language learning environment. It is not uncommon, for example, for bilingual Latino children to travel to their native countries during the summer or for entire school years, during which time they may speak only Spanish. As a result, these children's English abilities may not advance or may decline. Upon return, the children's Spanish abilities may regress while their English abilities improve and develop (Hammer et al., 2004). Thus, these periodic changes in the language learning environment can differentially affect bilingual children's language development.

## LARGER COMMUNITY

The larger community can also impact bilingual children's language abilities. In places such as Canada and Europe where bilingual children may speak two majority languages, bilingualism is generally supported by the community, the educational system, and the government. However, in the United States, the vast majority of individuals who speak two languages are from minority groups, and their native languages are often not valued and in some communities are stigmatized (Hammer, et al., 2004). Non-English and bilingual speakers often experience discrimination at work and in the larger community (Arriagada, 2005). For example, a well-known restaurant in Philadelphia recently received national attention for requiring their customers to speak only English. As a result of such experiences, families may convey to their children that use of English in public circles is required and that use of their native language is restricted to the home, where families strive to maintain their language (Vidal-Ortiz, 2004).

Of course, in communities where there are large concentrations of speakers of a minority language and where members of the culture have positions of status in the community, acceptance of the minority language and bilingualism is greater. Consequently, families may feel comfortable using their native language in the community as well as at home. This provides children with the message that their native language is valued by the larger community, which in turn may encourage children to speak their native language outside their home.

The educational system also greatly impacts bilingual children's language abilities. Generally speaking, the educational system in the United States promotes usage of English, while providing no or limited support to children's first languages when they are not English. Traditionally, preschool programs such as Head Start and Even Start have had policies that support English language development but do not focus on the promotion of a home language other than English. Many elementary and secondary schools provide minimal bilingual programming or support for native language learning while children are learning English. In extreme cases, such as in California, Arizona, and Massachusetts, legislation has been passed that eliminates bilingual education. These policies and practices have significant implications for children's language learning, as it is generally accepted that children who come to school not knowing English typically require 2–3 years to develop conversational skills in their second language and 5–7 years to develop academic abilities in English (Cummins, 1981). Related to this, children use their knowledge of their first language when learning and acquiring knowledge in a second. Therefore, if children's native language development is not supported while they are learning a second language, children may be in danger of losing competencies in their native language as well as not fully developing their abilities in English.

## DIALECTICAL DIFFERENCES

All the factors previously described may impact bilingual children's language competencies differentially and result in varying proficiencies in their first and second languages. In addition, the dialect(s) bilingual children speak also need to be considered, not because the dialect will impact the children's language proficiencies, but because the dialects spoken may lead to individual differences in the characteristics of the children's productions. Such information needs to be considered so that dialectical differences are not mistaken for language impairments.

For example, the Spanish language, like all languages, has numerous dialects. The dialects spoken by Spanish-speaking children are influenced by the dialect spoken in their country of origin and/or by the dialect spoken in their community in the United States. Dialects can vary greatly from the standard variety of Spanish, which is spoken in Spain and typically taught in language classes in schools in the United States. Within the United States, the Mexican dialect of Spanish is spoken by the largest number of speakers, followed the Puerto Rican and Cuban dialects. Like all languages, dialects of Spanish contrast in phonology, vocabulary, and grammatical patterns. A thorough discussion of the characteristics of the dialects of Spanish is beyond the scope of the chapter. (The reader is referred to

Butt & Benjamin, 2000; Penny, 2002; Pousada & Poplack, 1982; Sanchez, 1994; and Silva-Corvalán, 1995.) However, given that the dialect of Spanish that a child speaks may result in individual differences in the characteristics of the child's Spanish language (and the subsequent impact that may have on the perception of the adequacy of the child's language), it is important for an SLP to be aware of what those characteristics may be.

In addition, the dialect of English that bilingual children speak may also impact the children's English productions. For instance, Latino children who live in areas where there are large numbers of speakers of African American English may acquire features of African American English. Therefore, individual differences in children's English language development can also be expected; not all learners of English should be assumed to be learning features of standard American English only.

## SUMMARY

All of the factors previously discussed contribute to individual differences in the development of bilingual children's language competencies. That is, the children's generational status, length of time in country, parents' and siblings' language usage, gender, age and amount of exposure to the second language, and the larger community all have the potential to impact children's proficiencies in each language. Because not every child's life experience is the same, it should be expected that bilingual children may achieve different levels of competence in their two languages. For example, some children may become fluent in both of their languages. Others may not receive sufficient exposure to either language and become limited bilinguals. Other children may be Spanish-dominant and have minimal knowledge of English, and still others may become English-dominant and have minimal knowledge of their native language (Portes & Rumbaut, 2001). In other words, a group of children may lose their native language abilities or may experience restricted development of their native language and fail to become proficient speakers of it. These differences in language proficiencies may present SLPs with challenges when determining whether or not a bilingual child has a speech-language disorder.

The following section discusses individual differences that have been observed in bilingual children's language development and addresses characteristics of language loss and language impairment. It also presents preliminary results of a longitudinal study of bilingual children's expressive language development. Because Spanish–English bilingual children constitute the largest bilingual population in the United States, the focus of the discussion will again be on this particular population.

## BILINGUAL CHILDREN'S LANGUAGE DEVELOPMENT

### TYPICAL BILINGUAL LANGUAGE DEVELOPMENT

Although there is a rich body of literature describing the course of English language development, there is limited research examining bilingual Spanish–English language development of children living in the United States. Moreover, the few studies that do exist generally rely on cross-sectional data samples and do not include detailed information about the children's length of exposure to English and other factors that may impact bilingual development. Although these studies provide needed information, they restrict our understanding of the typical patterns of bilingual language acquisition because they ignore the influence that the changing language learning environment has on children's language outcomes over time. Cross-sectional studies examine differences in children's performance between age groups, but discernible patterns of language development must be interpreted against the overall background of variability that is the hallmark of bilingual language acquisition. With that caveat in mind, a summary of the literature describing the typical patterns of semantic, syntactic, and narrative development in young children growing up bilingually is presented in the following sections.

## Semantic Development

A number of studies have examined semantic development in young bilingual Spanish- and English-speaking children. From this work, we know that vocabulary development across the two languages is quite similar. That is, infants and toddlers learning vocabulary in a bilingual environment follow developmental trajectories similar to those of their monolingual counterparts (Patterson, 1998; Pearson & Fernández, 1994). Bilingual children, exposed to a variety of bilingual environments, attained vocabulary milestones at points in development similar to those reported for monolingual children. For instance, young bilingual children, 10–30 months of age, had similar numbers of words in their vocabulary compared with monolingual children when their vocabularies in each language were combined (Pearson & Fernández, 1994). As a group, typically developing bilingual children are expected to reach specific semantic developmental milestones at about the same time monolinguals reach them. However, individual bilingual children, whose language learning experiences are uniquely shaped by a number of environmental factors discussed previously, may present patterns of semantic development in each language that vary from the average monolingual performance.

In fact, there is evidence to suggest that semantic development for bilingual children is often characterized by different patterns of growth between the two languages. These patterns, or individual differences, arise as a result of differences in the social contexts of language learning, as previously discussed. The timing of initial exposure to two languages and the levels of language input differ across bilingual children, which can lead to different rates of overall lexical development for each language (Patterson & Pearson, 2004; Pearson, Fernández, Lewedeg, & Oller, 1997). Studies of young typically developing bilingual children (Marchman & Martínez-Sussmann, 2002; Pearson et al., 1997) have demonstrated substantial associations between children's vocabulary size and the amount of exposure to two languages. For example, Pearson et al. examined the relationship between exposure to English and Spanish and the percentage of words known in each language in a group of children 9–30 months of age. The results were intuitive, indicating that children who had had more frequent exposure to English produced more words in English, whereas those who had received more exposure to Spanish produced more words in Spanish. Thus, the amount of exposure matters: it is related to vocabulary growth in that specific language (Pearson, 2002).

Recently, Oller, Pearson, and Cobo-Lewis (2007) found a different pattern of vocabulary growth in a group of school-age bilingual children living in Miami, Florida. The children's Spanish receptive vocabulary abilities were much better than their Spanish vocabulary productive abilities. In English, there was no receptive–productive vocabulary gap. The researchers concluded that the asymmetry in semantic development was the result of the gain in importance of English in peer communication, along with limited access to Spanish vocabulary for production. Although all of the children had been significantly exposed to Spanish early in life, the predominant tendency was for children to speak and to hear other children speaking English. Oller et al. attributed their findings to the patterns of exposure to Spanish and English rather than the amount of exposure to each language.

Thus, children's exposure to Spanish and English over time is important to consider when assessing children's semantic development. In addition, the proficiency that bilingual children demonstrate may be influenced by the tasks used to assess children's semantic development. Children who are exposed to two languages may be exposed to different vocabulary as well as to different uses for that vocabulary in each of their two languages (Peña & Kester, 2004). Bilingual children have been shown to be more successful on some semantic tasks in English than other tasks in Spanish. Peña, Bedore, and Rappazzo (2003) found that bilingual children (ages 4 years 5 months to 7 years 0 months) performed better on tasks in Spanish when they were required to name or identify the functions of items and better in English when responding to tasks requiring them to name and identify similarities and differences between two objects. The investigators concluded that the combination of test language and semantic task influenced the bilingual children's semantic performance. This research has implications for assessment of semantic knowledge in bilingual children with respect to task selection and test language.

## Syntactic Development

As with bilingual children's semantic development, it is important to understand bilingual children's syntactic development in both of their languages. Relatively few studies have examined the English syntactic development in typically developing bilingual children. One study has documented the sequence and timing of English morphological development in Spanish–English bilingual children. Bland-Stewart and Fitzgerald (2001) reported on their findings concerning English morphological development gleaned from spontaneous language samples produced in English by 15 bilingual Hispanic preschoolers, between ages 2 years 6 months and 5 years 0 months. The children were placed in one of three groups according to mean length of utterance (MLU): Group 1 (*n* = 6), MLU 3.0–3.4; Group 2 (*n* = 3), MLU 3.5–3.9; and Group 3 (*n* = 6), MLU 4.0–4.4.

Emergent use of Brown's 14 grammatical morphemes was observed across the three MLU groups, but mastery of the morphemes was not attained at the same ages as those expected for children who are learning to speak standard American English only. The children in the Bland-Stewart and Fitzgerald (2001) study also demonstrated different rates of accuracy in the use of the grammatical morphemes across the three MLU subgroups. For example, regular past tense was used with 59% accuracy for Group 1, 62% accuracy for Group 2, and 34% accuracy for Group 3. Unfortunately, individual differences within each MLU subgroup were unexamined and unique error patterns produced by individual children were not analyzed by the authors. Therefore, it is currently unclear how an individual child's language learning environment (e.g., amount of exposure to English) may influence the rate and course of English morphological development.

Similarly, Dale (1980) examined children's Spanish and English development of grammatical morphemes from kindergarten through third grade. The children's knowledge of morphological rules was assessed using a morphology measure administered in both Spanish and English. The results indicated that similarities and differences existed in the bilingual and monolingual children's English grammatical development. Similar to monolingual English development, present progressive -*ing* was mastered early. In addition, plural noun -*z* and possessive singular -*z* occurred accurately earlier in children's development, whereas the grammatical morphemes including plural -*əz*, present tense third person singular, and past -*əd* were mastered much later in development for both monolingual children and the bilingual participants. In general, these results seemed to indicate that Spanish–English bilingual children followed a sequence of acquisition similar to that of monolingual English children. However, it appeared that the bilingual group exhibited a lower percentage of accuracy and a younger age of acquisition across all morphemes compared with the monolingual data.

With regard to bilingual children's Spanish syntactic development, a general pattern has been identified that is consistent with what has been reported for monolingual Spanish-speaking children. Bilingual children as young as 20 months begin using the present, preterit, infinitives, and imperatives, and with lower frequencies the progressive and periphrastic future morphological markers (R. Anderson, 1995; Bedore, 1999; Gathercole, Sebastian, & Soto, 1999). The acquisition of the Spanish verb system is gradual (Childers, Fernández, Echols, & Tomasello, 2001; Gathercole et al.; Serrat & Aparici, 2001), with bilingual children in the early stages of development acquiring primarily one form for each verb. That is, bilingual children produce specific Spanish verbs with specific inflections. Jacobsen and Schwartz (2002) evaluated the spontaneous language samples of Spanish–English children between the ages of 4 years 2 months and 5 years 4 months and their ability to use verb tenses in Spanish. Results suggested that children produced present indicative, preterit, periphrastic future, progressive, imperfect, and present subjective forms. The participants also demonstrated minimal use of the present perfect and the past subjunctive form.

As children acquire increasing numbers of verbs in their vocabulary, tense/ aspect inflection is used with more verb types and more person and number morphological markers (Jackson-Maldonado, 2004). Children who are learning both English and Spanish display grammatical skills in a given language that are strongly tied to vocabulary growth in that language (Marchman, Martínez-Sussmannn, & Dale, 2004). SLPs must be cognizant of the highly systematic and specific relationship between tense/aspect and semantics in bilingual children's language acquisition.

## Narrative Development

Studies of bilingual children's narrative skills have illustrated the range of individual differences in measures of English productivity and sentence organization. Muñoz, Gillam, Peña, and Gulley-Faehnle (2003) examined narratives produced by 4- and 5-year-old Latino preschool children, who were predominately English-speaking, from a low-socioeconomic status community. Narratives were collected in English, but the children were allowed to code switch between English and Spanish. The measures of productivity (e.g., total words, total different words) and sentence organization (e.g., number of C-units, mean length of C-units in words, percentage of grammatically acceptable C-units) suggested that children's English narratives did not differ significantly by age (cf. Loban, 1976).

Four- and five-year-old children did not differ on the total number of words (TNW) and total number of different words (TDW) that were included in their stories. However, there was significant variability within the group of 5-year-old children. Considerable within-group variability also was apparent in sentence organization for the older children. Muñoz et al. (2003) suggested that the variability reflected individual differences in children's skill level when learning to tell stories. The clinical utility of the productivity measures, in particular, for bilingual children appears to be unclear because of the variability in performance among typically developing children.

The effect of language on Spanish–English bilingual children's production of narratives has also been examined (Fiestas & Peña, 2004). Children ranging in age from 4 years 0 months to 6 years 11 months produced two narratives elicited using a wordless picture book and a static picture. Children told stories of equal complexity in Spanish and English in the wordless picture book task. There were differences between the Spanish and English narratives with regard to the children's use of specific story grammar components. Children used more attempts and initiating events in Spanish, while producing more consequences in English. The authors suggested that these differences could be attributed to individual differences in exposure to stories and the vocabulary of storytelling in school as compared with storytelling at home.

Recently, Uccelli and Páez (2007) examined the developmental patterns of narrative skills in a longitudinal sample of 24 Spanish–English bilingual children from low-socioeconomic status backgrounds. On average, the children showed significant change in English narrative quality measures, whereas in Spanish, only story scores (e.g., production of story elements, story sequence, and perspective) showed improvement from kindergarten to first grade. Bilingual children's ability to organize a story continued to improve over time in Spanish. Vocabulary and narrative quality measures were positively associated within language at kindergarten and first grade. That is, children with larger Spanish vocabularies tended to have higher scores on the Spanish narrative quality measures. In addition, children who had higher story scores in Spanish tended to have higher story scores in English. Uccelli and Páez's research highlights the complex relationships at play in the language development of bilingual children.

Studies of narrative production by bilingual children highlight the differences in performance between English and Spanish production. For example, Gutiérrez-Clellen (2002) examined the narratives of typically developing 7- to 8-year-old bilingual children of Mexican American descent. Spontaneous narrative samples, in Spanish and English, were collected using wordless picture books. Comparisons on the proportion of grammatical utterances indicated no significant differences between the two languages. However, Gutiérrez-Clellen noted large individual differences in children's recall of a multiepisodic narrative that was read to them and in the responses to questions about the story. Some children demonstrated better performance in Spanish and some showed the opposite pattern. Therefore, reliable and valid estimates of bilingual children's narrative ability must be obtained from data collected in English and Spanish.

Together, these studies have implications for clinical practice. The findings from the Fiestas and Peña (2004) study suggest that the use of a wordless picture book, as opposed to a static picture, serves as a valid and relevant task to assess bilingual children's narrative skills in English and Spanish. When assessing narrative productivity, the findings from the Uccelli and Páez (2007) investigation lend support for the use of TDW as a sensitive developmental measure for describing children's narrative development. TNW did not describe meaningful developmental changes for bilingual children, a finding that parallels the results obtained by Muñoz et al. (2003). The results from the Gutiérrez-Clellen (2002) study highlight the importance of eliciting narratives in both English and Spanish.

Although these studies remind clinicians that the course of English and Spanish language development is variable for bilingual children, additional research is needed to examine the individual differences in semantic, syntactic, and narrative development that emerge from the contributions of environmental factors. Moreover, information describing the sequence and timing of the development of specific English and Spanish syntactic structures for bilingual children is crucial to guide clinicians in assessing language skills to distinguish between patterns of typical language development and language loss, as well as language impairments.

## LANGUAGE LOSS OR LANGUAGE IMPAIRMENT?

Although there is abundant research on the characteristics of English-speaking children with language disorders, research on English-Spanish bilingual children with language disorders is limited. There is some initial evidence that suggests the linguistic skills of a Spanish–English bilingual child with specific language impairment (SLI) are qualitatively different from those of a bilingual child with normal language development (Restrepo & Kruth, 2000).

Case studies describing and comparing the language characteristics of two bilingual children, one with SLI and one with normal language development, documented the differences in grammatical characteristics observed in a bilingual child with SLI (Restrepo & Kruth, 2000). Language data collected using spontaneous language samples revealed that the bilingual child with SLI produced significantly more morphosyntactic errors and less variety of grammatical forms and sentence types in English and Spanish compared with the child with normal language skills. The child with SLI produced a greater number of grammatical errors per T-unit (i.e., an utterance that consists of an independent clause and associated dependent clauses) and a limited repertoire of sentence types, verb types, prepositions, and pronouns compared with the child with normal language development. For example, the child with SLI produced one preposition consistently (*on*), whereas the child with normal language skills consistently produced a variety of prepositions (e.g., *for, of, to, down,* and *out*). Moreover, a verb type count revealed a limited vocabulary for the child with SLI, and other data pointed to the production of very few complex sentence structures for the child with SLI. Different linguistic profiles emerged for bilingual children who were identified with SLI compared with bilingual children who were typically developing.

Restrepo and Kruth (2000) also suggested, on the basis of a case study, that bilingual children with SLI may be particularly vulnerable to first-language loss. The bilingual child with SLI seemed to experience a more rapid loss of skills in her first language compared with the typically developing bilingual child. Continued exposure to English seemed to have a deleterious effect on the MLU calculated from this child's language sample, even though the child with SLI continued to communicate with her family in her first language. Within a year's time, her production of various grammatical forms and sentences, along with sentence complexity, significantly decreased.

## Language Loss

The linguistic features associated with language loss are important for SLPs to consider when assessing the language skills of a bilingual child. Language loss occurs in a context in which minimal support is given for the use and maintenance of a child's first language (L1). Thus, the domains of the child's L1 become restricted and the child begins to interact more frequently in contexts where the second language (L2) is spoken (Petrovic, 1997). While the L1 is relegated to restricted contexts, the degree of language loss is associated with the amount of L2 exposure (Isurin, 2000).

Researchers have argued that the features of language loss mirror patterns observed in monolingual children with language disorders, primarily SLI (R. Anderson, 1999). Monolingual children with SLI are characterized as having language learning deficits in the absence of neurological or emotional impairment, hearing loss, or cognitive deficit (Leonard, 1998). Monolingual English-speaking children with SLI exhibit difficulties with inflectional morphology that are very similar to those of children learning a second language (R. Anderson, 1999).

Although there are a limited number of investigations examining grammatical patterns of language loss, a number of specific grammatical patterns seem to characterize first language loss of an English–Spanish bilingual child. First, gender agreement and person/number morphology appear to be particularly vulnerable to loss (R. Anderson, 1999). Children experiencing an L1 loss frequently make errors in gender agreement, often using a masculine article with a feminine noun. R. T. Anderson's (2001) analysis of the verb forms used by two children indicated that most of their errors occurred in the use of the correct person and/or number. Second, bilingual children experiencing an L1 loss use aspectual distinctions less frequently across time. Spanish verbs are inflected with aspects of tense, mood, aspect, person, and number. Over time, bilingual children may less frequently use aspectual distinctions, and one form (e.g., preterit tense) becomes the dominant form, even in contexts in which the alternate form is obligatory (e.g., imperfect tense). Third, bilingual children transfer L2 syntactic structure to L1 (R. Anderson, 1999). That is, a child may use English word order while speaking Spanish, despite the fact that the word order is unacceptable in the Spanish grammatical system; for example, an adjective may be placed before rather than after the noun being described.

Vocabulary use is an aspect of language that can also be affected by language loss (Isurin, 2000). At the earliest stages, bilingual children may begin to lose their ability to retrieve words, leading to an eventual loss of lexical items. Isurin studied a child who abruptly lost contact with her L1 and was placed in a strictly English-speaking environment. In past research on bilinguals, certain word categories appeared to be more vulnerable to attrition than others; for example, words that are used infrequently were more likely to be lost than more commonly used words. However, Isurin found that in cases where contact with the L1 was abruptly ended, frequency of use did not appear to impact retention. The unexpected retention of these low-frequency words was attributed to delayed acquisition of similar concepts in the L2. Still, it has been found in other studies that in bilingual children who continue to receive input simultaneously from both languages, low-frequency words seemed to cause more retrieval problems and disappear faster from the vocabulary repertoire (Silva-Corvalán, 1995; Weltens & Grendel, 1993).

Another word category examined by Isurin (2000) was cross-linguistic similarity. In general, words with similar phonation and meaning in both languages, often known as cognates, have been reported as one of the least affected categories. Results on this word category also contrasted with past studies. With the aforementioned child whose L1 input was abruptly ended, Isurin found that cognates were poorly accessed in the L1 and were frequently replaced by the L2 equivalent. This may indicate that depending on the amount of input, cognateness may actually cause confusion in lexical access, rather than facilitating retrieval.

The grammatical and semantic patterns associated with language loss are examples of the variability in bilingual children's language skills that may result from environmental and social factors. Variability in bilingual language development seems to be the rule rather than the exception. It is the job of SLPs to discriminate language differences from language disorders to correctly determine which children need additional support in language acquisition. A significant amount of research has been conducted regarding the language acquisition of monolingual children, and although still limited, data regarding bilingual speakers is on the increase (R. Anderson, 1995). Clinicians need information about the typical patterns of bilingual language acquisition over time to make well-informed clinical decisions, including how best to assess differences in English and Spanish competencies in young bilingual language learners and the extent of individual variability that can be expected in normal bilingual language development.

## PRELIMINARY RESULTS FROM AN ONGOING LONGITUDINAL STUDY

Furthermore, longitudinal investigations are needed to describe the contributions of specific environmental variables on English language development in young bilingual language learners. A recent report from our own ongoing longitudinal study examined the individual differences in semantic and syntactic measures in a sample of typically developing Spanish–English bilingual preschoolers attending English-immersion Head Start programs (Rodríguez, Winslow, Hammer & Miccio, 2008). We collected information about when and where children were exposed to Spanish and English and subsequently divided the children into two groups. The first group was composed of children who lived in homes where both English and Spanish were both spoken; in other words, these children had had previous opportunities to interact in English prior to entering school. These children were considered simultaneous language learners and for the purpose of this study were known as the HEC children. The second group was composed of children who lived in homes in which Spanish was the primary language; in other words, they were not required to interact in English until entering school. These children were considered sequential language learners and for the purpose of this study were known as the SEC children. Comparisons of the language development of the two groups of children were made over time.

The language patterns of a subset of 12 children who participated in the larger longitudinal study are described in the following section. Conversational language samples were elicited from the children in the fall and spring of the children's 2 years in Head Start. The goal was to analyze changes in bilingual children's productive competencies in Spanish by focusing on (a) syntactic complexity, (b) lexical diversity, and (c) verb morphology. Two specific findings illustrated the variability in language skills resulting from differences in the children's language learning contexts. The first finding was the influence of language input on the skills and productivity of the children in Spanish. The analysis of the percentages of complete and intelligible utterances, syntactic complexity, lexical diversity, and errors indicated that children who were exposed to Spanish only at home prior to school entry (i.e., the SEC group) demonstrated better performance in Spanish when compared to children in the HEC group. This finding may be the result of these children living in homes that were supportive of Spanish language development. In addition, the SEC children began Head Start with higher average levels of productivity than the HEC children when they entered Head Start. This difference was maintained throughout the children's 2 years in Head Start, with the SEC children continuing to exhibit greater productivity, syntactic complexity, and lexical diversity than the HEC group at every sampling time.

In addition, members of the SEC group demonstrated measurable increases in their Spanish language competencies during the summer months, when they spent more time at home, where Spanish was spoken. Recall that the children attended English-immersion Head Start classes. This result demonstrates the role that input from the home environment plays in supporting children's language development.

The second main finding was the significant individual variation present within each group. Even though the children in both groups had many characteristics in common, such as dialect, socioeconomic status, and geographic location, their Spanish language competencies varied greatly within each group. Specifically, two children in each of the groups exhibited dramatic increases and decreases in their Spanish language productivity over time, leading to changes in syntactic complexity and lexical diversity. Especially in the SEC group, these children appeared to be particularly sensitive to changes in the amount of Spanish language input they received. Specifically, the children made increases in productivity and lexical diversity during the summer months when they were at home and experienced decreases during the school years.

The individual differences in bilingual children's language development contributed to the complexity in distinguishing language disorders from language differences within a bilingual population. One of the primary roles of SLPs with this population is to assess children's language skills to determine the presence/absence of a language disorder. When assessing children's language skills, SLPs typically compare children's performance to that of speakers of the same language background. However, we continue to lack sufficient normative information necessary to ascertain whether a bilingual child's rate of language acquisition is similar to that of a monolingual child. Moreover, the impact that environmental factors (e.g., generational status, length of time in the United States, etc.) have on individual children's language development is not fully known. Such information is greatly needed by SLPs when assessing bilingual children's language development. In the following section, considerations for assessing bilingual children are presented given the current, limited state of knowledge.

## CLINICAL IMPLICATIONS

To accurately assess the language abilities of bilingual children, SLPs need to gather information from multiple sources. A primary source of information comes from interviews of family members and educators who have knowledge of the children's language abilities as well as language experiences. Hammer (1998) has recommended that semistructured interviews be conducted with the children's family members. Semistructured interviews differ from structured interviews in that the SLP develops a list of guide questions that cover topics that will be addressed during the interview; however, the questions are not asked in a preset order. Rather, the SLP follows the family's lead and has a conversation with the family. Throughout the course of the interview, the SLP covers the desired topics as they arise in the conversation. In addition, emphasis is placed on developing a rapport with the family by learning and acknowledging their views and perspectives about their children's abilities and needs.

When interviewing families of bilingual children, SLPs can use the interview as an opportunity to learn about the family's and child's language background. Specifically, information can be elicited about the generational status of the child, the length of time the child and family have lived in the United States, and the child's and family's travels and stay in their home country. In addition, information can be obtained about the specific dialect the family speaks, the languages used between family members and the child, the age at which the child was exposed to the two languages, and potential changes in language exposure that have occurred during the child's life. The interview is also an excellent opportunity to gain information about the child's language abilities in both languages, as well as the family's concerns about the child's language development, their beliefs about language development, and the efforts they have made to promote their children's language abilities. Such information can be built upon when developing an intervention plan, if the child requires therapeutic services (Hammer, 1998).

If the child attends day care and/or is enrolled in an educational program, it is also important for the SLP to interview key caregivers, teachers, and assistants. Questions may be asked about the language learning environment (e.g., the languages spoken by the adults and children the child has contact with during activities of daily living, the language of formalized instruction, the caregivers' beliefs about bilingual language development), the child's language competencies as demonstrated in the environment, and any concerns that the caregivers or teachers may have regarding the child's ability to communicate successfully. In addition, teachers or classroom assistants who speak the child's native language can be an invaluable source of information and can provide information about the child's native language abilities as well as the child's developing abilities in English. When possible, caregivers and teachers can provide helpful information by comparing the competencies of the targeted child with the abilities of other children with similar language backgrounds and experiences.

In addition to data collected through interviews, observations of the child interacting at home and in school can provide valuable information. Data can be obtained about the languages used by individuals and other children who interact with the child, and by the child when communicating with others in his or her environment. In addition, information about the child's competencies in Spanish and English can be gathered as the SLP observes the child interacting with key family members, teachers, and peers. In addition to providing information about the child's language proficiency, such observations will provide the SLP with information about the support the environment currently provides for the child's two languages, the amount of exposure that the child has to the languages, and the opportunities the child has to use those languages throughout the day.

Naturally, a more formal language assessment should be conducted in both languages, so that a complete understanding of the child's language system can be obtained. This is true regardless of the child's proficiency in either language. If the child is bilingual, it is necessary to obtain a complete picture of that child's abilities in both languages. If the child speaks a non-English language and has minimal exposure to English, it is important to test the child in the first language to determine whether there is a bona fide language impairment. It is also important to obtain baseline measures of the child's English language abilities so that changes in those abilities can be captured as the child's exposure to and usage of English increases over time, just as might be done for any individual learning a second language. In addition, bilingual children's language abilities should be monitored regularly to document language growth as well as to look for signs of language loss. Such information will be valuable in differentiating between children who are losing their first language abilities and children who have a language impairment.

Because of the limited number of language tests specifically developed for use with bilingual children, concerns about the standardization samples of existing measures, and the likelihood of test bias, standardized tests should be used with caution. Instead, alternate, nonbiased assessment approaches should be used. For example, a contrastive analysis can be employed to assist the SLP differentiate between differences in language production that are due to the child's dialect and differences that are due to a language disorder. This approach can be used when assessing a Spanish–English bilingual child's abilities in either language, as the child may not speak the "standard" dialect of Spanish or English (McGregor, Williams, Hearst, & Johnson, 1997).

Procedures for conducting a contrastive analysis are as follows. First, the SLP becomes familiar with the language variety or dialect that the child speaks. This can be done by consulting the published literature. For example, there are numerous sources that discuss the differences among the various dialects of Spanish and that provide valuable information to SLPs. Another way of learning about a dialect is to compare the child's production to that of the child's family members. Productions that are similar to family members' productions reflect the family's dialect and not a disorder. Local norms can also be developed for specific tasks or tests; however, such efforts are time consuming and require the efforts of multiple individuals in order to be developed.

Second, the SLP collects expressive language samples from the child. Such data may come from items on standardized tests, informal tasks, and collection of spontaneous language samples.

Next, the SLP identifies all patterns that are nonstandard. Once these patterns are identified, the patterns are compared with the characteristics of the child's dialect. Patterns that are dialectical indicate that a disorder is not present, whereas patterns that are not typically found in the child's dialect may be indicative of a language impairment.

Finally, the SLP combines the results of the contrastive analysis with other sources of data (e.g., interviews, observations) to determine whether or not a language impairment is present (McGregor et al., 1997). In many cases, a dynamic assessment may be performed to provide the SLP with additional data from which to make a diagnosis. A dynamic assessment is a procedure based on Vygotsky's theory of the zone of proximal development, which represents the difference between the child's performance on a given task without assistance from an adult or more capable peer and the child's performance when provided with support for learning. Therefore, the goal of a dynamic assessment is "to establish the amount of change that can be induced during interactions with the examiner during the assessment process" (Gutiérrez-Clellen & Peña, 2001, p. 212).

Essentially, a dynamic assessment follows a test–teach–retest sequence. Initially, the SLP tests the child's language ability in a particular area and then targets a selected ability using unstructured mediation activities and teaching probes. The length of mediation varies by child and the structure that is targeted. It may last one or two sessions, or it may involve multiple sessions carried out over a number of weeks. Once the remediation is complete, the child is then retested, a qualitative analysis of the child's responses is performed, and the child's modifiability is rated using a Likert-type scale. Examples of modifiability include the child's ability to attend to a task, self-regulate, use the adult as a reference, and transfer a newly taught skill to a novel task. In addition, the child's responsiveness to remediation and the intensity of effort used by the SLP to cause change may also be evaluated. A child who is able to attend to the task, employ skills taught to a new situation, internalize learning strategies, and respond to remediation is likely to be a typical language learner. On the other hand, a child who requires that much more effort be employed in teaching, who does not respond to remediation although supports are in place, and who has difficulty attending to tasks most likely has a language learning impairment (Gutierrez & Peña, 2001).

Data from all of these sources are then combined to assist the SLP determine whether differences in the bilingual child's language abilities are simply due to individual differences in language development or are due to a language impairment. When making such a determination, it is essential to remember that in the case of a bilingual child, a bona fide language impairment will be observed in both languages. If it is not, additional information needs to be gathered to determine the presence or absence of an impairment. If questions still remain, the SLP may want to consider enrolling the child in diagnostic therapy. A child without a language impairment is likely to make rapid gains in diagnostic therapy, whereas a child with a true language impairment will take longer to display gains in language abilities.

As the result of a careful and thorough assessment of a bilingual child's language abilities, appropriate diagnostic decisions can be made and misdiagnoses can be avoided. Without such efforts, bilingual children who have typical language development may be stigmatized when incorrectly diagnosed as having problems learning language and requiring special education services. This may compound the stigma that bilingual children often experience, which is the view that being an ELL signifies deficiency simply because the child did not grow up in an English-speaking household. These views, in turn, can result in lowered expectations for the children's academic performance. Alternatively, without a thorough and accurate assessment, bilingual children with language impairments may not be diagnosed properly, because the children's language patterns and development are attributed to the fact that the child is bilingual. Instead, with a comprehensive and dynamic assessment of the children's competencies in both languages, appropriate services can be provided to the children that will maximize their learning potential.

## REFERENCES

Anderson, R. (1995). Spanish morphological and syntactic development. In H. Kayser (Ed.), *Bilingual speech-language pathology: A Hispanic focus* (pp. 41–73). San Diego, CA: Singular Publishing Group.

Anderson, R. (1999). Impact of first language loss on grammar in a bilingual child. *Communication Disorders Quarterly, 21*(1), 4–16.

Anderson, R. T. (2001). Lexical morphology and verb use in child first language loss: A preliminary case study investigation. *International Journal of Bilingualism, 5*, 377–401.

Arriagada, P. (2005). Family context and Spanish-language use: A study of Latino children in the United States. *Social Science Quarterly, 83*, 599–619.

Bedore, L. (1999). The acquisition of Spanish. In O. L. Taylor & L. Leonard (Eds.), *Language acquisition across North American: Cross-cultural and cross-linguistic perspectives* (pp. 157–207). San Diego, CA: Singular Publishing Group.

Bland-Stewart, L. M., & Fitzgerald, S. M. (2001). Brown's 14 grammatical morphemes by bilingual Hispanic preschoolers: A pilot study. *Communication Disorders Quarterly, 22*, 171–186.

Butler, Y., & Hakuta, K. (2004). Bilingual and second language acquisition. *The handbook of bilingualism* (pp. 114–144). Malden, MA: Blackwell.

Butt, J., & Benjamin, C. (2000). *A new reference grammar of modern Spanish* (3rd ed.). Chicago: NTC Publishing Group.

Childers, J. B., Fernández, A. N., Echols, C. H., & Tomasello, M. (2001). Experimental investigations of children's understanding and use of verb morphology: Spanish and English speaking 2½- and 3-year-old children. In M. Almgren, A. Berrena, M. J. Ezeizabarrena, I. Idiazabal, & B. MacWhinney (Eds.), *Research in child language acquisition: Proceedings of the 8th Conference of the International Association for the Study of Child Language* (pp. 104–127). Somerville, MA: Cascadilla Press.

Cummins, J. (1981). The role of primary language development in promoting educational success for language minority students. In California State Department of Education (Ed.), *Schooling and Language Minority Students: A Theoretical Framework* (pp. 3–49). Los Angeles: Evaluation, Dissemination and Assessment Center, California State University.

Dale, P. (1980). *Acquisition of English and Spanish morphological rules by bilinguals.* Unpublished doctoral dissertation, University of Florida.

De Von Figueroa, Ramey, Keltner, & Lanzi. (2006). Variations in Latino parenting practices and their effects on child cognitive developmental outcomes. *Hispanic Journal of Behavioral Sciences, 28*, 102–144.

Fiestas, C. E., & Peña, E. D. (2004). Narrative discourse in bilingual children: Language and task effects. *Language, Speech, and Hearing Services in Schools, 35*, 155–168.

Flannagan, D., Baker-Ward, L., & Graham, L. (1995). Talk about preschool: Patterns of topic discussion and elaboration related to gender and ethnicity. *Sex Roles, 32*, 1–15.

Gathercole, V. M., Sebastian, E., & Soto, P. (1999). The early acquisition of Spanish morphology: Across-the-board or piecemeal knowledge? *International Journal of Bilingualism, 2*, 72–89.

Genesee, F. (2004). What do we know about bilingual education for majority-language students? In T. Bhatia & W. Ritchie (Eds.), *The handbook of bilingualism* (pp. 547–576). Malden, MA: Blackwell.

Genesee, F., Paradis, J., & Crago, M. (2004). *Dual language development and disorders.* Baltimore: Brookes Publishing.

González, A., Umana-Taylor, A., & Bamaca, M. (2006). Familial ethnic socialization among adolescents of Latino and European descent. *Journal of Family Issues, 27*, 184–207.

Grosjean, F. (1989). Neurolinguists, beware! The bilingual is not two monolinguals in one. *Brian and Language, 36*, 3–15.

Gutiérrez-Clellen, V., & Peña, L. (2001). Dynamic assessment of diverse children: A tutorial. *Language, Speech, and Hearing Services in Schools, 32*, 212–224.

Gutiérrez-Clellen, V. F. (2002). Narratives in two languages: Assessing performance of bilingual children. *Linguistics and Education, 13*, 175–197.

Hakuta, K. (1994). Distinguishing among proficiency, choice, and attitudes in questions about language for bilinguals. In G. Lamberty & C. Garcia Coll (Eds.), *Puerto Rican women and children* (pp. 191–209). NY: Plenum Press.

Hammer, C. S. (1998). Toward a 'thick description' of families: Using ethnography to overcome the obstacles to providing family-centered services. *American Journal of Speech-Language Pathology, 9*, 1–22.

Hammer, C. S., Lawrence, F. R., & Miccio, A. W. (2007). Bilingual children's language abilities and reading outcomes in Head Start and kindergarten. *Language, Speech, and Hearing Services in Schools, 38*, 237–248.

Hammer, C. S., Lawrence, F. R., & Miccio, A. W. (2008). Exposure to English before and after entry into Head Start: Bilingual children's receptive language growth in Spanish and English. *International Journal of Bilingual Education and Bilingualism, 11*(1), 30–56.

Hammer, C. S., Miccio, A. W., & Rodríguez, B. (2004). Bilingual language acquisition and the child socialization process. In B. Goldstein (Ed.), *Bilingual language development and disorders in Spanish-English speakers.* Baltimore: Paul H. Brookes.

Hurtado, A., & Vega, L. (2004). Shift happens: Spanish and English transmission between parents and their children. *Journal of Social Issues, 60*, 137–155.

Isurin, L. (2000). Deserted island or a child's first language forgetting. *Bilingualism: Language and Cognition, 3*(2), 151–166.

Jackson-Maldonado, D. (2004). Verbal morphology and vocabulary in monolinguals and emergent bilinguals. In B. Goldstein (Ed.), *Bilingual language development and disorders in Spanish-English speakers* (pp. 131–161). Baltimore: Brookes Publishing Co.

Jacobsen, P. F., & Schwartz, R. G. (2002). Morphology in incipient bilingual Spanish-speaking preschool children with specific language impairment. *Applied Psycholinguistics, 23*, 23–42.

Leonard, L. B. (1998). *Children with specific language impairment.* Cambridge, MA: Massachusetts Institute of Technology Press.

Loban, W. D. (1976). *Language development kindergarten through grade 12* (Research Rep. No. 18). Urbana, IL: National Council of Teachers of English.

Marchman, V. A., & Martinez-Sussman, C. (2002). Concurrent validity of caregiver/parent report measures of language for children who are learning both English and Spanish. *Journal of Speech, Language, and Hearing Research, 45*, 983–997.

Marchman, V. A., Martínez-Sussmann, C., & Dale, P. S. (2004). The language-specific nature of grammatical development: evidence from bilingual language learners. *Developmental Science, 7*, 212–224.

McGregor, K., Williams, D., Hearst, S., & Johnson, A. (1997). The use of contrastive analysis in distinguishing differences from disorder: A tutorial. *American Journal of Speech-Language Pathology, 6*, 45–56.

McLaughlin, B. (1984). Early bilingualism: Methodological and theoretical issues. In M. Paradis & Y. Lebrun (Eds.), *Early bilingualism and child development* (pp. 19–45). Lisse, the Netherlands: Swets and Zeitlinger.

Meisel, J. (1994). Code-switching in young bilingual children: The acquisition of grammatical constraints. *Studies in Second Language Acquisition, 16*, 413–439.

Muñoz, M. L., Gillam, R. B., Peña, E. D., & Gulley-Faehnle, A. (2003). Measures of language development in fictional narratives of Latino children. *Language, Speech, and Hearing Services in Schools, 34*, 332–342.

Office of English Language Acquisition. (2007). *The growing numbers of limited English proficient students*. Washington, DC: United States Government Printing Office.

Oller, D. K., & Eilers, R. E. (2002). *Language and literacy in bilingual children*. Tonawanda, NY: Multilingual Matters.

Oller, D. K., Pearson, B. Z., & Cobo-Lewis, A. B. (2007). Profile effects in early bilingual language and literacy. *Applied Psycholinguistics, 28*, 191–230.

Patterson, J. L. (1998). Expressive vocabulary development and word combinations of Spanish-English bilingual toddlers. *American Journal of Speech-Language Pathology, 7*, 46–56.

Patterson, J. L., & Pearson, B. Z. (2004). Bilingual lexical development: Influences, contexts, and processes. In B. A. Goldstein (Ed.), *Bilingual language development and disorders in Spanish-English speakers* (pp. 77–104). Baltimore: Paul H. Brookes Publishing Co.

Pearson, B. Z. (2002). Bilingual infants. In M. Suarez-Orozco & M. Paez (Eds.), *Latino remaking America* (pp. 306–320). Los Angeles: University of California Press and David Rockefeller Center for Latin American Studies, Harvard University.

Pearson, B. Z., & Fernández, S. C. (1994). Patterns of interaction in the lexical growth in two languages of bilingual infants and toddlers. *Language Learning, 44*, 617–653.

Pearson, B. Z., Fernández, S., Lewedeg, V., & Oller, D. K. (1997). The relation of input factors to lexical learning by bilingual toddlers. *Applied Psycholinguistics, 18*, 41–58.

Peña, E., Bedore, L. M., & Rappazzo, C. (2003). Comparison of Spanish, English, and bilingual children's performance across semantic tasks. *Language, Speech, and Hearing Services in the Schools, 34*, 5–16.

Peña, E., & Kester, E. S. (2004). Semantic development in Spanish-English bilinguals. In B. A. Goldstein (Ed.), *Bilingual language development and disorders in Spanish-English speakers* (pp. 105–128). Baltimore: Paul H. Brookes Publishing Co.

Penny, R. (2002). *A history of the Spanish language*. Cambridge, United Kingdom: Cambridge University Press.

Petrovic, J. E. (1997). Balkanization, bilingualism, and comparisons of language situations at home and abroad. *Bilingual Research Journal, 21*, 103–124.

Portes, A., & Hao, L. (1998). E pluribus unum: Bilingualism and loss of language in the second generation. *Sociology of Education, 71*, 269–294.

Portes, A., & Hao, L. (2002). The price of uniformity: Language, family and personality adjustment in the immigrant second generation. *Ethnic and Racial Studies, 25*, 889–912.

Portes, A., & Rumbaut, R. G. (2001). *Legacies: The story of the immigrant second generation.* Los Angeles: University of California Press.

Portes, A., & Schauffler, R. (1994). Language and the second generation: Bilingualism yesterday and today. *International Migration Review, 28*, 640–661.

Pousada, A., & Poplack, S. (1982). No case for convergence: The Puerto Rican Spanish verb system in a language-contact situation. In J. Fishman & G. Keller (Eds.), *Bilingual education for Hispanic students in the United States* (pp. 207–237). New York: Teachers College Press.

Restrepo, M. A., & Kruth, K. (2000). Grammatical characteristics of a Spanish-English bilingual child with specific language impairment. *Communication Disorders Quarterly, 21*, 66–76.

Rodríguez, B., Winslow, A., Hammer, C., & Miccio, A. W. (2008, June). *Bilingual children's English and Spanish expressive language skills: A focus on individual differences in syntactic complexity, lexical diversity, and verb morphology.* Poster presentation at the National Head Start's 9th Research Conference, Washington, DC.

Sanchez, R. (1994). The Spanish of Chicanos. In R. Sanchez (Ed.), *Chicano discourse: Socio-historic perspectives* (pp. 98–138). Houston, TX: Arte Público Press.

Serrat, E., & Aparici, M. (2001). Morphological errors in early language acquisition: Evidence from Catalan and Spanish. In M. Almgren, A. Berrena, M. J. Ezeizabarrena, I. Idiazabal, & B. MacWhinney (Eds.), *Research in child language acquisition: Proceedings of the 8th Conference of the International Association for the Study of Child Language* (pp. 1260–1277). Somerville, MA: Cascadilla Press.

Silva-Corvalán, C. (1995). S*panish in four continents: Studies in language contact and bilingualism.* Washington, DC: Georgetown University Press.

United States Department of Education. (2002). *Survey of the states' limited English proficient students and available educational programs and services.* Washington, DC: United States Government Printing Office.

Uccelli, P., & Páez, M. M. (2007). Narrative and vocabulary development of bilingual children from kindergarten to first grade: Developmental changes and associations among English and Spanish skills. *Language, Speech, and Hearing Services in Schools, 38*, 225–236.

Veltman, C. (1981). Anglicization in the United States: The importance of parental nativity and language practice. *International Journal of Society and Language, 32*, 65–84.

Veltman, C. (1983). Anglicization in the United States: Language environment and language practice of American adolescents. *International Journal of the Sociology of Language, 44*, 99–114.

Veltman, C. (1988). Modeling the language shift process of Hispanic Immigrants. *International Migration Review, 22*, 545–562.

Vidal-Ortiz, S. (2004). Puerto Ricans and the politics of speaking Spanish. *Latino Studies, 2*, 254–258.

Weltens, B., & Grendel, M. (1993). Attrition of vocabulary knowledge. In R. Schreuder & B. Weltens (Eds.), *The bilingual lexicon* (pp. 135–156). Amsterdam: John Benjamins.

Zentella, A. (1997). *Growing up bilingual.* Malden, MA: Blackwell Publishers.

# 5 Perspectives on Individual Differences in Preschool Children With Specific Language Impairment

*Judith Vander Woude*

## INTRODUCTION

As clinicians and researchers, we know that preschool children come to the therapeutic setting with individual characteristics that may positively or negatively affect the success of treatment, yet few empirical studies have systematically studied how those characteristics contribute to the effectiveness of treatment for children with language disorders. Children with language disorders have significant difficulty with the comprehension and/or use of spoken and written language in comparison with their peers (American Speech-Language-Hearing Association, 1993). A language disorder can also be associated with other disabilities, such as autism, Down syndrome, significant hearing loss, or traumatic brain injury; or a language disorder can be a specific language impairment (SLI) with no obvious cause. SLI has been defined conventionally with exclusionary criteria because of its extremely heterogeneous nature; as such, it is generally accepted that children with SLI exhibit significantly poorer language skills in comparison with their typically developing peers in the absence of significant sensory and neurodevelopmental deficits and that their nonverbal cognition must be within or above the average range (cf. Leonard, 1998; Rice & Warren, 2004). In this chapter, I focus on how individual characteristics may influence the success of interventions for preschool children with SLI.

## INDIVIDUAL FACTORS DEFINED

The heterogeneous nature of SLI presents at least five complicating factors for defining the condition and determining treatment approaches. First, children with SLI might exhibit deficits in some or only one of the language domains, such as in only phonology or pragmatics, or in any other combinations of the other language areas (e.g., syntax, morphology). For example, evidence from longitudinal data supports these SLI subtypes: phonological-only, semantic-pragmatic, lexical-syntactic, or phonological-syntactic impairments (e.g., Conti-Ramsden & Botting, 1999; Rapin et al., 1996; Rice & Warren, 2004; also see Tomblin, Xhang, Weiss, Catts, & Ellis Weismer, 2004, for an excellent discussion of subtypes).

To further complicate the heterogeneity issue, a second factor is that children with SLI show relative strengths or weaknesses in their receptive and expressive language proficiency across the different language domains (Leonard, 1998). For instance, one child may largely present delays in only expressive syntax, whereas another may have delays in both receptive and expressive syntax. We know that in general, children with receptive and expressive SLI have poorer long-term outcomes after treatment than children with expressive-only SLI do (Law, Garrett, & Nye, 2004; Stothard, Snowling, Bishop, Chipchase, & Kaplan, 1998). Thus, for many children, initial identification and subsequent treatment of specific receptive and/or expressive weaknesses across the different domains is critical for effective intervention over the long term.

A third complicating factor is that children with SLI follow their own language maturational trajectories, even though they seem to acquire language developmental milestones in relatively the same order as their typically developing peers. For instance, overwhelming evidence has indicated that children diagnosed with SLI take a longer time to acquire grammatical tense markers in comparison with their peers (see Rice & Warren, 2004, for a discussion). We also know that for children with typically developing language, great individual variation in language development has been demonstrated. For instance, the median number of words in 12-month-old children's expressive, single-word vocabularies is 6 words, with a range of 0–52 words, and for 16-month-old children, the median number of different words produced is 40, with a range of 0–347 words, via parental reports (Bates et al., 1994). Although the variance in language milestones decreases significantly by the age of 4 years for children with typically developing language, it stands to reason that children with SLI will show even greater individual variations and for a longer period of time, given the nature of SLI.

A fourth complicating factor, related to variability, is distinguishing between children with SLI and children who are considered to be late talkers. Late talkers are usually defined as children younger than 3 years old who display primarily expressive language delays without other significant developmental delays in comparison with their age-mates. However, late talkers, like children diagnosed with SLI, are also more likely to have poorer motor, adaptive, and psychosocial skills compared to their peers (e.g., Zubrick, Taylor, Rice, & Slegers, 2007). Late talkers as a group tend to have better language outcomes than children with SLI, although they continue to show relatively weaker language skills than their typically developing peers later in their development (Dale, Price, Bishop, & Plomin, 2003; Paul, 2000; Paul, Murray, Clancy, & Andrews, 1997; Rescorla, 1989, 2002).

Rescorla (2005) recently reported on the outcomes of adolescents who were identified as late talkers at the age of 2 years. She found that adolescents diagnosed as late talkers when preschoolers exhibited significantly poorer syntax, vocabulary, verbal memory, and reading comprehension skills in comparison with their typically developing peers, even though their language and literacy skills were still within the normal range. Rescorla's (2005) results were consistent with her previous longitudinal study of late talkers at age 9 years (Rescorla, 2002). As such, Rescorla (2005) suggested "it is possible that providing late talkers with activities to improve language processing, phonological discrimination, verbal memory, and word retrieval might help to forestall future language weaknesses relative to typically developing children from the same backgrounds" (p. 469). Thus, even though late talkers have better outcomes than children with SLI, they may benefit from early, proactive treatment.

A fifth and final complicating child factor is that children with SLI exhibit other individual differences that have the potential to positively or negatively contribute to the effectiveness of interventions for children diagnosed with SLI. These differences may be related to children's personal conversational styles and the home environments that are supportive of language stimulation. Conversational styles and the home environment characteristics are often mentioned as confounds in the literature, usually in the discussion sections of intervention studies (e.g., Kouri, 2005), or in textbooks focusing on treatment (e.g., McCauley & Fey, 2006; N. Nelson, 1998; Paul, 2007). Despite the acknowledgement that these factors are relevant to the understanding of treatment success, few well-designed studies that test individual effects on different types of treatment presently exist. Until our clinical expertise and data base prove otherwise, accounting for children's unique characteristics is viewed as essential by master clinicians for making good clinical decisions when treating preschool children with SLI.

Given this background, in this chapter I first discuss clinical treatment decisions as related to evidence-based practice (EBP) principles and three common treatment approaches for preschool children with SLI. Second, I describe three specific child characteristics (children's language maturation, conversational style, and supportive home environment) relative to clinical decisions for treatment. Finally, I speculate on how documenting individual differences in future research might contribute to what we presently know about providing successful intervention for preschool-age children diagnosed with SLI.

## CLINICAL TREATMENT DECISIONS

Obviously, the primary purpose of treatment for preschool children with SLI is to both accelerate and accomplish language learning in the most efficient manner. Said another way, we want children's gains to reflect the greatest possible development in the least amount of time because of the treatment we provide. At a minimum, we want that acceleration to be greater than what we could expect from maturation alone. To achieve efficient language learning, we must know children's relative strengths and weaknesses. In addition to completing comprehensive assessments to determine children's relative linguistic strengths and weaknesses, speech-language pathologists (SLPs) must also document children's individual characteristics beyond their specific language abilities. Once they have gathered all relevant data on children, SLPs need to analyze and prioritize the data they collected in light of EBP principles to select the most effective treatment approaches and specific targets for each child. Underlying the last statement is the belief that intervention is not a "one-size-fits-all" proposition.

## EBP

EBP provides a systematic process to help us select the most efficient treatment approaches and targets for children. Four steps for implementing EBP are (a) developing a clinical question, (b) searching for evidence, (c) critically evaluating available evidence, and (d) using the evidence to make a clinical decision (cf. Dollaghan, 2005; Gillam & Gillam, 2006; Johnson, 2006; Justice & Fey, 2004; also see the American Speech-Language-Hearing Association's 2005 online policy document). Thus, EBP, as applied to speech-language pathology, incorporates the results of the best available research with clinicians' expertise and client preferences when clinical decisions are made.

SLPs are generally well equipped to make clinical decisions based on approaches they learned in graduate school, their own clinical experience, or advice from trusted colleagues and experts; however, as of yet, many clinicians do not use the results of research as part of their clinical decision-making process. According to a survey of 240 SLPs (Zipoli & Kennedy, 2005), the majority of the respondents reported they supported the concept of EBP, but approximately half of the SLPs indicated that they did not have the time and resources to access evidence-based resources to develop their own analyses of available literature. To test the time needed to answer one clinical question using the four EBP steps, Brackenbury, Burroughs, and Hewitt (2008) found that it took three university faculty members between 3 and 7 hours to complete the four recommended steps for one question each. They concluded that SLPs more than likely do not have the time and resources needed to implement EBP routinely in its present state. They did, however, provide several suggestions to make the task easier, such as forming EBP clubs and using reference librarians to help find research evidence.

In addition to a lack of time and resources to answer clinical questions, another important issue that is repeate 'v discussed in the literature on EBP for speech-language pathology is the lack ⌐ ı substantial body of well-designed intervention studies to subject to EBP analy is. Even though more well-designed studies have appeared recently, especially in lan ɪge disorders (e.g., R. B. Gillam et al., 2008; Leonard, Camarata, Brown, & Ca.ɪ ɪrata, 2004; Leonard, Camarata, Pawlowska, Brown, & Camarata, 2006, 2008a), more empirical work is still needed to determine which types of treatment ar proaches work best. In particular, we need carefully designed work that especially addresses the effects of particular child characteristics on different treatment approaches.

## TYPES OF TREATMENT APPROACHES

Three main types of treatment approaches for children with SLI are usually taught in graduate courses and discussed in the literature. They are clinician-directed, child-centered, and hybrid approaches (e.g., Fey, 1986; Paul, 2007; Weiss, 2001). Clinician-directed treatment, as the term suggests, is treatment that is controlled primarily by the clinician. It is based on operant conditioning techniques that include long-established practices for using temporal sequences of antecedent events (e.g., verbal, picture, or object stimuli presented just before or during the client's responses), client responses to the antecedent event, and consequent events (e.g., reinforcement for the clients' responses). The sequence was designed to elicit many desired targets effectively within the least amount of time. For instance, one temporal sequence for working on increasing a preschool child's use of common nouns is as follows: (a) the clinician shows the child a toy fire truck and says, "What's this?" (*antecedent event*); (b) the child says, "fire truck" (*client response*); and (c), the clinician says, "Yes! It's a fire truck!" (*consequent event*).

In contrast to clinician-directed approaches, child-centered approaches include the use of more naturalistic, reactive language stimulation techniques in play or in typical daily routines. The clinician selects specific targets related to the children's needs and then provides a variety of models to focus the child on the learning of those targets usually by response to something the child says or does. Common conversational strategies for providing models for preschool children are *parallel talk*, *expansions*, *extensions*, and *recasts* (see Paul, 2007, for full descriptions). For *parallel talk*, while engaged in a motivating activity, adults talk about what the children are doing. For example, if the activity is baking cookies together, the adult would describe what the child is doing by commenting on his or her actions (e.g., "You're stirring the dough"). For *expansions*, the adult responds to something a child has said and adds additional syntax forms or lexical details to make the child's utterance more adult-like. For example, when the child says, "This yummy!" the adult could reply, "Yes, it is yummy!" *Extensions* are similar to expansions, except they are responses that add additional meaning to the child's utterances. Using the previous example of "this yummy," the adult could expand the child's utterance with, "Yeah, the dough has chocolate chips." *Recasts* are also much like expansions except that the adult uses the child's previous utterance to make a different type of sentence. For instance, again using the same example of a child utterance ("this yummy"), the adult now responds with, "Is that dough yummy?" or could reply in jest, "It isn't yummy." Consistent uses of all of these types of interactional devices have been associated with young children's increased sentence length and grammatical growth (see Fey, 1986; N. Nelson, 1998; Paul, 2007).

A third major approach for treatment is the hybrid approach. Specific hybrid approaches share features of both clinician-directed and child-centered approaches (see Fey, 1986). In contrast to child-centered approaches, hybrid approaches usually focus on one language goal at a time, and the clinician carefully chooses the materials and activities to fit that goal. However, as in child-centered approaches, naturalistic conversational contexts are used to elicit children's spontaneous responses. Two common types of hybrid approaches often discussed in the literature are focused stimulation (see Ellis Weismer & Robertson, 2006, for a review) and enhanced milieu teaching (see Hancock & Kaiser, 2006). Focused stimulation provides children with many models of the targets that address a specific language goal in conversational contexts, usually during a play activity. Thus, if we return to the child-centered example of baking cookies, the clinician would select specific targets to repeatedly model. For example, if the goal is to increase the child's vocabulary, the clinician may repeatedly model the words *dough* and *mix* in a variety of utterances throughout the activity.

Enhanced milieu teaching combines arranging the child's environment, using responsive interactions, and employing milieu teaching strategies, such as modeling, time delays, and incidental teaching. For example, an adult may also use natural time delays (commonly referred to as *wait-time*), during which the adult pauses and then waits for the child to respond, and if the child does not respond, the adult then models the child's turn. Incidental teaching takes advantage of children's spontaneous initiations to naturally encourage the incorporation of new language behaviors in appropriate contexts.

In many research studies, clinician-directed treatments have been proven to be effective (see Fey, 1986; Peterson, 2004, for reviews); however, not all studies support their conclusions. Others have shown better results with more naturalistic approaches, both child-centered and hybrid approaches, particularly for treatment with young children with SLI (e.g., Cole & Dale, 1986; Fey, Cleave, & Long, 1997; Fey, Cleave, Long, & Hughes, 1993; Fey & Loeb, 2002; K. E. Nelson, Camarata, Welsh, Butkovsky, & Camarata, 1996). Most importantly, several studies show that client-directed approaches are better at facilitating the generalization of language skills to other contexts and settings (e.g., Gillum, Camarata, Nelson, & Camarata, 2003; Hughes, 1985; Peterson, 2004).

## SPECIFIC CHILD CHARACTERISTICS

Choosing the most effective type of treatment approach for a particular child involves integrating and analyzing multiple factors, and as Paul (2006) and Nelson (1998) both suggest, clinicians should flexibly, yet systematically, adopt a variety of approaches as needed to meet the specific language goals and objectives in a developmental period. Furthermore, given recent emphasis on EBP, clinicians should also base their treatment choices on available evidence for the efficacy of a particular treatment approach. As such, some approaches may be more effective for children with different rates of language maturation, conversational styles, or types of home environments. In this section, I have addressed these three specific child characteristics that I believe should be considered when making clinical decisions for treatment. These child characteristics were chosen after an extensive review of intervention studies for preschool children with SLI. Language maturation, conversational styles, and home environments were the most frequent planned variables or ex post facto confounds mentioned in the discussions of these studies.

## LANGUAGE MATURATION

Children's rates of language maturation have been shown to be related to provision of effective treatment. As stated in the first section, we know that preschool children with SLI by and large follow the normal sequence of language development milestones, although at a slower rate than their age-matched peers. However, their developmental trajectories in particular language areas can be quite different from those of their peers. For example, preschool children diagnosed with SLI have significantly more difficulty learning new morphosyntactic skills than their typically developing peers. In particular, children with SLI take much longer to consistently and spontaneously use grammatical tense markers, such as regular past tense -*ed*, irregular past tense, third-person singular -*s*, and copular and auxiliary *be* and *do* forms, in comparison with younger language-matched children matched for mean length of utterance (e.g., Hadley & Holt, 2006; Rice, 2004; Rice & Wexler, 1996; Rice, Wexler, & Cleave, 1995).

Evidence from intervention studies suggests that children's scope of language knowledge may play an important role in the effectiveness of an intervention. To illustrate, in a series of three studies, Leonard and colleagues evaluated the effectiveness of a treatment program designed to increase the use of tense and agreement morphemes by preschool children with SLI (Leonard et al., 2004; Leonard et al., 2006; Leonard, Camarata, Pawlowska, Brown, & Camarata, 2008b). For these studies, one group's treatment goals focused on increasing the children's use of the third-person singular verb marker -*s,* and the other group's treatment goals concentrated on increasing their use of the auxiliaries *is, are,* and *was*. In addition, the children's use of past tense -*ed* was assessed and monitored without specifically being treated. Generalization effects for each group's respective untreated conditions (i.e., use of auxiliaries and the use of past tense by children receiving treatment focused on third-person singular verb marker) were documented. As reported by Leonard et al (2004), after 48 treatment sessions, children in both groups showed significant, although modest, gains in their use of treatment targets due to the intervention, although no child achieved 100% mastery. In addition, children in both groups showed gains on their use of untreated morphemes. Leonard et al. (2004) suggested that the children's relative lack of mastery could be explained by the need for more treatment sessions and/or lack of language maturation. They proposed that some of the children were still treating the forms as optional rather than obligatory (see Rice, 2004, for a discussion of the optional infinitive theory); therefore, they might not have been ready to master the forms, given their poor foundation of prerequisite language competence at that point in time.

The second study in the series examined the effects of twice as many treatment sessions as the first study (48 more sessions, for a total of 96 sessions) using the same procedures with 18 of the same preschool children in the first study and the addition of 7 new participants (Leonard et al., 2006). The preschool children with SLI, as a group, again made modest gains toward mastery of the treated morphemes. The gains, however, depended on the children's previous use of the target morpheme. Those children, who used the morphemes an average of approximately 30% of the time after the first 48 treatment sessions, subsequently used the target morpheme an average of approximately 50% of the time after the additional 48 sessions. Children who did not use the target morpheme at all before beginning the second set of 48 sessions only used the targets an average of approximately 25% of the time post-treatment. Leonard et al. (2006) proposed again that the participants' language maturation may have played a role in the relative success of the intervention.

The third study in the series examined the enduring effects of the treatment 1 month after completing 96 treatment sessions under three conditions of focused facilitation: third person singular, auxiliary, and general language stimulation with no specific morpheme targets (Leonard et al., 2008b). The children in the third person singular and auxiliary groups continued to show modest gains 1 month after the end of treatment; the children in the general language stimulation group also made gains on the morpheme targets, but significantly less than the groups that specifically targeted the morphemes. Leonard et al. (2008) again proposed that maturation may play a role and suggested that future research may determine what factors predict children's readiness to acquire agreement and tense morphemes during treatment.

When discussing preschool children's lack of significant gains in their intervention study, Fey and Loeb (2002) also emphasized the importance of children's underlying language maturation. They evaluated the effectiveness of using inverted yes–no questions (e.g., "Is Daddy driving the truck?") as adult recasts for children's omissions of auxiliaries (e.g., "Daddy driving the truck") with 3-year-old children with SLI and 2-year-old children with typically developing language during play. None of the children were using the auxiliary *is* or *will* at the beginning of treatment, and after treatment, neither the typically developing nor language-delayed groups showed significant growth in their use of the two auxiliaries. Fey and Loeb speculated that the intervention might have been more effective had the two featured grammatical forms already started to appear in the children's conversations before treatment, which, in turn, would signal children's readiness to acquire those forms in intervention.

Taking children's language maturation or competence into account is not a new concept in treatment decisions. For typically developing children, it has been demonstrated that new knowledge builds on the old knowledge they already possess (Brown, 1973; Karmiloff-Smith, 1996; K. A. Nelson, 1996; Piaget, 1954), and it has also been demonstrated that children's old knowledge does not necessarily need to be within the same domains of language to foster new knowledge in different language domains, as per the linguistic theory of *bootstrapping* (Morgan & Demuth, 1996). Bootstrapping represents the idea that children can more effectively master new knowledge of one domain by building on what they have already mastered in another domain. For example, children's current phonological development has been shown to predict or facilitate lexical development (Schwartz & Leonard, 1982; Schwartz, Leonard, Loeb, & Swanson, 1987). In another example, children's lexical gains have been shown to be closely related to their syntax knowledge and vice versa, as syntax gains have been shown to closely coordinate with children's current lexical knowledge (Bates & Goodman, 1997; Bedore & Leonard, 2000; Dale, Dionne, & Plomin, 2000; Moyle, Ellis Weismer, Evans, & Lindstrom, 2007). Furthermore, Hancock and Kaiser (2006) have recommended using the enhanced milieu approach only after children are able to imitate verbally, are able to use at least 10 words to communicate, and have mean lengths of utterances between 1.0 and 3.5 morphemes.

If we recognize the importance of bootstrapping in predicting children's readiness for language learning, and thus pay attention to children's individual rates of maturation, it seems logical to use children's relative strengths in one or more language domains to facilitate growth in others where learning is proceeding more slowly. To effectively use children's relative strengths in one or more language domains, we need to know children's existing skills in all language domains before selecting targets for another (i.e., selecting target words for vocabulary growth that include phonemes the child has in his or her repertoire). As such, we can select developmentally appropriate targets for children only if we know their particular developmental profiles at specific points in time. The findings of intervention studies thus far appear to argue that effective clinical decisions require careful documentation of children's language maturation across all domains before and during treatment by using both baseline and ongoing dynamic assessment procedures for the duration of therapeutic interventions.

## CONVERSATIONAL STYLES

Language maturation, however, is not the only child characteristic related to treatment effectiveness for SLI. One important part of young children's social world is participating in conversations, since even very young children begin learning from others in conversational contexts. As such, given a sociocultural perspective, children can learn social skills through language and can also learn language through socialization (Schieffelin & Ochs, 1986). At first glance, this relationship seems deceptively simple, but in truth, the bidirectional nature of language and socialization is complex. For example, the purpose, topic, and context of conversations, along with other variables, such as the participants' ages, familiarity, relative status, language proficiency, and frames of mind at a particular point in time, may influence the nature of particular conversations. Furthermore, the participants' conversational styles based on their relative levels of assertiveness and responsiveness may vary from one individual to the next or from one conversational dyad to the next (Fey, 1986). Assertiveness refers to how readily people engage conversational partners by initiating new topics or turns, and responsiveness refers to how readily people respond to their conversational partners by, for example, appropriately answering questions, staying on topic, and responding to requests for clarification.

Children with SLI demonstrate different conversational styles, much like children who are typically developing (Fey, 1986); however, it is conceivable that some conversational styles may be more conducive to effective interventions for SLI and others can make treatment more challenging. Indeed, most beginning SLPs have a story or two about particularly challenging preschool children in therapy. Often the challenging behaviors were related to conversational style, based on the clinicians' and children's relative levels of assertiveness and responsiveness expressed during the treatment session.

Fey's (1986) description of four distinct conversational styles has provided a useful system for characterizing children's varying levels of assertiveness and responsiveness. The styles are as follows: (a) *active conversationalists,* who exhibit high assertive and high responsive conversational participation; (b) *passive conversationalists,* who exhibit low assertive and high responsive participation; (c) *inactive communicators,* who exhibit both low assertive and low responsive participation; and (d) *verbal noncommunicators,* who exhibit high assertive and low responsive participation. Children's styles of conversational participation can be identified by coding transcribed language samples gathered in different situations and then computing the ratio of assertive and responsive communicative acts contained in both the child's and conversation partner's language samples, or just the amount of time it takes to collect 100 child utterances when recording a language sample can indicate the children's general responsiveness or assertiveness levels. In addition to language samples, the use of structured parental reports, such as Girolametto's (1997) rating scale of young children's conversational skills, can help clinicians to identify children's respective styles.

Although many SLPs have assumed that children with SLI usually fall into the inactive communicator category, characterized by being both less assertive and less responsive conversationalists, the evidence for this is not definitive. Some researchers have reported that children with SLI are less assertive and/or responsive than their age- or language-matched peers, whereas others have reported no differences among the groups. Conti-Ramsden and Friel-Patti (1983), for example, found that children with SLI in their study were less assertive when conversing with their mothers in comparison with younger language-matched peers. Others have reported that when conversing with their age-mates with typical language development, children with SLI were less likely to be assertive conversationalists (Brinton, Fujiki, Spencer, & Robinson, 1997; Craig & Washington, 1993; Liiva & Cleave, 2005) and were less likely to be responsive than their chronological age-matched peers and/or language age-matched peers (e.g., Brinton & Fujiki, 1982; Hadley & Rice, 1991).

Results of other studies, however, have shown that children with SLI were just as assertive or responsive as their typically developing peers, particularly compared with younger language-matched peers. For example, Fey and Leonard (1984) found that 4–6-year-old children with SLI were just as assertive as their chronological age-matched peers when conversing with adults, chronological age-matched peers, and language age-matched peers. They did suggest, however, given the heterogeneity of the SLI population, that conversational styles may be useful for distinguishing among subgroups of SLI. In a comparative study of conversational replies with children at the 1-word stage, Leonard (1986) found that 2–3-year-old children with expressive SLI were as responsive as younger typically developing children (range from 1 year 5 months to 1 year 11 months) when conversing with adults. Leonard proposed that children with SLI can be active conversationalists when the interaction does not require extensive syntactic abilities. The differences in results among the studies may have been due to differences in conversational partners and their respective conversational styles, the age and language maturation of the children with SLI, and the personal predispositions for particular conversational styles in the children, in spite of their language impairment.

It is conceivable, moreover, that children with SLI may change their conversational styles over time. They may have more difficulty being active conversationalists as the difficulty of the linguistic tasks increases, or they may become more active conversationalists as their language skills improve. Conti-Ramsden and Gunn (1986), for instance, reported on developmental changes in conversational skills for a preschool child with SLI. The child responded during conversation much earlier than he initiated conversations. Then, as his language skills improved, he began initiating conversations by labeling or describing items and events before he began making requests. Thus, his conversational style changed over time and depended on his relative language ability at particular points in time.

Therefore, it is too simplistic to state that children with SLI are usually inactive communicators. Although it may be true that some children with SLI display primarily one type of conversation style across different communicative contexts, it seems more likely that children with SLI may display different types of conversational styles with different conversational partners depending on their language maturation, the severity of the language impairment, and different subtypes of SLI.

Conversational styles have been mentioned as possible complicating factors ex post facto in discussion sections of intervention studies for children with SLI or early language delays (e.g., Rosinski-McClendon & Newhoff, 1987; Sorensen & Fey, 1992; Ellis Weismer, Murray-Branch, & Miller, 1993), or when treatment suggestions are outlined in resource texts for clinicians (e.g., Fey, 1986; Fujiki & Brinton, 1995; Paul, 2007; Weiss, 2001). To illustrate, Ellis Weismer, Murray-Branch and Miller compared the effectiveness of two intervention approaches, modeling alone and modeling plus evoked production, for improving the vocabulary development of late talkers between 27 and 28 months old. The children were taught different sets of words in an alternating treatment design. Results showed that the effectiveness of the two treatments varied across the subjects. One child showed a better outcome for the modeling-only approach, another child showed better results with the modeling plus evoked production approach, and the third child did not show significant gains under either approach. The authors speculated that the children's conversational styles may have predicted each child's response to treatment. The child who responded the best to the modeling-only approach was a child who was highly assertive and responsive. Thus, because his productions were optional under the modeling-only approach, the authors stated that he may have been more likely to contribute to the conversation under that condition. In contrast, the child who did best under the modeling plus evoked production condition had significant difficulty with phonology and thus seemed to need the extra production practice that the modeling plus evoked production condition offered. The third child who did not show gains under either condition was described as "reticent to interact verbally, and when faced with a teaching situation in which there were frequent expectations for productions, he often gave no response" (p. 35). It stands to reason, then, that the differences in the children's response to treatment may have been due, in part, to a mismatch between their respective conversational styles and the treatment approaches.

In a more direct approach to understanding the effects of conversational styles on preschoolers with language impairment, Weiss and Nakamura (1992) observed the conversational styles of three preschoolers with typically developing language who were recruited as peer models for seven children with SLI in a preschool classroom practicing reverse mainstreaming. Results indicated that the peer models, as a group, engaged the adults in the classroom as conversational partners more frequently than they engaged their peers with SLI. This observation was consistent with other studies that also found decreased classroom interactions between children with typically developing language and those with language impairment (DeKroon, Kyte, & Johnson, 2002; Gertner, Rice, & Hadley, 1994; Hadley & Rice, 1991; Rice, Sell, & Hadley, 1991). Most germane to this discussion, however, is the observation that the peer models showed varying levels of assertiveness and responsiveness as part of their personal conversational styles by demonstrating style differences across different conversational partners. For example, one of the peer models in the Weiss and Nakamura study was more assertive in conversations with children with SLI but less assertive in conversations with adults. Given this observation, the authors suggested that when recruiting new peer models for the classroom, clinicians and teachers should determine the peer models' relative levels of assertiveness and responsiveness in addition to ensuring that their language proficiency is within the average range. Weiss and Nakamura also noted that peer modeling would be most successful when classroom personnel worked to match the peer models' styles to best fit the needs of their classmates with SLI.

Brinton and Fujiki (1989, 1994, 2005) have supported the use of conversational contexts to facilitate children's acquisition of language. They emphasized the importance using "the contextually rich framework available in conversation to support the skills targeted throughout the course of intervention" (Brinton & Fujiki, 1994, p. 63). Furthermore, Brinton and Fujiki (1994) offered specific treatment suggestions for working with children diagnosed with SLI who are inactive communicators (low levels of assertiveness and responsiveness) and verbal noncommunicators (high assertiveness and low responsiveness). For an inactive communicator, for example, they suggested finding the best situation in which the child successfully takes turns, verbally or nonverbally, and then working on facilitating turns in an age-appropriate highly motivating structured situation, such as peek-a-boo or card matching games. Once the child demonstrates more use of assertive and responsive conversation acts in the structured situation, they suggested moving to less-structured conversational contexts to further encourage the child's assertive and responsive participation. For a verbal noncommunicator, the activities would be similar, except that the focus would be on learning how to respond by intentionally giving turns to conversational partners. These suggestions are based on the belief that children spend the majority of their day with caregivers, teachers, and people other than clinicians; therefore, improving the quality of their access to and active participation in conversations will likely lead to more opportunities for learning language in natural, everyday contexts. There should be additional academic and social benefits for preschoolers resulting from an improvement in their conversation competencies.

It makes good intuitive sense to use conversations as the basis for intervention with preschool children. Conversations are an essential part of children's social lives and are used to regulate most social behavior, such as seeking attention from adults and peers, engaging in play, learning rules for participating in different situations, and developing attachments and friendships with others. It is no surprise, then, that many older children with SLI report having difficulty socially, such as feeling lonely, shy, afraid to join in, having few or no friends, or feeling hostility toward others (e.g., Craig & Washington, 1993; Qi & Kaiser, 2004). Consideration of children's conversational abilities in the clinical decision-making process and designing treatments that address their specific needs at the preschool level may prevent, or alleviate, the negative social consequences that older children with SLI might experience (see Brinton & Fujiki, Chapter 2).

The key to using more natural clinical conversations as the context for an intervention strategy is familiarity with both the child and the child's communicative partners. Clinicians need to know how the child communicates with different conversational partners in different situations across different settings at different times in their development. Although we as clinicians need much more empirical data to know what works therapeutically for particular children, we can use expert opinions, such as those expressed by Brinton and Fujiki (1994) and others (e.g., Fey, 1986; N. Nelson, 1998; Paul, 2007), to guide our clinical decisions when taking children's conversational styles into account.

## HOME ENVIRONMENT

Just as children's rates of language maturation and particular conversation styles may shape SLPs' treatment decisions, children's home environments should also influence SLPs' choice of treatment strategies. Children with SLI come to the therapeutic setting with vastly different experiences in their home environments. Issues of caregiver sensitivity and responsiveness, maternal education, and socioeconomic status in a child's home environment are associated with children's rate of language acquisition during the preschool years. Given the relationships of typical language acquisition with these variables, it is likely then that preschool children with SLI may be even more vulnerable to their effects. Thus, children's particular home environments should be considered when making clinical decisions for preschoolers with SLI. Therefore, clinicians need to account for and directly address disparities in children's home environments when working with them. This section addresses how caregiver sensitivity and responsivity, maternal education, and socioeconomic status may or may not be facilitative of language development in general. These three factors are interrelated and thus difficult to address separately. Maternal education predicts families' socioeconomic status (e.g., Burchinal, Campbell, Bryant, Wasik, & Ramey, 1997), and both less maternal education and low socioeconomic status have been associated with less caregiver responsivity and less frequent language input for children (Hammer, Tomblin, Zhang, & Weiss, 2001; Hart & Risley, 1995; Landry, Smith, Swank, & Miller-Loncar, 2000; Stanton-Chapman, Chapman, Bainbridge, & Scott, 2002).

Caregivers represent a critical part of nurturing home environments, whether they are the children's parents, grandparents, older siblings, or daycare providers. We know that in general, caregivers who provide frequent and stimulating learning experiences contribute to better language, cognitive, and academic outcomes for their young children (Bradley, Corwyn, Burchinal, Pipes McAdoo, & Garcia Coll, 2001; Burchinal et al., 1997; Tamis-LeMonda, Shannon, Cabrera, & Lamb, 2004). Stimulating learning experiences include caregiver sensitivity and responsiveness, such as answering children's questions or responding to their comments; offering early literacy experiences, such as book sharing; and taking the child on a variety of outings, such as going shopping, going to the park, and visiting libraries and museums. As a general rule, young children whose caregivers respond to their emotional and communicative needs in a positive, nurturing manner have better linguistic and cognitive outcomes than children with less responsive and nurturing caregivers (National Institute of Child Health and Human Development Early Child Care Research Network, 2000, 2002).

Some studies have found that children from low-income families, as a group, have weaker language skills on average than children from middle-income families (Hart & Risley, 1995; Heath, 1982; Horton-Ikard & Ellis Weismer, 2007; O'Neil-Pirozzi, 2003, 2006; Qi & Kaiser, 2004; Snow, Dubber, & De Blauw, 1982). In their longitudinal study of 42 young children, Hart and Risley found that children from working-class and professional families heard significantly more and different words and received greater encouragement for producing new words than children from families receiving welfare. As a result, the children who experienced more language input exhibited greater vocabulary gains than the children who were exposed to less frequent input. Hart and Risley concluded that when parents provide their young children with the opportunity to hear many different words and expressions and also prompt them to use those words and expressions, the children then practice them more frequently. Consequently, the children's use of the newly practiced words leads to parental approval, along with additional prompts for more practice. In other words, frequent language input encourages children's responsiveness and practice, and then in turn, children's responsiveness encourages more parental input.

In another study of the effects of socioeconomic status, Hammer and Weiss (1999) studied the play and communicative interactions between two groups of six African American mother–infant dyads, one group consisting of low-income mothers with an average of 11.8 years of education and the other of middle-income mothers with an average of 14.7 years of education. The investigators found few differences between groups regarding the children's play and communicative behaviors. All of the children used vocalizations and some words to communicate.

Unlike the results of Hart and Risley's (1995) study, the mothers in both groups used similar amounts of speech with their young children, and they reduced their utterance lengths, much like the conversations of white middle-class mothers, as described by Snow (1977). However, additional analyses of the mothers' communicative interactions revealed some potentially important differences between the two groups. In spite of the fact that the mothers in both groups had similar amounts of speech, over twice as many of the mothers' vocalizations and verbalizations were addressed to their children in the middle-income group in comparison with the vocalizations and verbalizations by mothers in the low-income group. In addition, the children in the middle-income group used twice as many vocalizations during play as the children in the low-income group, which in turn provided more opportunities for their mothers to respond verbally to their young children. Among the clinical implications of this study was evidence that to predict the effectiveness of treatments recommending caregiver–child conversations, we need to look at more than just frequency of language input and focus as well on the interactional quality of the parent–child communication.

In a study that compared the relative effects of responsivity education and prelinguistic milieu teaching interventions on the language development of young children with developmental delays, Yoder and Warren (1998, 2001) found that pretreatment maternal responsivity and maternal education were related to the effectiveness of each treatment approach. Responsivity education teaches parents to follow their children's lead and to respond to children's attempts to communicate. Prelinguistic milieu teaching uses natural communicative prompts during routine play contexts to help children learn how to use communication intentions such as requesting a turn, or joint attention to an object or person. For children whose mothers were very responsive and had at least 3–4 years of college, the prelinguistic milieu teaching approach was the most effective. For children whose mothers were less responsive and less educated, the responsivity education approach was the most effective. These results suggested that it would be important for SLPs to include responsivity education for caregivers in treatment programs for prelinguistic children with parents who are relatively less responsive and/or less educated.

More recently, Horton-Ikard and Ellis Weismer (2007) found that children from low-income families were able to learn novel word meanings on a fast-mapping task just as well as their peers from middle-income homes. They suggested that fast mapping of novel words could be used to differentiate between young children who have had less exposure to language because of low-socioeconomic status backgrounds and those children who have bona fide language impairments. The results of their study provided important evidence for using alternative measures to identify children who are genuinely in need of treatment because of language deficits.

Since most SLPs will have at least some children from low-income families on their caseloads, they need to be aware of some of the stressors that families in poverty face and avoid unwarranted negative judgments of parenting practices. As Snow, Dubber, and DeBlauw (1982) suggested, mothers of low-income families spend much of their time out of necessity providing for the physical needs of their children and coping with undue stress given their family situations. As such, it is no surprise that children who are homeless, for example, have been shown to be at particular risk for language delays, given their tenuous living situations (O'Neil-Pirozzi, 2003, 2006). Effective treatment approaches are more likely to facilitate the language growth of children with SLI from low-income families if they are designed to provide layers of collaborative support across agencies for their caregivers and teachers.

The clinical implications of these findings do not always lead to clear-cut solutions, given the complexity of family structures, pressures, and stressors and the children's caregivers' personal characteristics. Nevertheless, since frequency of language input seems to be a common factor in many of the studies of children from low-income homes, it makes sense to select treatment approaches designed to increase children's exposure to rich interactions. The approach may include a wide variety of vocabulary with a full range of supportive facilitative utterances such as recasts, prompts that elicit imitations or requests for information, expansions of the children's utterances, or comments that provide more information for children (e.g., Fey, 1986; Fey & Loeb, 2002; Girolametto, Pearce, & Weitzman, 1996; Girolametto, Weitzman, & Greenberg, 2003; Girolametto, Weitzman, Lefebvre, & Greenberg, 2007).

As stated earlier in this chapter, adults who spend the most time with children with SLI should be trained to use facilitative language techniques, whether they are parents, daycare providers, or Head Start teachers. However, as van Kleeck (1994) cautioned, we need to make sure that the suggestions we make for families fit their cultural ways of communicating. For example, for some cultures in the United States, (e.g., African American or Hispanic) verbally displaying one's knowledge by answering "known information" questions, meaning that the person who is asking the question already knows the answer, may not be part of the language socialization practices of that community (see also van Kleeck, 2003). An adult asking a child "What's this?" while pointing to a picture both adult and child can see may result in the child ignoring the adult or refusing to respond. Thus, we need to choose effective interventions that authentically fit children's cultural ways of communicating, as well as work on strategies that create bridges of understanding for communicative norms across communities.

A treatment context that may help adults provide a wide variety of vocabulary with a full range of supportive facilitative utterances for preschoolers with SLI is shared book reading, an important preliteracy activity for preschool children in general. Children with SLI not only represent heterogeneous home environments in general, but more specifically they may present with differing quantities and qualities of preliterate experiences as preschoolers. The relationships between engaging in preliterate activities and developing children's knowledge about their world and facilitating their language development have been well documented in the literature (for a review, see Dickinson & McCabe, 2001).

Given substantial evidence of less-direct caregiver language input overall in the homes of low-income families, it stands to reason that children from low-income families may also experience fewer preliteracy opportunities, such as shared book reading, in their homes. Indeed, results of the Early Childhood Longitudinal Study on kindergarten children (West, Kristin, & Reaney, 2000) found that only 36% of parents with a low socioeconomic status shared books with their preschool children in comparison with 69% of parents with high socioeconomic status. Pellegrini and Galda (2003) suggested that given their limited financial resources, less book sharing in the families with low incomes may be due to a lack of literacy props, including books, which are typically valued and present in middle-class homes and schools. The authors reported observing book-sharing behaviors with more indigenous texts, such as comics and advertisements in low-income homes. Finally, they observed that mothers sometimes had difficulty reading the books to their children, given their own literacy deficits, which in turn affected the quality of and the children's participation in the book-sharing event (Pellegrini, Perlmutter, Galda, & Brody, 1990).

Even so, caregivers with limited education can still be supported in efforts to read with their young children. We can help parents of very young children at risk for SLI learn how to make sharing books part of their daily routines. We know that when parents read to their young children as frequently as possible at the earliest ages possible (given prerequisite joint attention skills, most 6-month-old children can participate in book sharing), children later show better language skills than those children whose parents read less frequently and began reading to their children at an older age (e.g., Bus, 2003; DeBaryshe, 1993).

We can specifically teach caregivers of children with SLI how to have book-sharing conversations that help to increase their children's understanding and use of new vocabulary (Arnold, Lonigan, Whitehurst, & Epstein, 1994; Dale, Crain-Thoreson, Notari-Syverson, & Cole, 1996; Whitehurst et al., 1988). When parents use *wh-* questions during book-sharing conversations (e.g., "What is this?" "What is he doing now?" or "Why did he do that?") that require answers with lexical content, their children have more opportunities to formulate the answers and practice using new vocabulary in supportive conversational contexts. Parents also have structured opportunities in natural and routine contexts to expand, recast, and praise their children's responses (see Zevenbergen & Whitehurst, 2003, for specific suggestions).

In a study of 2- and 3-year-old children and their mothers with limited educations, Bus, Sulzby, and Kaderavek (cited in Bus, 2003) found that if mothers began sharing books with their infants before the age of 14 months, when the children were 2–3 years of age, they were better able to talk about the characters and events and use actual phrases and vocabulary when retelling the stories they had repeatedly read in comparison with children of the same age whose mothers began reading to them after 14 months of age. Bus (2003) maintained that early experiences with book sharing will enable children to better internalize the information from the stories, thereby giving them the tools to recognize story structure templates with greater ease.

The nurturing dyadic nature of a book-sharing conversation makes it an ideal activity for contributing to children's positive participation in stimulating learning activities with their caregivers that are important for language development. Furthermore, books give children and adults the possibility of transcending their immediate environments, even those with limited resources, by providing characters, scenes, vocabulary, and concepts in the text and pictures. Adults can learn how to be sensitive and responsive to their children's linguistic and other needs and thus provide children with multiple opportunities for learning. Also, because we cannot assume that all young children with SLI will fully engage in book-sharing conversations without the structure provided by caregivers, preschool teachers, and other more sophisticated language users, SLPs should probably err on the side of providing support for book-sharing conversations to all of the preschool children on their caseloads. Taken together, these experiences provide children with early foundations in language skills related to later social and academic expectations.

## WHERE DO WE GO FROM HERE?

In this chapter, I have presented some of the child characteristics related to effective or not so effective treatment of preschool language impairments, along with an overview of EBP and common treatment approaches. Of course there are many more child characteristics to consider (cognitive differences, processing deficits, attention behaviors, and bilingualism issues, to name a few) whose effects on the success of treatment may be at least as great as those I have discussed. However, I chose to present three major issues, individual language maturation rates, conversational styles, and home environments, that need continued attention both in our clinical practice and when we design intervention studies. Although more research is addressing the role of individual characteristics, it is time to move beyond primarily mentioning those factors ex post facto as confounds in the empirical literature. Although we know that it is difficult to control all individual factors in large-scale clinical studies, we also know that other legitimate research designs, such as case studies and single-subject designs that use alternating treatments with the same child, can provide much information on the relationship between an individual child's language-learning characteristics and particular treatment approaches. Although case studies and single-subject research designs may not always command the same weight or respect in the research community as large-scale clinical studies, clearly they each have a important role in helping us understand what works for particular children. In summary, I encourage us to keep reminding ourselves that effectively assessing and treating preschool children with language impairment is not a simple, straightforward endeavor. Instead, we need to use our knowledge of the literature, expert opinions, and dynamic assessment procedures throughout clinical decision making because the relative effects of an individual difference discovered at initial diagnosis may be ameliorated over time.

## REFERENCES

American Speech-Language-Hearing Association. (1993). *Definitions of communication disorders and variations* [Relevant paper]. Available from http://www.asha.org/policy

American Speech-Language-Hearing Association. (2005). *Evidence-based practice in communication disorders* [Position statement]. Available from http://www.asha.org/docs/html/PS2005-00221.html

Arnold, D. H., Lonigan, C. J., Whitehurst, G. J., & Epstein, J. N. (1994). Accelerating language development through picture book reading: Replication and extension to a videotape training format. *Journal of Educational Psychology, 86*, 235–243.

Bates, E., & Goodman, J. (1997). On the inseparability of grammar and the lexicon: Evidence from acquisition, aphasia, and real-time processing. *Language and Cognitive Processes, 12*, 507–584.

Bates, E., Marchman, V., Thal, D., Fenson, L., Dale, P., Reznick, J. S., et al. (1994). Developmental and stylistic variation in the composition of early vocabulary. *Journal of Child Language, 21*, 85–123.

Bedore, L. M., & Leonard, L. B. (2000). The effects of inflectional variation on fast mapping of verbs in English and Spanish. *Journal of Speech, Language, and Hearing Research, 43*(1), 21–33.

Brackenbury, T., Burroughs, E., & Hewitt, L. E. (2008). A qualitative examination of current guidelines for evidence-based practice in child language intervention. *Language, Speech, and Hearing Services in the Schools, 39*(1), 78–88.

Bradley, R. H., Corwyn, R. F., Burchinal, M., Pipes McAdoo, H., & Garcia Coll, C. (2001). The home environments of children in the United States part II: Relations with behavioral development through age thirteen. *Child Development, 72*(6), 1868–1886.

Brinton, B., & Fujiki, M. (1982). A comparison of request-response sequences in the discourse of normal and language-disordered children. *Journal of Speech and Hearing Disorders, 47*(1), 57–62.

Brinton, B., & Fujiki, M. (1989). *Conversational management with language-impaired children: Pragmatic assessment and intervention.* Rockville, MD: Aspen.

Brinton, B., & Fujiki, M. (1994). Ways to teach conversation. In J. F. Duchan, L. E. Hewitt, & R. M. Sonnenmeier (Eds.), *Pragmatics: From theory to practice.* Englewood Cliffs, NJ: Prentice Hall.

Brinton, B., & Fujiki, M. (2005). Social competence in children with language impairments: Making connections. *Seminar in Language Disorders, 26*, 151–159.

Brinton, B., Fujiki, M., Spencer, J. C., & Robinson, L. A. (1997). The ability of children with specific language impairment to access and participate in an ongoing interaction. *Journal of Speech, Language, and Hearing Research, 40*(5), 1011–1025.

Brown, R. (1973). *A first language: The early stages.* Cambridge, MA: Harvard University Press.

Burchinal, M. R., Campbell, F. A., Bryant, D. M., Wasik, B. H., & Ramey, C. T. (1997). Early intervention and mediating processes in cognitive performance of children of low-income African American families. *Child Development, 68*(5), 935–954.

Bus, A. G. (2003). Social-emotional requisites for learning to read. In A. van Kleeck & S. A. Stahl (Eds.), *On reading books to children: Parents and teachers* (pp. 3–15). Mahwah, NJ: Lawrence Erlbaum Associates.

Cole, K. N., & Dale, P. S. (1986). Direct language instruction and interactive language instruction with language delayed preschool children: A comparison study. *Journal of Speech and Hearing Research, 29*(2), 206–217.

Conti-Ramsden, G., & Botting, N. (1999). Classification of children with specific language impairment: Longitudinal considerations. *Journal of Speech, Language, and Hearing Research, 42*(5), 1195–1204.

Conti-Ramsden, G., & Friel-Patti, S. (1983). Mothers' discourse adjustments to language-impaired and non-language-impaired children. *Journal of Speech and Hearing Disorders, 48*(4), 360–367.

Conti-Ramsden, G., & Gunn, M. (1986). The development of conversational disability: A case study. *British Journal of Disorders of Communication, 21*(3), 339–351.

Craig, H. K., & Washington, J. A. (1993). Access behaviors of children with specific language impairment. *Journal of Speech and Hearing Research, 36*(2), 322–337.

Dale, P. S., Crain-Thoreson, C., Notari-Syverson, A., & Cole, K. (1996). Parent-child book reading as an intervention technique for young children with language delays. *Topics in Early Childhood Special Education, 16*, 213–235.

Dale, P. S., Dionne, G. E., T., & Plomin, R. (2000). Lexical and grammatical development: A behavioral genetic perspective. *Journal of Child Language, 27*, 619–642.

Dale, P. S., Price, T. S., Bishop, D. V. M., & Plomin, R. (2003). Outcomes of early language delay: I. Predicting persistent and transient language difficulties at 3 and 4 years. *Journal of Speech, Language, and Hearing Research, 46*(3), 544–560.

DeBaryshe, B. D. (1993). Joint picture-book reading correlates of early oral language skill. *Journal of Child Language, 20*, 455–461.

DeKroon, D. M. A., Kyte, C. S., & Johnson, C. J. (2002). Partner influences on the social pretend play of children with language impairments. *Language, Speech, and Hearing Services in the Schools, 33*(4), 253–267.

Dickinson, D. K., & McCabe, A. (2001). Bringing it all together: The multiple origins, skills, and environmental supports of early literacy. *Learning Disabilities Research and Practice, 16*(4), 186–202.

Dollaghan, C. (2005). Evidence-based practice in communication disorders: What do we know, and when do we know it? *Journal of Communication Disorders, 37*(5), 391–400.

Ellis Weismer, S., Murray-Branch, J., & Miller, J. F. (1993). Comparison of two methods for promoting productive vocabulary in late talkers. *Journal of Speech and Hearing Research, 36*(5), 1037–1050.

Ellis Weismer, S., & Robertson, S. (2006). Focused stimulation approach in language intervention. In R. J. McCauley & M. E. Fey (Eds.), *Treatment of language disorders in children* (pp. 175–202). Baltimore: Paul Brookes Publishing.

Fey, M. E. (1986). *Language intervention with young children.* San Diego, CA: College-Hill Press.

Fey, M. E., Cleave, P. L., & Long, S. H. (1997). Two models of grammar facilitation in children with language impairments: Phase 2. *Journal of Speech, Language, and Hearing Research, 40*(1), 5–19.

Fey, M. E., Cleave, P. L., Long, S. H., & Hughes, D. L. (1993). Two approaches to the facilitation of grammar in children with language impairment: An experimental evaluation. *Journal of Speech and Hearing Research, 36*(1), 141–157.

Fey, M. E., & Leonard, L. B. (1984). Partner age as a variable in the conversational performance of specifically language-impaired and normal-language children. *Journal of Speech and Hearing Research, 27*(3), 413–423.

Fey, M. E., & Loeb, D. F. (2002). An evaluation of the facilitative effects of inverted yes-no questions on the acquisition of auxiliary verbs. *Journal of Speech, Language, and Hearing Research, 45*(1), 160–174.

Fujiki, M., & Brinton, B. (1995). Social competence and language impairment in children. In R. V. Watkins & M. L. Rice (Eds.), *Specific language impairments in children.* Baltimore: Paul Brookes Publishing.

Gertner, B. L., Rice, M. L., & Hadley, P. A. (1994). Influence of communicative competence on peer preferences in a preschool classroom. *Journal of Speech and Hearing Research, 37*(4), 913–923.

Gillam, R. B., Loeb, D. F., Hoffman, L. M., Bohman, T., Champlin, C. A., Thibodeau, L., et al. (2008). The efficacy of Fast Forword language intervention in school-age children with language impairment: A randomized controlled trial. *Journal of Speech, Language, and Hearing Research, 51*(1), 97–119.

Gillam, S. L., & Gillam, R. B. (2006). Making evidence-based decisions about child language intervention in schools. *Language, Speech, and Hearing Services in the Schools, 37*(4), 304–315.

Gillum, H., Camarata, S., Nelson, K. E., & Camarata, M. N. (2003). A comparison of naturalistic and analog treatment effects in children with expressive language disorder and poor preintervention imitation skills. *Journal of Positive Behavior Interventions, 5*(3), 171–178.

Girolametto, L. (1997). Development of a parent report measure for profiling the conversational skills of preschool children. *American Journal of Speech-Language Pathology, 6*(4), 25–33.

Girolametto, L., Pearce, P. S., & Weitzman, E. (1996). Interactive focused stimulation for toddlers with expressive vocabulary delays. *Journal of Speech and Hearing Research, 39*(6), 1274–1283.

Girolametto, L., Weitzman, E., & Greenberg, J. (2003). Training day care staff to facilitate children's language. *American Journal of Speech-Language Pathology, 12*(3), 299–311.

Girolametto, L., Weitzman, E., Lefebvre, P., & Greenberg, J. (2007). The effects of in-service education to promote emergent literacy in child care centers: A feasibility study. *Language, Speech, and Hearing Services in the Schools, 38*(1), 72–83.

Hadley, P. A., & Holt, J. K. (2006). Individual differences in the onset of tense marking: A growth-curve analysis. *Journal of Speech, Language, and Hearing Research, 49*(5), 984–1000.

Hadley, P. A., & Rice, M. L. (1991). Conversational responsiveness of speech- and language-impaired preschoolers. *Journal of Speech and Hearing Research, 34*(6), 1308–1317.

Hammer, C. S., Tomblin, J. B., Zhang, X., & Weiss, A. L. (2001). Relationship between parenting behaviours and specific language impairment in children. *International Journal of Language and Communication Disorders, 36*(2), 185–205.

Hammer, C. S., & Weiss, A. L. (1999). Guiding language development: How African American mothers and their infants structure play interactions. *Journal of Speech and Hearing Research, 42*(5), 1219–1233.

Hancock, T. B., & Kaiser, A. P. (2006). Enhanced milieu teaching. In R. J. McCauley & M. E. Fey (Eds.), *Treatment of language disorders in children*. Baltimore: Paul Brookes Publishing.

Hart, B., & Risley, T. R. (1995). *Meaningful differences in the everyday experiences of young American children*. Baltimore: Paul Brookes Publishing.

Heath, S. B. (1982). What no bedtime story means: Narrative skills at home and at school. *Language in Society, 11*, 49–76.

Horton-Ikard, R., & Ellis Weismer, S. (2007). A preliminary examination of vocabulary and word learning in African American toddlers from middle and low socioeconomic status homes. *American Journal of Speech-Language Pathology, 16*(4), 381–392.

Hughes, D. L. (1985). *Language treatment and generalization: A clinician's handbook*. San Diego, CA: College-Hill Press.

Johnson, C. J. (2006). Getting started in evidence-based practice for childhood speech-language disorders. *American Journal of Speech-Language Pathology, 15*(1), 20–35.

Justice, L. M., & Fey, M. E. (2004). Evidence-based practice in schools: Integrating craft and theory with science and data. *The ASHA Leader, 30–32*(4–5).

Karmiloff-Smith, A. (1996). *Beyond modularity: A developmental perspective on cognitive science*. Cambridge, MA: Massachusetts Institute of Technology Press.

Kouri, T. A. (2005). Lexical training through modeling and elicitation procedures with late talkers who have specific language impairment and developmental delays. *Journal of Speech, Language, and Hearing Research, 48*(1), 157–171.

Landry, S. H., Smith, K. E., Swank, P. R., & Miller-Loncar, C. L. (2000). Early maternal and child influences on children's later influences on children's later independent cogntive and social functioning. *Child Development, 71*, 358–375.

Law, J., Garrett, Z., & Nye, C. (2004). The efficacy of treatment for children with developmental speech and language delay/disorder: A meta-analysis. *Journal of Speech, Language, and Hearing Research, 47*(4), 924–943.

Leonard, L. B. (1986). Conversational replies of children with specific language impairment. *Journal of Speech and Hearing Research, 29*(1), 114–119.

Leonard, L. B. (1998). *Children with language impairment*. Cambridge, MA: Massachusetts Institute of Technology Press.

Leonard, L. B., Camarata, S. M., Brown, B., & Camarata, M. N. (2004). Tense and agreement in the speech of children with specific language impairment: Patterns of generalization through intervention. *Journal of Speech, Language, and Hearing Research, 47*(6), 1363–1379.

Leonard, L. B., Camarata, S. M., Pawlowska, M., Brown, B., & Camarata, M. N. (2006). Tense and agreement morphemes in the speech of children with specific language impairment during intervention: Phase 2. *Journal of Speech, Language, and Hearing Research, 49*(4), 749–770.

Leonard, L. B., Camarata, S. M., Pawlowska, M., Brown, B., & Camarata, M. N. (2008a). The acquisition of tense and agreement morphemes by children with specific language impairment during intervention: Phase 3. *Journal of Speech, Language, and Hearing Research, 51*(1), 120–125.

Leonard, L. B., Camarata, S. M., Pawlowska, M., Brown, B., & Camarata, M. N. (2008b). The acquisition of tense and agreement morphemes by children with specific language impairment during intervention: Phase 3. *Journal of Speech, Language, and Hearing Research, 51*, 120–125.

Liiva, C. A., & Cleave, P. L. (2005). Roles of initiation and responsiveness in access and participation for children with specific language impairment. *Journal of Speech, Language, and Hearing Research, 48*(4), 868–883.

McCauley, R. J., & Fey, M. E. (2006). *Treatment of language disorders in children*. Baltimore: Paul Brookes Publishing.

Morgan, C., & Demuth, K. (Eds.). (1996). *Signal to syntax: Bootstrapping from speech to grammar in early acquisition*. Mahwah, NJ: Lawrence Erlbaum Associates.

Moyle, M. J., Ellis Weismer, S., Evans, J. L., & Lindstrom, M. J. (2007). Longitudinal relationships between lexical and grammatical development in typical and late-talking children. *Journal of Speech, Language, and Hearing Research, 50*(2), 508–528.

National Institute of Child Health and Human Development Early Child Care Research Network. (2000). The relation of child care to cognitive and language development. *Child Development, 71*, 960–980.

National Institute of Child Health and Human Development Early Child Care Research Network. (2002). Early child care and children's development prior to school entry: Results from the NICHD study of early child care. *American Educational Research Journal, 39*, 133–164.

Nelson, K. A. (1996). *Language in cognitive development: The emergence of the mediated mind*. Cambridge, United Kingdom: Cambridge University Press.

Nelson, K. E., Camarata, S. M., Welsh, J., Butkovsky, L., & Camarata, M. (1996). Effects of imitative and conversational recasting treatment on the acquisition of grammar in children with specific language impairment and younger language-normal children. *Journal of Speech and Hearing Research, 39*, 850–859.

Nelson, N. (1998). *Childhood language disorders in context: Infancy through adolescence* (2nd ed.). Boston: Allyn & Bacon.

O'Neil-Pirozzi, T. M. (2003). Language functioning of residents in family homeless shelters. *American Journal of Speech-Language Pathology, 12*, 229–242.

O'Neil-Pirozzi, T. M. (2006). Comparison of context-based interaction patterns of mothers who are homeless with their preschool children. *American Journal of Speech-Language Pathology, 15*(3), 278–288.

Paul, R. (2000). Predicting outcomes of early expressive language delay: Ethical implications. In D. V. M. Bishop & L. B. Leonard (Eds.), *Speech and language impairments in children: Causes, characteristics, intervention and outcome* (pp. 185–209). Howe, United Kingdom: Psychology Press.

Paul, R. (2007). *Language disorders from infancy through adolescence: Assessment and intervention* (3rd ed.). St. Louis, MO: Mosby Elsevier.

Paul, R., Murray, C., Clancy, K., & Andrews, D. (1997). Reading and metaphonological outcomes in late talkers. *Journal of Speech, Language, and Hearing Research, 40*(5), 1037–1047.

Pellegrini, A. D., & Galda, L. (2003). Explicating the context of joint book reading. In A. v. Kleeck & S. A. Stahl (Eds.), *On reading books to children: Parents and teachers* Mahwah, NJ: Lawrence Erlbaum Associates.

Pellegrini, A. D., Perlmutter, J. C., Galda, L., & Brody, G. H. (1990). Joint reading between black Head Start children and their mothers. *Child Development, 61*, 443–453.

Peterson, P. (2004). Naturalistic language teaching procedures for children at risk for language delays. *The Behavior Analyst Today, 5*, 404–424.

Piaget, J. (1954). *The construction of reality in the child*. New York: Basic Books.

Qi, C. H., & Kaiser, A. P. (2004). Problem behaviors of low-income children with language delays: An observation study. *Journal of Speech, Language, and Hearing Research, 47*(3), 595–609.

Rapin, I., Allen, D. A., Aram, D., Dunn, D., Fein, D., Morris, R., et al. (1996). Classification issues. In I. Rapin (Ed.), *Preschool children with inadequate communication* (pp. 190–228). London: MacKeith.

Rescorla, L. (1989). The language development survey: A screening tool for delayed language in toddlers. *Journal of Speech and Hearing Disorders, 54*(4), 587–599.

Rescorla, L. (2002). Language and reading outcomes to age 9 in late-talking toddlers. *Journal of Speech, Language, and Hearing Research, 45*(2), 360–371.

Rescorla, L. (2005). Age 13 language and reading outcomes in late-talking toddlers. *Journal of Speech, Language, and Hearing Research, 48*(2), 459–472.

Rice, M. L. (2004). Growth models of developmental language disorders. In M. L. Rice (Ed.), *Developmental language disorders: From phenotype to etiologies*. Mahwah, NJ: Lawrence Erlbaum Associates.

Rice, M. L., Sell, M. A., & Hadley, P. A. (1991). Social interactions of speech, and language-impaired children. *Journal of Speech and Hearing Research, 34*(6), 1299–1307.

Rice, M. L., & Warren, S. F. (Eds.). (2004). *Developmental language disorders: From phenotypes to etiology*. Mahwah, NJ: Lawrence Erlbaum Associates.

Rice, M. L., & Wexler, K. (1996). Toward tense as a clinical marker of specific language impairment in English-speaking children. *Journal of Speech and Hearing Research, 39*(6), 1239–1257.

Rice, M. L., Wexler, K., & Cleave, P. L. (1995). Specific language impairment as a period of extended optional infinitive. *Journal of Speech and Hearing Research, 38,* 850–863.

Rosinski-McClendon, M. K., & Newhoff, M. (1987). Conversational responsiveness and assertiveness in language-impaired children. *Language, Speech, and Hearing Services in the Schools, 18,* 53–62.

Schieffelin, B. B., & Ochs, E. (Eds.). (1986). *Language socialization across cultures.* New York: Cambridge University Press.

Schwartz, R. G., & Leonard, L. B. (1982). Do children pick and choose? An examination of phonological selection and avoidance in early lexical acquisition. *Journal of Child Language, 14,* 411–418.

Schwartz, R. G., Leonard, L. B., Loeb, D. F., & Swanson, L. (1987). Attempted sounds are sometimes not: An expanded view of phonological selection and avoidance. *Journal of Child Language, 14,* 411–418.

Snow, C. E. (1977). The development of conversation between mothers and babies. *Journal of Child Language, 4,* 1–22.

Snow, C. E., Dubber, C., & De Blauw, A. (1982). Routines in mother-child interaction. In L. Feagans & D. Farran (Eds.), *The language of children reared in poverty: Implications for evaluation and intervention* (pp. 53–72). New York: Academic Press.

Sorensen, P., & Fey, M. E. (1992). Informativeness as a clinical principle: What's really new? *Language, Speech, and Hearing Services in the Schools, 23*(4), 320–328.

Stanton-Chapman, T. L., Chapman, D. A., Bainbridge, N. L., & Scott, K. G. (2002). Identification of early risk factors for language impairment. *Research in Developmental Disabilities, 23*(6), 390–405.

Stothard, S. E., Snowling, M. J., Bishop, D. V. M., Chipchase, B. B., & Kaplan, C. A. (1998). Language-impaired preschoolers: A follow-up into adolescence. *Journal of Speech, Language, and Hearing Research, 41*(2), 407–418.

Tamis-LeMonda, C. S., Shannon, J. D., Cabrera, N. J., & Lamb, M. E. (2004). Fathers and mothers at play with their 2- and 3-year-olds: Contributions to language and cognitive development. *Child Development, 75*(6), 1806–1820.

Tomblin, J. B., Zhang, X., Weiss, A., Catts, H., & Ellis Weismer, S. (2004). Dimensions of individual differences in communication skills among primary grade children. In M. L. Rice & S. F. Warren (Eds.), *Developmental language disorders: From phenotypes to etiologies* (pp. 53–76). Mahwah, NJ: Lawrence Erlbaum Associates.

van Kleeck, A. (1994). Potential cultural bias in training parents as conversational partners with their children who have delays in language development. *American Journal of Speech-Language Pathology, 3,* 67–78.

van Kleeck, A. (2003). Research on book sharing: Another critical look. In A. van Kleeck, S. A. Stahl, & E. B. Bauer (Eds.), *On reading books to children.* Mahwah, NJ: Lawrence Erlbaum Associates.

Weiss, A. L. (2001). *Preschool language disorders resource guide: Specific language impairment.* San Diego, CA: Singular Thomson Learning.

Weiss, A. L., & Nakamura, M. (1992). Children with normal language skills in preschool classrooms for children with language impairments: Differences in modeling styles. *Language, Speech, and Hearing Services in the Schools, 23,* 64–70.

West, J., Kristin, D., & Reaney, L. M. (2000). *The kindergarten year: Findings from the early childhood longitudinal study, kindergarten class of 1998–99.* Washington, DC: National Center for Education Statistics, U.S. Department of Education. NCES 2001–023.

Whitehurst, G. J., Falco, F. L., Lonigan, C. J., Fischel, J. E., Debarysche, N. D., Valdez-Menchacha, M. C., et al. (1988). Accelerating language development through picture book reading. *Developmental Psychology, 24,* 552–559.

Yoder, P. J., & Warren, S. F. (1998). Maternal responsivity predicts the prelinguistic communication intervention that facilitates generalized intentional communication. *Journal of Speech, Language, and Hearing Research, 41*(5), 1207–1219.

Yoder, P. J., & Warren, S. F. (2001). Relative treatment effects of two prelinguistic communication interventions on language development in toddlers with developmental delays vary by maternal characteristics. *Journal of Speech, Language, and Hearing Research, 44,* 224–237.

Zevenbergen, A. A., & Whitehurst, G. J. (2003). Dialogic reading: A shared picture book reading intervention for preschoolers. In A. van Kleeck, S. A. Stahl & E. B. Bauer (Eds.), *On reading books to children: Parents and teachers.* Mahwah, NJ: Lawrence Erlbaum Associates.

Zipoli, R. P., Jr., & Kennedy, M. (2005). Evidence-based practice among speech-language pathologists: Attitudes, utilization, and barriers. *American Journal of Speech-Language Pathology, 14,* 208–220.

Zubrick, S. R., Taylor, C. L., Rice, M. L., & Slegers, D. W. (2007). Late language emergence at 24 months: An epidemiological study of prevalence, predictors, and covariates. *Journal of Speech, Language, and Hearing Research, 50,* 1562–1592.

# 6 Individual Differences in Underlying Oral Language Competencies Associated With Learning to Read
## *Implications for Intervention*

*Linda S. Larrivee and Emily S. Maloney*

## INTRODUCTION: LINGUISTIC FOUNDATIONS OF LEARNING TO READ

Although reading is a complex linguistic and cognitive activity, it comes easily to most children without extraordinary instruction (e.g., Perfetti, 1985). As a result, it is sometimes difficult to appreciate the numerous cognitive and linguistic skills involved in learning to read. Researchers have often divided reading skills into two skill categories: word recognition and comprehension (e.g., Hoover & Gough, 1990). Word recognition, which involves both decoding (sounding out) and word identification, is the ability to quickly and accurately identify written words. Skilled word recognition involves orthographic processing, as well as the use of sound–letter correspondence rules (Coltheart, 1981; Seidenberg, Walters, Barnes & Tanenhaus, 1984). In short, word recognition allows us to translate print into language. Comprehension, on the other hand, is the ability to interpret the linguistic information at the word, sentence, and discourse levels (Kintsch & Van Dijk, 1978; Sticht, 1979; Sticht & James, 1984).

Although most children seem to learn to read easily, some do not. During the past century, a large body of research has examined reading disabilities and predictors of reading disabilities (Galaburda, 1985; Geschwind, 1985; Hinshelwood, 1917; Huey, 1968; Schiffman, 1962; Orton, 1925). Specifically, for many years, researchers have attempted to explain why some children learn to read so easily whereas others failed even with the same instruction as those who succeeded. At one time, difficulties in such areas as vision and visual-spatial ability, among others, were suggested as causes of reading disabilities (e.g., Catts & Kamhi, 2005). However, it is now well accepted by researchers and practitioners that reading is a language-based skill (see Adams, 1990). Several breakthroughs have occurred in reading research during the past several years contributing to this change of perspective. Indeed, spoken language (listening and speaking) has many similarities to written language (reading and writing). Although written language is not simply an offshoot of spoken language, they do have similar linguistic and cognitive bases (Kamhi & Catts, 2005). For example, phonology, the way that sounds are organized within a language to convey differences in meaning, is obviously an important component of oral language communication. It is also important to the development of reading, especially through the contributions of phonological awareness and phonics. To acquire sound–letter correspondence rules, readers must be familiar with the sounds of their native language. Competencies in the area of morphology (word structure) and syntax (word sequence within sentences) are also important for reading because to comprehend written language, one must understand the basic underlying language structure. Similarly, semantics (vocabulary within the language), and word finding are as important for both word recognition and for reading comprehension. Thus, any aspect of oral language with which children struggle may also be difficult for them as they learn to read.

Metalinguistic skills are also important for reading. Metalinguistic awareness involves the ability to focus on linguistic form apart from the content of a message (e.g., Hakes, 1982, 1984; Pratt & Grieve, 1984; van Kleeck, 1982). Language comprehension and production have been described as transparent (Cazden, 1972, 1975). In other words, the forms of language lead us to the message content. Individual sentences do not stand in isolation but are integrated into a meaningful message through text-level processing. This is generally an automatic process that is executed rapidly and requires little attention (Hakes, 1984). In contrast, metalinguistic ability has been described as opaque. This implies that metalinguistic performance is a focus on the language forms apart from their context and content. Likely, it is the metalinguistic aspects of all areas of language, including phonology, morphosyntax, and semantics, that are most important to reading ability.

Many children with primary language impairments (LIs) often have difficulty learning to read. Given the close association between oral and literate language competencies, it is probably not surprising that for children diagnosed with LI, their difficulties in oral language are likely related to their difficulties in written language. To enhance the effectiveness of the treatment they provide, speech-language pathologists (SLPs) can identify children's specific areas of linguistic and metalinguistic weaknesses so that they can impact both oral and written language development. This chapter examines several aspects of oral language and how deficits in these areas relate to deficits in written language. Implications for individualized intervention are discussed.

## PHONOLOGICAL AWARENESS: LINKS TO WORD RECOGNITION

Phonological awareness has been defined as awareness of the sound system of language (e.g., Catts, 1991; Hakes, 1982; Stanovich, 1988; Tunmer & Nesdale, 1985). It involves the awareness that words are composed of phonemes and syllables. Having this awareness enables one to identify words that rhyme or have the same beginning or ending sounds. Phonological awareness also allows one to conceive of a word as being made up of syllables and phonemes.

Numerous studies have shown that phonological awareness is related to reading (e.g., Bradley & Bryant, 1985; Catts, 1991, 1993; Gillon & Dodd, 1994; Larrivee & Catts, 1999; Lundberg, Olofsson & Wall, 1980; MacLean, Bryant & Bradley, 1988; Mann & Liberman, 1984; Scarborough, 1991). Studies comparing good and poor readers have demonstrated a close relationship between phonological awareness and reading ability. These studies have shown that good readers perform well on tasks measuring phonological awareness, whereas poor readers perform poorly on these tasks (Bradley & Bryant, 1978; Fox & Routh, 1980). In addition, phonological awareness, measured before formal reading instruction, has been shown to be predictive of later reading ability (Bradley & Bryant, 1983, 1985; Bryant, Bradley, MacLean, & Crossland, 1989; Catts, 1991; Stanovich, Cunningham & Cramer, 1984).

Phonological awareness is a metalinguistic skill. Language skills likely predict metalinguistic ability. Therefore, performance in speech-sound production can be expected to relate to performance in phonological awareness. For example, children with good phonological production, or articulation, should have good phonological awareness, and children with poor phonological production should have poor phonological awareness. Several studies have investigated this relationship. Children who exhibit mild expressive phonological disorders, or articulation errors, in preschool do not later have associated reading difficulties (Catts, 1993). These children have no greater risk for difficulties developing reading skills than children with good speech and language skills. However, children with difficulties with expressive phonology alone may be at increased risk if these problems continue upon entry into kindergarten and first grade (Bird, Bishop, & Freeman, 1995; Bishop & Adams, 1990; Larrivee & Catts, 1999). Children with moderate to severe phonological disorders have a somewhat different outcome (Larrivee & Catts, 1999). Most importantly, children with difficulties in both expressive phonology along with oral LIs in areas of semantics and/or morphosyntax are at far greater risk than children with expressive phonological disorders alone (Justice & Schuele, 2004; see also Larrivee & Schuele, 2005). Thus, the key to poor phonological awareness and poor reading is likely concomitant LI (i.e., semantic and/or morphosyntactic).

## SEMANTICS AND MORPHOSYNTAX: LINKS TO WORD RECOGNITION AND READING COMPREHENSION

### VOCABULARY AND WORD RETRIEVAL

Typically developing children acquire approximately 2,000–3,000 new words each year during their school years for a total of more than 40,000 words by high school graduation (e.g., Nagy & Scott, 2000). As these words are acquired, they must be stored so that they can be retrieved as needed. Storage and retrieval are separate but related processes, and word finding is dependent upon both.

Vocabulary growth and organization are important for both speakers and readers in their need to quickly access appropriate words to use and comprehend. For example, in a longitudinal study examining children from kindergarten through seventh grade, Wolf and colleagues (e.g., Wolf, 1991; Wolf, Bally, & Morris, 1986) found that naming speed in young children was a strong predictor of word recognition and that word recall as measured by confrontational naming was a strong predictor of later reading comprehension. Similarly, Snyder and Downey (1991) examined word retrieval skills in children with reading disabilities compared with children with normal reading achievement. The researchers found that the children with reading disabilities differed significantly from the children with normal reading achievement on both the time and accuracy of word retrieval. In addition, performance on word retrieval measures, along with performance on sentence completion tasks, best accounted for reading comprehension ability for younger children with reading disabilities. In an examination of children with good versus poor reading comprehension, Cain and Oakhill (2006) found that poor receptive and expressive vocabulary skills predicted poor growth in reading ability.

Children with LI often have difficulty with vocabulary development and word recall (Dollaghan, 1998; McGregor, Newman, Reilly, & Capone, 2002). In fact, late onset of vocabulary development is often an early sign of LI in children (Rice, Oetting, Marquis, Bode, & Pae, 1994; Watkins, Kelly, Harbers, & Hollis, 1995). Because children with LIs often also have difficulty in reading acquisition, assessment and intervention for these children must take into account their vocabulary and word retrieval skills.

Some researchers have found that typical receptive vocabulary tests, such as the Peabody Picture Vocabulary Test-Third Edition (PPVT-III) (Dunn & Dunn, 1997), do not capture the true vocabulary ability of children with LIs. McGregor et al. (2002) administered the PPVT-III to a group of children with LIs. Although the mean standard score was 89, these children demonstrated limited semantic knowledge on other types of probes examining their semantic storage and retrieval. The researchers found a link between semantic knowledge and naming performance. They suggested that intervention should focus on increasing robustness of semantic representations. In other words, they stated that it is not necessarily the size of children's vocabulary that impacts retrieval, but rather the completeness of the stored lexical items. Although several published materials are available for such an intervention approach, it is also unlikely that intervention based on rapid naming will improve word retrieval.

Many researchers have found that children with deficits in both phonological awareness and naming abilities have difficulty learning to read (see Allor, 2002, for a review). Interestingly, researchers have indicated that children's phonological awareness ability may be related to their semantic ability. For example, Walley and colleagues (Garlock, Walley, & Metsala, 2001; Metsala & Walley, 1998; Walley, 1993; Walley, Metsala, & Garlock, 2003) suggested that phonological awareness arises from lexical reorganization in late preschool and into early school years as children's vocabulary increases. They hypothesized that increases in children's vocabulary leads to phonological representations that become increasingly specified at the phoneme level. Application of this research to children with speech-language impairments may provide insight into the mechanisms that underlie deficient phonemic awareness and related deficits in reading ability. It may explain the differing outcomes for children with phonological disorders alone and children with both phonological and other language deficits.

## MORPHOSYNTAX

As previously discussed, reading comprehension draws on a variety of language skills, including word recognition and vocabulary knowledge. Clearly, children use their knowledge of the meanings of words to understand what they read. However, reading comprehension, as with language comprehension, requires that children integrate the meanings of single words at the sentence and text levels. Many children with specific language impairment demonstrate deficits in the area of morphosyntactic skills. These children often have difficulty comprehending sentences as they become longer and more grammatically complex. Children's language comprehension skills provide the basis for the children's comprehension of text. Consequently, children who demonstrate difficulties in grammatical understanding in the oral dimension will likely encounter difficulties with reading comprehension as well. In addition, children use a variety of structural cues when listening to speech or when reading text to figure out the meaning of unknown words. A variety of studies have examined both the relationship between morphosyntactic skills and reading comprehension, as well as how children use morphosyntactic skills to assist with word recognition and inference of word meaning.

A growing body of research has examined the relationship between reading comprehension and a wide range of oral language skills (e.g., Catts, Adlof, & Weismer, 2006; Nation, Clarke, Marshall, & Durand, 2004). These studies have shown that poor comprehenders have deficits in oral language skills, includ-ing grammatical understanding. For example, Nation et al. investigated the oral language skills of 8-year-old children with impaired reading comprehension. A variety of tasks were used to assess morphosyntactic skills. Nation et al. found that poor comprehenders had relative weaknesses across broad language skills, including morphosyntax. In another study examining the language abilities of children with specific reading comprehension deficits, Catts et al. also found that poor comprehenders demonstrated weaknesses in grammatical understanding. Again, these deficits were present within the larger context of deficits in broad language skills. Specifically, the poor comprehenders scored near the 30th per-centile in grammatical understanding, which was slightly better than their scores in the 20th percentile in receptive vocabulary. Catts et al. pointed out that although these deficits may be mild in nature, they may lead to difficulties understanding text-length material. These findings are consistent with several other studies indi-cating that poor comprehenders demonstrate weak grammatical understanding in addition to deficits in broader language skills (Cragg & Nation, 2006; Gillon & Dodd, 1994; Snyder & Downey, 1991; Stothard & Hulme, 1992). (See Cain & Oakhill, 2006, and Smith, Macaruso, Shankweiler, & Crain, 1989, for contrasting findings.)

## MORPHOLOGICAL AWARENESS AND READING

As with other forms of metalinguistic awareness, morphological awareness becomes increasingly important as children learn to read. Morphological awareness refers to the ability to reflect upon and manipulate morphemes and use word formation rules (Kuo & Anderson, 2006). Research on morphological awareness and reading has focused mainly on inflections (e.g., Brittain, 1970; Carlisle & Nomanbhoy, 1993; Casalis & Louis-Alexandre, 2000) and derivations (e.g., Carlisle, 2000; Champion; 1997; Fowler & Liberman; 1995; Leong, 1989; see Kuo & Anderson [2006] for overview of empirical studies on morphological awareness and reading). Inflectional morphology involves adding prefixes or suffixes to words to mark grammatical function. For example, a verb may be marked by inflectional morphemes to indicate past tense (*play* becomes *played*). Inflectional morphology is typically acquired by the early elementary grades (e.g., Berko, 1958). Research suggests that awareness of inflectional morphology may have an impact on reading (e.g., Brittain, 1970). However, the correlation between awareness of inflectional morphology and reading appears to be present in the early elementary grades, which is likely because inflectional morphology is acquired by the age of 6 or 7 years (Berko, 1958; Derwing & Baker, 1977).

In contrast to inflectional morphology, derivational morphology develops throughout the school years and into adulthood. Derivational morphology involves the addition of a morpheme to change the meaning (i.e., *understand/misunderstand*) and/or part of speech (i.e., *develop/development*) of a word. Some derived forms, referred to as nonneutral forms, alter the phonological representation of the word (i.e., *sign/signature*). Tasks involving nonneutral forms tend to be more difficult for children (Carlisle & Nomanbhoy, 1993). Although children in the early elementary grades begin to develop understanding of derivational morphology, the largest growth of derivational morphology skills occurs between Grade 4 and Grade 8 (Nippold, 2007). Moreover, as children get older, they will encounter an increasing number of morphologically complex words in text, particularly in mathematics, science, and social studies textbooks (Henry, 2003; Nippold, 2007). Children who exhibit weakness in morphological awareness will encounter difficulty as they are exposed to these more difficult words.

Recent studies suggest that awareness of derivational morphology is important to reading development as children get older. Studies comparing morphological awareness skills in good and poor readers generally suggest that poor readers perform more poorly on morphological awareness tasks than good readers (Champion, 1997; Fowler & Liberman, 1995; Leong, 1989; Shankweiler et al., 1995). Poor readers seem to have particular difficulty with tasks involving nonneutral derived forms that involve phonological changes from the base form (Fowler & Liberman, 1995; Shankweiler et al., 1995). Additional research suggests that morphological awareness is predictive of later reading skill (e.g., Carlisle, 1995; Casalis & Louis-Alexandre, 2000). More recently, studies have indicated a specific relationship between children's morphological awareness and decoding skills (e.g., Carlisle, 2000; Mahony, Singson, & Mann, 2000), as well as reading comprehension (e.g., Carlisle, 2000; Mahony, 1994). Mahony et al. (2000) found that performance on a morphological awareness task requiring students to determine whether pairs of words were related to each other was related to decoding skill for third-, fourth-, fifth-, and sixth-grade students. This finding suggests that children's awareness of the components of words and knowledge of the meaning of the components influences decoding skills.

Carlisle (2000) conducted a study to determine whether morphological aware-ness was related to reaching achievement, including word reading and reading comprehension for third and fifth graders. The children's morphological aware-ness was assessed using three tasks: decomposition of derived words in order to finish a sentence, production of a derived word to finish a sentence, and a vocabu-lary task that required defining morphologically complex words. The children's ability to read morphologically complex words and their comprehension at the word and passage levels was also evaluated. To investigate the relationship between morphological awareness and decoding skill, Carlisle included morphologically complex transparent and shift words, as well as words matched on base frequency but differing in surface frequency. Carlisle found that both third and fifth grad-ers performed significantly better on transparent words, in which the base words were clearly represented in the derived form, than on shift words, which involved phonological and/or orthographic changes. The results also showed that both third and fifth graders read high-frequency transparent words more accurately than low-frequency transparent words, suggesting that children at this age are not yet able to use knowledge of morphological cues to parse a difficult word into morphemes, even when they might have knowledge of the base. Furthermore, for both third and fifth graders, oral production of shift words during a morpho-logical awareness task was significantly related to reading of shift words, which Carlisle proposed may suggest awareness of the complex relations of shift words for reading. For both grade levels, scores on morphological structure tasks were significantly correlated with the word definition task. This finding suggests that children's ability to define morphologically complex words is related to their awareness of word structure. Results also showed that awareness of structure and meaning and the ability to read derived words contributed significantly to reading comprehension. However, the contribution was more significant for the fifth graders than for the third graders.

Additional research is needed to determine the specific relationship between morphological awareness and reading. It is possible that the relationship between morphological awareness and reading may be reciprocal, because orthographic representations of words may assist with understanding morphological structure (Carlisle, 1988; Fowler & Liberman, 1995; Templeton & Scarborough-Franks, 1985). Therefore, increased exposure to more morphologically complex words in print may facilitate improved morphological awareness. It is also impor-tant to consider the relationship between morphological awareness and other metalinguistic skills, such as phonological and syntactic awareness, as there is a clear overlap between these skills during the complex process of reading.

## SYNTACTIC AWARENESS AND READING COMPREHENSION

Clearly, children with deficits in reading comprehension often have underlying language deficits, including deficits in syntax. Of course, these findings are not surprising. Children's comprehension of sentence-level information involves both their comprehension of semantic information and their knowledge of sentence structure, or grammar. Furthermore, children's ability to comprehend at the sentence level is a prerequisite skill to comprehension at higher levels, including paragraphs and lengthier discourse.

More specifically, children's syntactic awareness skills are related to their reading ability (e.g., Nation & Snowling, 2000; Tunmer, Nesdale, & Wright, 1987; Willows & Ryan, 1986). Syntactic awareness, a type of metalinguistic awareness, refers to the ability to reflect upon and manipulate the internal grammatical structure of sentences (Tunmer et al., 1987). As with other forms of metalinguistic knowledge, syntactic awareness plays a role in literacy development (e.g., Tunmer et al; Willows & Ryan, 1986). As was mentioned previously, a component argued to contribute to the development of metalinguistic ability is language knowledge (Hakes, 1982). To reflect on language, it is assumed that one needs to have the ability to use language to communicate effectively. Therefore, children with good syntactic language skills should have good syntactic awareness, and children with poor syntactic skills should have poor syntactic awareness.

Tunmer et al. (1987) investigated syntactic awareness skills in good readers in second grade and poor readers in fourth grade who were matched for reading comprehension, reading fluency, decoding ability, and verbal intelligence. Tunmer et al. found that the young good readers scored significantly better than poor readers on two measures of syntactic awareness. These findings suggest that the older poor readers were developmentally delayed in syntactic awareness and that this delay may have affected reading development. Tunmer et al. also found that measures of syntactic awareness varied with reading level at each grade, with better readers performing better on syntactic awareness tasks. The authors concluded that these two findings suggest that syntactic awareness is causally related to learning to read. Nation and Snowling (2000) examined the nature of syntactic awareness skills in children with reading and language comprehension deficits compared with normally developing children matched for age, nonverbal ability, and decoding skills and found similar results to Tunmer et al. Syntactic awareness was measured by word order correction tasks. Overall, the poor comprehenders did not perform as well as normally developing children. Although passive sentences were more difficult for all children, they were particularly difficult for the poor comprehenders, suggesting that performance on word order correction tasks is sensitive to syntactic complexity. In addition, children demonstrated greater difficulty correcting word order in sentences that were reversible, indicating that semantic ambiguity also influences syntactic awareness. Nation and Snowling's findings suggest that although all children had more difficulty with sentences that were long, complex, and ambiguous, poor comprehenders showed a substantial degree of impairment compared with typically-developing children.

Syntactic awareness also seems to plays a role in children's ability to engage in the process of comprehension monitoring. Comprehension monitoring refers to children's ability to verify their understanding and make repairs when this understanding does not make sense (Perfetti, Landi, & Oakhill, 2005). When children are syntactically aware, they are able to check that their response to the words in a text conforms to the surrounding grammatical context (Tunmer et al., 1987). If a breakdown in comprehension occurs, children with difficulties in syntactic awareness may have difficulty detecting and/or using grammatical context to repair the error.

## SYNTACTIC AWARENESS AND WORD RECOGNITION

In addition to the role that syntactic awareness plays in comprehension of text and comprehension monitoring, syntactic awareness skills may play a more direct role in reading acquisition via their role in word recognition. Several researchers have suggested that syntactic awareness may influence children's ability to identify unfamiliar words by enabling them to use their knowledge of the constraints of sentential context (Catts & Kamhi, 2005; Nation & Snowling, 1998; Rego & Bryant, 1993; Tunmer & Hoover, 1992; Tunmer et al., 1987; Willows & Ryan, 1986). More specifically, grammatical morphemes may provide listeners and readers with information about the word class of an unfamiliar word. As Kamhi and Catts (2005) pointed out, grammatical morphemes provide information about word classes. For example, adverbs are marked by the inflections -*ly* and -*y,* and verbs are signaled by the inflections -*ed, -ing,* and -*en.* Therefore, it seems probable that children with good morphosyntactic awareness would be more likely to use contextual support, whereas children with poor morphosyntactic awareness might be at a disadvantage. See Clark and Clark (1997) for a review of studies demonstrating the influence of syntactic and morphologic knowledge on comprehension of sentences.

As some researchers have pointed out, it is difficult to differentiate between syntactic awareness and semantic awareness or vocabulary knowledge during tasks that evaluate children's ability to use context to identify unfamiliar words (Nation & Snowling, 2000; Rego & Bryant, 1993; Tunmer et al., 1987). It is likely that "poor comprehenders' impaired syntactic awareness is a manifestation of more general language processing difficulties, encompassing both semantic and grammatical weaknesses" (Nation & Snowling, 2000, p. 237).

Rego and Bryant (1993) conducted a study to determine the specific contributions that phonological awareness and syntactic and semantic awareness make to reading. They evaluated the phonological awareness and the syntactic and semantic awareness skills of 5-year-old children. The semantic and syntactic awareness tasks included a cloze task, a sentence anagram task, and a sentence completion task. During the cloze task, the children had to provide 10 missing words from within a story. The sentence anagram task required the children to listen to a jumbled sentence and repeat the sentence while putting the words in the correct order. The sentence completion task involved the children providing missing function and content words within sentences. Five months later, the children were given an invented spelling test and a contextual facilitation task to determine the contributions phonological and semantic/syntactic skills had on these skills. To develop the contextual facilitation task, Rego and Bryant used 10 words that the children were unable to read on a previous reading test and embedded them in a meaningful sentence. The children were verbally presented with the sentence and were then asked to read the previously unknown word. Results indicated a strong relationship between children's semantic and syntactic skills and their ability to use context in reading. The authors concluded that the more sensitive children are to semantic and syntactic categories, the better they will be at using semantic and syntactic cues in reading. To facilitate language-impaired children's use of contextual support to help them figure out unknown words, these children may need explicit instruction in semantic and syntactic awareness.

## SPECIFIC COMPREHENSION SUBSKILLS

It is evident that children with deficits across a range of language skills may have difficulties with literacy development. These difficulties may range from the sound level (phonology) to sentence-level processing (semantics/syntax). However, poor comprehenders' difficulties with reading comprehension may extend beyond problems in vocabulary and grammar. Many children may demonstrate deficits with inferential language skills. In addition, children with LIs may have difficulties at the discourse level of language processing. When children read narrative texts, they not only have to process the meanings of the words or sentences, they need to integrate the information at the paragraph or multiparagraph level to extract meaning from text. An increasing number of studies have examined the higher level processing skills in children who demonstrate poor reading comprehension. Children with poor comprehension skills often have difficulty with discourse-level skills, including making inferences, knowledge of story structure, and comprehension monitoring (Cain, 1996; Cain & Oakhill, 1996, 1999; Cain, Oakhill, Barnes, & Bryant, 20 ; Ehrlich & Redmond, 1997; Oakhill, Cain, & Bryant, 2003; Yuill & Oakhill, 1991). Some of these skills are more metacognitive than metalinguistic and thus beyor ' the scope of this chapter. An argument can be made that one of these skills, making inferences, appears to be fundamentally linguistic in nature.

Children with LIs often have difficu ty making inferences. Children's difficulty with inference-making is likely to impact their ability to comprehend discourse-level information, both orally and in text. Indeed, children who demonstrate poor reading comprehension have greater difficulty making inferences compared with normally achieving readers (e.g., Cain et al., 2001; Cain & Oakhill, 1999; Snyder & Downey, 1991). The process of making an inference requires that children go beyond what is explicitly stated to understand an intended message.

More specifically, answering questions that involve inferences requires children to relate the information they hear or read to their own background knowledge in order to extract meaning. Cain et al. suggest that poor comprehenders are unable to form a complete representation of text. That is, they may be able to understand information at a lower level but have difficulty producing a coherent integrated model. Cain et al. investigated the inference-making ability in 7- to 8-year-old good and poor comprehenders while controlling for the effect of background knowledge. Children were first taught a novel knowledge base, including a series of facts about an imaginary planet. Cain et al. then tested the children's acquisition of the knowledge base by a forced-choice picture recognition task and a verbal recall task. The children were then presented with story episodes, followed by questions assessing their ability to make two types of inference: coherence inferences, which are necessary to establish the links between premises in the text, and elaborative inferences, which enrich the text representation. The less skilled comprehenders generated significantly fewer inferences than the skilled comprehenders did, suggesting that even when these children had the necessary base knowledge, they were unable to make inferences as readily as their peers. A common source of inference difficulty for the poor comprehenders was a failure to retrieve the relevant textual premise. In contrast, the skilled comprehenders were often able to recall both the relevant textual premise and the knowledge base but had difficulty integrating the two. The problem for the poor comprehenders was not just in integrating the information; their problem occurred at an even more preliminary stage in the process. That is, they failed to recall the information that needed to be integrated in order to make the inference. The less skilled comprehenders generated significantly fewer inferences than the skilled comprehenders did, suggesting that even when these children had the necessary base knowledge, they were unable to make inferences as readily as their peers. Although this study demonstrated that children with poor reading comprehension are less skilled at making inferences from information presented orally, it is highly likely that they would have similar difficulty making inferences from text.

Van Kleeck, Vander Woude, and Hammet (2006) conducted a study examining the effects of a book-sharing intervention on the literal and inferential skills of language-impaired preschoolers in Head Start preschool programs. The 30 language-impaired preschoolers included in the study were divided into an intervention group and a control group. The 8-week intervention consisted of individual 15-minute book-sharing sessions two times per week. The two books used in the intervention were embedded with literal and inferential questions, as well as scripted prompts and answers to be used as needed. The questions related to either the text or the pictures in the books. Three different versions of questions were developed for each book, which allowed for repeated readings of the same two stories throughout the intervention. The results showed that children in the intervention group demonstrated greater growth in literal and inferential language skills than the control group. These findings provide evidence that book-sharing intervention can improve the literal and inferential language skills in preschoolers with LIs. As previously discussed, inferential language skills are important for reading comprehension, and the findings from this study suggest that intervention focusing on inferencing can be effective beginning in the preschool years.

## UNDERLYING ORAL LANGUAGE COMPETENCIES: IMPLICATIONS FOR INTERVENTION TO IMPACT READING SKILLS

### Phonological Awareness Deficits

Numerous training studies have shown that phonological awareness skills can be taught. Training in phonological awareness results in increased phonological awareness and in improved reading ability (Alexander, Anderson, Heilman, Voeller, & Torgesen, 1991; Ball & Blachman, 1988; Bradley & Bryant, 1983; Bryne & Fielding-Barnsley, 1989; Cunningham, 1990; Lie, 1991; Lundberg, Frost & Peterson, 1988; Treiman & Baron, 1983; Williams, 1980; Yopp, 1992). Several studies have found this to be true for children with LI. For example, Gillon (2000) used an integrated phonological awareness intervention approach for children with LI who had difficulty learning to read. The phonological awareness program consisted of the following components: rhyming activities, manipulation of sounds in isolation (based on Auditory Discrimination in Depth; Lindamood & Lindamood, 1975), identification of initial and final sounds in words, segmentation and blending of sounds in words, and grapheme-phoneme correspondence rules. Two groups of children, one group consisting of children with LI and the other consisting of children with typically developing language, participated in two 1-hour sessions per week for a total of 20 hours of training. Some of the children with LI received the integrated phonological awareness approach, and others participated in more traditional speech-language therapy. Children who received the integrated phonological awareness showed significantly more improvement in both phonological awareness and reading than did children who received the more traditional approach. In fact, children with LI who received the integrated approach performed similarly in phonological awareness and reading to the typically developing children after the intervention despite significant differences in this areas prior to the intervention. Interestingly, some of the children with LI also had articulation errors and the integrated approach was shown to improve their speech articulation as well. In a follow-up to this study, Gillon (2002) found that the integrated phonological awareness program led to sustained growth in phonological awareness and word recognition as well as strong phoneme-grapheme rules applied to spelling. In addition, Kirk and Gillon (2007) found that long-term benefits of the training included an ability to use morphological awareness in spelling complex words.

Choice of tasks for phonological awareness training may be an important consideration. Morais (1991) proposed two categories of phonological awareness: holistic and analytic. The first category, holistic phonological awareness, is used to judge the relationship between two utterances. In addition, holistic phonological awareness is used to "judge a number of suprasegmental properties of an utterance [and] may be sufficient to carry out tasks such as classification on the basis of overall similarity, rhyme appreciation, and the detection of mispronunciations" (p. 35). An oddity task likely requires a child to classify on the basis of similarity. A syllable segmentation task used calls for a judgment of suprasegmental properties (e.g., the rhythm of the word through the syllable divisions). Training tasks such as oddity (i.e., "Which word does not belong in this group?") may be beneficial for children whose linguistic deficits lie in the area of phonology or morphology.

The second category, analytic phonological awareness, allows one to consciously analyze, segment, and synthesize the parts of an utterance. Morais (1991) stated that the most complex type of analytic phonological awareness is needed to consciously isolate phonetic features of utterances. Blending and sound isolation tasks may require more conscious isolation of phonetic features. Blending tasks require children to listen to separate phonemes and put them together to make a word. In other words, children are asked to both analyze and synthesize phonetic units. Sound isolation requires that children analyze a phonetic unit (the initial or final sound of a word) and examine it as a possible part of a word. In other words, it is the opposite of the blending task. Thus, analytic phonological awareness, involving the processes of analyzing and synthesizing phonetic information, may require the same skills as semantic-syntactic language ability. Training tasks such as these may aid children whose difficulty with the linguistic system lies in semantic and/or morphosyntactic areas.

As previously mentioned, reading consists of both word recognition and comprehension skills. Phonological awareness is related more to word recognition skills in the early stages of reading instruction (Adams, 1990). Therefore, when children demonstrate deficits in word identification, intervention must include phonological awareness training. Several published materials are available (e.g., Adams, Foorman, Lundberg, & Beeler, 1998; Notari-Syverson, O'Connor, & Vadasy, 1998; O'Connor, Notari-Syverson, & Vadasy, 1998) that can be individualized to the needs of children working either in groups or one-to-one with SLPs.

## SEMANTICS AND MORPHOSYNTAX

Although there is good evidence of the link between semantic and morphosyntactic deficits and deficits in reading ability, there are relatively few intervention studies. Those that are available indicate that intervention for semantic and morphosyntactic deficits can have a positive impact on reading ability. For example, Gillon and Dodd (1995) investigated the efficacy of a program designed to remediate deficits of students with specific reading disability. Participants included children ages 10–12 identified as having a reading disability, with deficits in both reading comprehension and reading accuracy, and who also demonstrated phonological, semantic, and syntactic skills significantly inferior to matched good readers. The participants received a two-part intervention. One part was a phonological awareness component, which included activities similar to those of the Lindamood Phoneme Sequencing Program (Lindamood & Lindamood, 1998). The other part consisted of a semantic-syntactic program, which included the *Handbook of Exercises for Language Processing,* Volumes 1 and 4 (Lazzari & Peters, 1987, 1989). Activities included identifying a complete sentence, formulating compound and complex sentences, expanding sentences, combining information to make sentences, sentence cloze activities, and perceiving nonsense in sentences. A thematic approach to extend vocabulary and knowledge of sentence structure was also included, during which students selected a theme of interest and then were engaged in a brainstorming activity to think of nouns, verbs, adjectives, and adverbs associated with the theme. They were then asked to make sentences with combinations of theme words, including more complex sentences using conjunctions. The students then reflected on the quality of the sentences.

Results suggest remediation of students' underlying phonological, semantic, and syntactic processing deficits has a dramatic effect on both reading accuracy and reading comprehension. Prior to the intervention in the study, the students had been exposed to other remediations; therefore, the dramatic improvement in reading skills as a result of the study intervention could not be attributed simply to the conditions of the program (i.e., increased attention or more intensity of time on training). For some students, improved knowledge of sentence structure and word meanings in context appeared to be as important for reading comprehension as their improved phonological skills. However, some of the students with the more severe reading disabilities only benefited from the phonological training program in terms of gains in their reading performance. The authors suggested that these students may not be able to use their semantic and syntactic knowledge as a compensatory strategy because of the increased effort required for decoding. However, the results of this study suggest that the phonological and semantic-syntactic skills of students with reading disabilities can be improved significantly through direct intervention.

Other intervention studies generally support the finding that training in morphological awareness results in improved reading (e.g., Arnback & Elbro, 2000; Elbro & Arnback, 1996; Henry, 1988, 1993; see Baumann, Edwards, Boland, Olejnik, & Kame'enui, 2003, for contrasting findings). For example, Nunez, Bryant, and Olsson (2003) conducted an intervention study examining the effects of morphological and phonological training on word reading and spelling. The 7- and 8-year-olds in the study were divided into five groups: morphological training alone, morphological training with writing, phonological training alone, phonological training with writing, and a control group. The 12-week intervention included weekly small group sessions involving activities such as classification, analogies, and blending. Activities for morphological and phonological training were similar in nature (i.e., morphological tasks involved blending of stems and affixes to create a word, whereas phonological tasks involved blending onsets and rimes). The morphological and phonological groups required the children to provide oral responses, whereas the morphological and phonological training with writing required the children to say and write their answers. Results indicated that all four groups performed better than the control group on a standardized test of reading, which required children to read words that were increasingly long and less familiar to them. The morphological intervention resulted in progress in the use of morphological rules in spelling; however, there were no specific effects of intervention on the use of morphological rules in reading. Interestingly, the phonological intervention had no effect on the use of phonologically based spelling rules. The authors proposed that it was possible that the phonological distinction used as the focus of this study, which was related to long versus short vowels, may have been too difficult for the children in the study. The authors further suggested that it is possible that the children in the control group may have been receiving similar instruction in their classrooms. Nonetheless, the results of this study provide evidence that training in morphological awareness can affect positive change in reading performance.

Additional intervention studies are needed to determine the efficacy of various types of morphological, as well as syntactic and semantic training, along with the specific effects of this type of training on decoding and reading comprehension. In addition, future studies on intervention focusing on inferential language and the effects on reading comprehension will provide invaluable information to SLPs working with children with LIs and associated reading difficulties.

## CONCLUSION

Many children who are at risk for failure in reading are on SLPs' caseloads. Children with oral LIs are six times as likely to have difficulty reading than typical language peers and half of children who have reading disabilities in the early grades may have oral language deficits (Catts, Fey, Tomblin, & Zhang, 2002). Difficulties experienced by children with reading disabilities are likely related to their specific oral language deficits as well as their difficulty with metalinguistc ability. The areas of need can range from phonological awareness to word awareness to morphosyntactic awareness in any combination. Therefore, it is important to determine the specific areas of weakness to assist children who struggle with learning to read, because, as noted above, direct training in specific linguistic areas can lead to improvement in reading ability.

The National Reading Panel (NRP) report set the stage for evidence-based reading instruction (National Institute of Child Health and Human Development, 2000a, 2000b). Specifically, the NRP report suggested that phonemic awareness and vocabulary instruction should be part of the reading curriculum. Historically, vocabulary instruction has been a central part of SLPs' role when working with children with LIs. Similarly, over the past 10–15 years, SLPs have been aware of the importance of phonemic awareness and have increasingly incorporated it in intervention (Larrivee, Schuele, Hendrickson, & Craig, 2005).

Clearly, SLPs have a role in literacy learning (Schuele & Larrivee, 2004). The American Speech-Language-Hearing Association provided members with guidelines about their roles and responsibilities in literacy instruction (2001). Thus, not only should SLPs be involved in reading acquisition and remediation for the children on their caseloads, but they also must ensure that they provide instruction based on the needs of the individual.

Although not the primary reading instructors, SLPs can supplement and augment reading instruction given by classroom teachers. In doing so, SLPs can provide a unique contribution to efforts to enhance literacy instruction. One of SLPs' most unique and valuable skills is an ability to explore the linguistic strengths and needs of each child. SLPs can assess children to find their specific linguistic abilities and make connections between their linguistic difficulties and their problems learning to read. SLPs can look at a child from many different perspectives to consider where the child's difficulties lie, why the child has those difficulties, and what instructional strategies, scaffolding, and modifications can enhance the child's success (Vigil & van Kleeck, 1996).

Although SLPs are becoming increasingly involved in literacy instruction, intervention for children with LIs must focus on specific language deficits that contribute to reading problems. Skilled readers are exposed to new vocabulary and complex language. Therefore, the more these children read, the better their language skills become. In contrast, children with LIs who have poor decoding and/or comprehension skills read simpler texts and may read less often than skilled readers. Consequently, these children do not have the same access to the richness of vocabulary and language as skilled readers. This concept, referred to as the Matthew effect, suggests that the gap between the language skills of good and poor comprehenders will likely increase over time (e.g., Stanovich, 1986). Keeping this in mind, it is imperative that SLPs continue to provide treatment that targets specific linguistic skills. In addition, children with LIs who are struggling readers should not only read books at their reading level but should also have exposure to a wide range of literate language through book-sharing and read-aloud activities.

Indeed, SLPs' training and knowledge base allows them to make the link between oral and written language. Classroom curricula generally assume that children have a good foundation of oral language (vocabulary, grammar/syntax, discourse, etc.), but many children with LI do not have these skills. When working on oral language, SLPs can establish links with written language and vice versa. Regardless, the most important role of SLPs in literacy development is to individualize instruction on the basis of the children's specific language needs.

## REFERENCES

Adams, M. J. (1990). *Beginning to read: Thinking and learning about print*. Cambridge, MA: Massachusetts Institute of Technology Press.

Adams, M. J., Foorman, B. R., Lundberg, I., & Beeler, T. D. (1998). *Phonemic awareness in young children: A classroom curriculum*. Baltimore: Brookes Publishing Co.

Alexander, A., Anderson, H., Heilman, P., Voeller, K., & Torgesen, J. (1991). Phonological awareness training and remediation of analytic decoding deficits in a group of severe dyslexics. *Annals of Dyslexia, 41*, 193–206.

Allor, J. H. (2002). The relationships of phonemic awareness and rapid naming to reading development. *Learning Disability Quarterly, 25*, 47–57.

American Speech-Language-Hearing Association. (2001). Roles and responsibilities of speech-language pathologists with respect to reading and writing in children and adolescents (position statement, executive summary of guidelines, technical report). *ASHA Supplement, 21*, 17–27.

Arnback, E., & Elbro, C. (2000). The effects of morphological awareness training on the reading and spelling skills of young dyslexics. *Scandinavian Journal of Educational Research, 44,* 229–251.

Ball, E., & Blachman, B. (1988). Phoneme segmentation training: Effect on reading readiness. *Annals of Dyslexia, 38,* 208–225.

Baumann, J. F., Edwards, E. C., Boland, E., Olejnik, S., & Kame'enui, E. J. (2003). Vocabulary tricks: Effects of instruction in morphology and context on fifth-grade students' ability to derive and infer word meaning. *American Educational Research Journal, 40,* 447–497.

Berko, J. (1958). The child's learning of English morphology, *Word, 14,* 150–177.

Bird, J., Bishop, D. V. M., & Freeman, N. H. (1995). Phonological awareness and literacy development in children with expressive phonological impairments. *Journal of Speech and Hearing Research, 38,* 446–462.

Bishop, D. V. M., & Adams, C. (1990). A prospective study of the relationship between specific language impairment, phonological disorders, and reading retardation. *Journal of Child Psychology and Psychiatry, 21,* 1027–1050.

Bradley, L., & Bryant, P. (1978). Difficulties in auditory organization as a possible cause of reading backwardness. *Nature, 271,* 746–747.

Bradley, L., & Bryant, P. (1983). Categorizing sounds and learning to read: A causal connection. *Nature, 30,* 419–421.

Bradley, L., & Bryant, P. (1985). Rhyme and reason in reading and spelling. *International Academy for Research in Learning Disabilities Monograph Series* (Number 1). Ann Arbor, MI: University of Michigan.

Brittain, M. M. (1970). Inflectional performance and early reading achievement, *Reading Research Quarterly, 6,* 34–48.

Bryant, P., Bradley, L., & MacLean, M., & Crossland, J. (1989). Nursery rhymes, phonological skills, and reading. *Journal of Child Language, 16,* 407–428.

Bryne, B., & Fielding-Barnsley, R. (1989). Phonemic awareness and letter knowledge in the child's acquisition of the alphabetic principle. *Journal of Educational Psychology, 82,* 429–438.

Cain, K. (1996). Story knowledge and comprehension skills. In C. Cornoldi & J. V. Oakhill (Eds.), *Reading comprehension difficulties: Processes and remediation.* Mahwah, NJ: Lawrence Erlbaum Associates.

Cain, K., & Oakhill, J. V. (1996). The nature of the relation between comprehension skill and the ability to tell a story. *British Journal of Developmental Psychology, 14,* 187–201.

Cain, K., & Oakhill, J. V. (1999). Inference making and its relation to comprehension failure. *Reading & Writing, 11,* 489–503.

Cain, K., & Oakhill, J. (2006). Profiles of children with specific reading comprehension difficulties. *British Journal of Educational Psychology, 76,* 683–696.

Cain, Oakhill, Barnes, & Bryant (2001). Comprehension skill, inference-making ability, and their relation to knowledge. *Memory & Cognition, 29*(6), 850–859

Carlisle, J. F. (1988). Knowledge of derivational morphology and spelling ability in fourth, sixth, and eight graders. *Applied Psycholinguistics, 9,* 247–266.

Carlisle, J. F. (1995). Morphological awareness and early reading achievement. In L. Feldman (Ed.), *Morphological aspects of language processing* (pp. 189–209). Mahwah, NJ: Lawrence Erlbaum Associates.

Carlisle, J. F. (2000). Awareness of the structure and meaning of morphologically complex words: Impact on reading. *Reading and Writing: An Interdisciplinary Journal, 12,* 169–190.

Carlisle, J. F., & Nomanbhoy, D. F. (1993). Phonological and morphological awareness in first graders. *Applied Psycholinguistics, 14,* 177–195.

Casalis, S., & Louis-Alexandre, M. (2000). Morphological analysis, phonological analysis and learning to read French. *Reading and Writing, 12,* 303–335.

Catts, H. W. (1991). Early identification of dyslexia: Evidence from a follow-up study of speech-language impaired children. *Annals of Dyslexia, 41,* 163–177.

Catts, H. (1993). The relationship between speech-language impairments and reading disabilities. *Journal of Speech and Hearing Research, 36,* 948–958.

Catts, H. W., Adlof, S. M., & Weismer, S. E. (2006). Language deficits in poor comprehenders: A case for the simple view of reading. *Journal of Speech, Language, and Hearing Research, 49,* 278–293.

Catts, H., Fey, M., Tomblin, J. B., & Zhang, X. (2002). A longitudinal investigation of reading outcomes in children with language impairments. *Journal of Speech, Language, and Hearing Research, 45,* 1142–1157.

Catts, H. W., & Kamhi, A. G. (2005). Causes of reading disabilities. In H. W. Catts & A. G. Kamhi (Eds.), *Language and reading disabilities* (2nd ed., pp. 94–125). Boston: Allyn & Bacon.

Cazden, C. B. (1972). *Child language and education.* New York: Holt, Rinehart and Winston.

Cazden, C. B. (1975). Play with language and metalinguistic awareness: One dimension of language experience. In C. B. Winsor (Ed.), *Dimensions of language experience.* New York: Agathon Press.

Champion, A. (1997). Knowledge of suffixed words: A comparison of reading disabled and nondisabled readers. *Annals of Dyslexia, 47,* 29–55.

Clark, H., & Clark, E. (1997). *Psychology and language.* New York: Harcourt Brace Jovanovich.

Coltheart, M. (1981). Disorders of reading and their implications for models of normal reading. *Visible Language, 15,* 245–286.

Cragg, L., & Nation, K. (2006). Exploring written narrative in children with poor reading comprehension. *Educational Psychology, 26*(1), 55–72.

Cunningham, A. (1990). Explicit vs. implicit instruction in phonological awareness. *Journal of Experimental Child Psychology, 50,* 429–444.

Derwing, B. L., & Baker, W. J. (1977). The psychological basis of morphological rules. In J. MacNamara (Ed.), *Language, learning and thought.* New York: Academic Press.

Dollaghan, C. (1998). Spoken word recognition in children with and without specific language impairment. *Applied Psycholinguistics, 19,* 193–207.

Dunn, L. M., & Dunn, L. M. (1997). *The peabody picture vocabulary test-III.* Circle Pines, MN: American Guidance Services.

Ehrlich, M. F., & Remond, M. (1997). Skilled and less skilled comprehenders: French children's processing of anaphoric devices in written texts. *British Journal of Developmental Psychology, 15,* 291–309.

Elbro, C., & Arnbak, E. (1996). The role of morpheme recognition and morphological awareness in dyslexia. *Annals of Dyslexia, 46,* 209–240.

Fowler, A., & Liberman, I. Y. (1995). The role of phonology and orthography in morphological awareness. In L. Feldman (Ed.), *Morphological aspects of language processing* (pp. 157–188). Hillsdale, NJ: Erlbaum.

Fox, B., & Routh, D. (1980). Phonemic analysis and severe reading disability. *Journal of Psycholinguistic Research, 9,* 115–119.

Galaburda, A. M. (1985). Developmental dyslexia: A review of biological interactions. *Annals of Dyslexia, 35,* 21–33.

Garlock, V., Walley, A., & Metsala, J. (2001). Age-of-acquisition, word frequency, and neighborhood density effects on spoken word recognition by children and adults. *Journal of Memory and Language, 45,* 468–492.

Geschwind, N. (1985). Biological foundations. In F. H. Duffy and N. Geschwind (Eds.), *Dyslexia: A neuroscientific approach to clinical evaluation.* Boston: Little, Brown and Co.

Gillon, G. (2000). The efficacy of phonological awareness intervention for children with spoken language impairment. *Language, Speech, and Hearing Services in the Schools, 31*, 126–141.

Gillon, G. (2002). Follow-up study investigating the benefits of phonological awareness intervention for children with spoken language impairments. *Language, Speech, and Hearing Services in the Schools, 37*, 381–400.

Gillon, G., & Dodd, B. (1994). A prospective study of the relationship between phonological, semantic and syntactic skills of specific reading disability. *Reading and Writing, 6*(4), 321–345.

Gillon, G., & Dodd, B. (1995). The effects of training phonological, semantic, and syntactic processing skills in spoken language on reading ability. *Language, Speech, and Hearing Services in Schools, 26*, 58–68.

Hakes, D. T. (1982). The development of metalinguistic abilities: What develops? In S. Kuczaj (Ed.), *Language development: Vol. 2. Language, thought and culture* (pp. 163–210). Hillsdale, NJ: Erlbaum.

Hakes, D. T. (1984). *Metalinguistic awareness in children: Theory, research, and implications.* Berlin, Germany: Springer-Verlag.

Henry, M. K. (1988). Beyond phonics: Integrated decoding and spelling instruction based on word origin and structure. *Annals of Dyslexia, 38*, 258–275.

Henry, M. K. (1993). Morphological structure: Latin and Greek roots and affixes as upper grade code strategies. *Reading and Writing: An interdisciplinary Journal, 5*, 227–241.

Henry, M. K. (2003). *Unlocking literacy: Effective decoding and spelling instruction.* Baltimore: Brookes.

Hinshelwood, J. (1917). *Congenital word blindness.* London: H. K. Lewis.

Hoover, W. A., & Gough, P. B. (1990). The simple view of reading. *Reading and Writing: An Interdisciplinary Journal, 2*, 127–160.

Huey, E. B. (1968). *The psychology and pedagogy of reading.* Cambridge, MA: Massachusetts Institute of Technology Press. (Original work published 1908)

Justice, L., & Schuele, C. M. (2004). Phonological awareness: Description, assessment, and intervention. In J. Bernthal & N. Bankson (Eds.), *Articulation and phonological disorders* (5th ed., pp. 376–405). Boston, MA: Allyn & Bacon.

Kamhi, A. G., & Catts, H. W. (2005). Language and reading: Convergences and divergences. In H. Catts & A. G. Kamhi (Eds.), *Language and reading disabilities* (2nd ed., pp. 1–25). Boston: Allyn & Bacon.

Kintsch, W., & Van Dijk, T. A. (1978). Toward a model of text comprehension and production. *Psychological Review, 85*, 363–394.

Kuo, L., & Anderson, R. C. (2006). Morphological awareness and learning to read: A cross-language perspective. *Educational Psychologist, 41*, 161–180.

Larrivee, L. S., & Catts, H. W. (1999). Early reading achievement in children with expressive phonological disorders. *American Journal of Speech-Language Pathology, 8*, 22–32.

Larrivee, L. S., & Schuele, C. M. (2005). Literacy acquisition in children with preschool speech and language impairments. *Frequences, 17*, 31–37.

Larrivee, L. S., Schuele, C. M., Hendrickson, B., & Craig, J. (2005, November). *SLPs' role in literacy acquisition: Results of a survey.* Presented at national meeting of the American Speech-Language-Hearing Association, San Diego, CA.

Lazzari, A., & Peters, P. (1987). *Handbook for exercises in language processing, Volume 1.* East Moline, IL: Linguisystems.

Lazzari, A., & Peters, P. (1989). *Handbook for exercises in language processing, Volume 4.* East Moline, IL: Linguisystems.

Leong, C. K. (1989). Productive knowledge of derivational rules in poor readers. *Annals of Dyslexia, 39,* 94–115.

Lie, A. (1991). Effects of a training program for stimulating phonological awareness in preschool children. *Reading Research Quarterly, 26,* 234–250.

Lindamood, P., & Lindamood, P. (1975). *Auditory discrimination in depth* (Rev. ed.). Allen, TX: DLM Teaching Resources.

Lindamood, P., & Lindamood, P. (1998). *LiPS: The Lindamood® phoneme sequencing program for reading, spelling, and speech* (3rd ed.). Upper Saddle River, NJ: Pearson.

Lundberg, I., Frost, J., & Peterson, O. (1988). Effects of an extensive program of stimulating phonological awareness in preschool children. *Reading Research Quarterly, 23,* 263–284.

Lundberg, I., Olofsson, J., & Wall, S. (1980). Reading and spelling skills in the first school years predicted from phonemic awareness skills in kindergarten. *Scandinavian Journal of Psychology, 21,* 159–173.

Maclean, M., Bryant, P., & Bradley, L. (1988). Rhymes, nursery rhymes, and reading in early childhood. In K. E. Stanovich (Ed.), *Children's reading and the development of phonological awareness.* Detroit, MI: Wayne State University Press.

Mahony, D. (1994). Using sensitivity to word structure to explain variance in high school and college level reading ability. *Reading and Writing: An Interdisciplinary Journal, 6,* 19–44.

Mahony, D., Singson, M., & Mann, V. (2000). Reading ability and sensitivity to morphological relations. *Reading and Writing: An Interdisciplinary Journal, 12,* 191–218.

Mann, V. A., & Liberman, I. Y. (1984). Phonological awareness and verbal short-term memory. *Journal of Learning Disabilities, 17,* 592–598.

McGregor, K. K., Newman, R. M., Reilly, R. M., & Capone, N. C. (2002). Semantic representation and naming in children with specific language impairment. *Journal of Speech, Language, and Hearing Research, 45,* 998–1014.

Metsala, J., & Walley, A. (1998). Spoken vocabulary growth and the segmental restructuring of lexical representations: Precursors to phoneme awareness and early reading ability. In J. Metsala & L. Ehri (Eds.), *Word recognition in beginning literacy* (pp. 89–120). Mahwah, NJ: Erlbaum.

Morais, J. (1991). Phonological awareness: A bridge between language and literacy. In D. J. Sawyer & B. J. Fox (Eds.), *Phonological awareness in reading: The evolution of current perspectives* (pp. 31–72). Berlin, Germany: Springer-Verlag.

Nagy, W. E., & Scott, J. A. (2000). Vocabulary processes. In M. Kamil, P. Mosenthal, P. Pearson, & R. Barr (Eds.), *Handbook of reading research* (Vol. 3, pp. 269–284). Mahwah, NJ: Lawrence Erlbaum Associates.

Nation, K., Clarke, P., Marshall, C. M., Durand, M. (2004). Hidden language impairments in children: Parallels between poor reading comprehension and specific language impairment? *Journal of Speech, Language, and Hearing Research, 47,* 199–211.

Nation, K., & Snowling, M. J. (1998). Individual differences in contextual facilitation: Evidence from dyslexia and poor reading comprehension. *Child Development, 69,* 996–1011.

Nation, K., & Snowling, M. J. (2000). Factors influencing syntactic awareness skills in normal readers and poor comprehenders. *Applied Psycholinguistics, 21,* 229–241.

National Institute of Child Health and Human Development. (2000a). *Report of the National Reading Panel. Teaching children to read: An evidence-based assessment of the scientific research literature on reading and its implications for reading instruction* (NIH Publication No. 00-4769). Washington, DC: U.S. Government Printing Office.

National Institute of Child Health and Human Development. (2000b). *Report of the National Reading Panel. Teaching children to read: An evidence-based assessment of the scientific research literature on reading and its implications for reading instruction: Report of the Subgroups* (NIH Publication No. 00-4754). Washington, DC: U.S. Government Printing Office.

Nippold, M. (2007). *Later language development: School-age children, adolescents, and young adults* (3rd ed.). Austin, TX: Pro-Ed.

Notari-Syverson, A., O'Connor, R. E., & Vadasy, P. F. (1998). *Ladders to literacy: A preschool activity book*. Baltimore: Brookes Publishing Co.

O'Connor, R. E., Notari-Syverson, A., & Vadasy, P. F. (1998). *Ladders to literacy: A kindergarten activity book*. Baltimore: Brookes Publishing Co.

Nunez, T., Bryant, P., & Olsson, J. (2003). Learning morphological and phonological spelling rules: An intervention study. *Scientific Studies of Reading, 7*, 289–307.

Oakhill, J. V., Cain, K., & Bryant, P. E. (2003). The dissociation of word reading and text comprehension: Evidence from component skills. *Language and Cognitive Processes, 18*(4), 443–468.

Orton, S. T. (1925). Word-blindness in school children. *Archives of Neurology and Psychiatry, 14*, 581–615.

Perfetti, C. A. (1985). *Reading ability*. New York: Oxford University Press.

Perfetti, C. A., Landi, N., & Oakhill, J. (2005). The acquisition of reading comprehension skills. In M. Snowling & C. Hulme (Eds.), *The science of reading: A handbook* (pp. 227–247). Oxford, United Kingdom: Blackwell Publishing.

Pratt, C., & Grieve, R. (1984). The development of metalinguistic awareness: An introduction. In W. E. Tunmer, C. Pratt, & M. L. Herriman (Eds.), *Metalinguistic awareness in children*. Berlin, Germany: Springer-Verlag.

Rego, L. L. B., & Bryant, P. E. (1993). The connection between phonological, syntactic and semantic skills and children's reading and spelling. *European Journal of Psychology of Education, 8*, 235–246.

Rice, M., Oetting, J., Marquis, J., Bode, J., & Pae, S. (1994). Frequency of input effects on word comprehension of children with specific language impairment. *Journal of Speech and Hearing Research, 37*, 106–122.

Scarborough, H. S. (1991). Early syntactic development of dyslexic children. *Annals of Dyslexia, 41*, 207–220.

Schiffman, G. (1962). Dyslexia as an educational phenomenon. In J. Money (Ed.), *Reading disability: Progress and research needs in dyslexia* (pp. 45–50). Baltimore: The Johns Hopkins University Press.

Schuele, C. M., & Larrivee, L. S. (2004). What's my job? Differential diagnosis of the speech-language pathologist's role in literacy learning. *Perspectives on Language, Learning, and Education, 11*(3), 4–7.

Seidenberg, M. S., Walters, G. S., Barnes, M. A., & Tanenhaus, M. K. (1984). When does irregular spelling or pronunciation influence word recognition? *Journal of Verbal Learning and Verbal Behavior, 23*, 383–404.

Shankweiler, D., Crain, S., Katz, L., Fowler, A. E., Liberman, A. E., Brady, S. A., et al. (1995). Cognitive profiles of reading disabled children: Comparison of language skills in phonology, morphology and syntax. *Psychological Science, 6*, 149–156.

Smith, S. T., Macaruso, P., Shankweiler, D., & Crain S. (1989). Syntactic comprehension in young poor readers. *Applied Psycholinguistics, 10*, 429–454.

Snyder, L. S., & Downey, D. M. (1991). The language-reading relationship in normal and reading-disabled children. *Journal of Speech and Hearing Research, 34*, 129–140.

Stanovich, K. E. (1986). Matthew effects in reading: Some consequences of individual differences in the acquisition of literacy. *Reading Research Quarterly, 21*, 360–407.

Stanovich, K. (1988). *Children's reading and the development of phonological awareness.* Detroit, MI: Wayne State University Press.

Stanovich, K. E., Cunningham, A., & Cramer, B. (1984). Assessing phonological awareness in kindergarten children: Issues of task comparability. *Journal of Experimental Child Psychology, 38*, 175–190.

Stothard, S. E., & Hulme, C. (1992). Reading-comprehension difficulties in children: The role of language comprehension and working memory skills. *Reading and Writing, 4*, 245–256.

Sticht, T. G. (1979). Applications of the audread model to reading evaluation and instruction. In L. B. Resnick and P. A. Weaver (Eds.), *Theory and practice of early reading* (Vol. 1, pp. 209–226). Hillsdale, NJ: Erlbaum.

Sticht, T. G., & James, J. H. (1984). Listening and reading. In P. D. Pearson (Ed.), *Handbook of reading research* (pp. 293–317). New York: Longman.

Templeton, S., & Scarborough-Franks, L. (1985). The spelling's the thing: Knowledge of derivational morphology in orthography and phonology among older students. *Applied Psycholinguistics, 6*, 371–389.

Treiman, R., & Baron, J. (1983). Phonemic analysis training helps children benefit from spelling-sound rules. *Memory and Cognition, 11*, 382–389.

Tunmer, W. E., & Hoover, W. A. (1992). Cognitive and linguistic factors in learning to read. In P. Gough, L. Ehri, & R. Treiman (Eds.), *Reading acquisition* (pp. 175–214). Hillsdale, NJ: Erlbaum.

Tunmer, W. E., & Nesdale, A. R. (1985). Phonemic segmentation skill and beginning reading. *Journal of Educational Psychology, 77*, 417–427.

Tunmer, W. E. Nesdale, A. R., & Wright, A. D. (1987). Syntactic awareness and reading acquisition. *British Journal of Developmental Psychology, 5*(1), 25–34.

van Kleeck, A. (1982). The emergence of linguistic awareness: A cognitive framework. *Merrill Palmer Quarterly, 28*, 237–265.

van Kleeck, A., Vander Woude, J., & Hammett, L. (2006). Fostering literal and inferential language skills in head start preschoolers with language impairment using scripted book-sharing discussions. *American Journal of Speech-Language Pathology, 15*, 85–95.

Vigil, A., & van Kleeck, A. (1996). Clinical language teaching: Theories and principles to guide our responses when children miss our language targets. In M. Smith & J. Damico (Eds.), *Childhood language disorders* (pp. 64–96). New York: Thieme.

Walley, A. (1993). The role of vocabulary development in children's spoken word recognition and segmentation ability. *Developmental Review, 13*, 286–350.

Walley, A., Metsala, J., & Garlock, V. (2003). Spoken vocabulary growth: Its role in the development of phoneme awareness and early reading ability. *Reading and Writing: An Interdisciplinary Journal, 16*, 5–20.

Watkins, R. V., Kelly, D. J., Harbers, H. M., & Hollis, W. (1995). Measuring children's lexical diversity: Differentiating typical and impaired language learners. *Journal of Speech, Language, and Hearing Research, 28*, 1349–1355.

Williams, J. (1980). Teaching decoding with an emphasis on phoneme analysis and phoneme blending. *Journal of Educational Psychology, 72*, 1–15.

Willows, D. M., & Ryan, E. B. (1986). The development of grammatical sensitivity and its relationship to early reading achievement. *Reading Research Quarterly, 21*(3), 253–266.

Wolf, M. (1991). Naming speed and reading. The contribution of the cognitive neurosciences. *Reading Research Quarterly, 26*(2), 123–141.

Wolf, M., Bally, H., & Morris, R. (1986). Automaticity, retrieval processes, and reading: A longitudinal study in average and impaired readers. *Child Development, 57,* 988–1000.

Yopp, H. (1992). Developing phonological awareness in young children. *The Reading Teacher, 45,* 696–703.

Yuill, N. M., & Oakhill, J. V. (1991). *Children's problems in text comprehension: An experimental investigation.* Cambridge, United Kingdom: Cambridge University Press.

# 7 Individual Differences in Intervention Response in Children and Adults With Autism Spectrum Disorders

*Lynne E. Hewitt*

## BEYOND LABELS: SELECTING APPROPRIATE INTERVENTIONS FOR INDIVIDUALS WITH AUTISM SPECTRUM DISORDERS

Understanding of the particular challenges faced by individuals with autism and autism spectrum disorder (ASD) has come a long way in the past 20 years. Individual differences are a hallmark of these disorders, and thus considering unique characteristics of each individual is always a primary concern when planning for support of people on the spectrum. Autism is diagnosed in terms of three core characteristics: communicative impairment, social impairment, and a restricted repertoire of interests and activities (American Psychiatric Association [APA], 1994). These characteristics can apply to a highly verbal but pragmatically challenged individual with a strong fascination for Disney movies, which he discusses with anyone who will listen. They can equally well be applied to a child with quite different behavioral and cognitive characteristics. Thus, another child diagnosed with ASD might be nonverbal and socially passive, having a primary interest in flicking light switches on and off and opening and shutting doors. It is evident to any clinician that a child who is highly verbal but pragmatically challenged has needs that are completely different from those of a nonverbal child. These two examples show that the core aspects of autism can be manifested in widely diverse ways, a diversity that makes it impossible to base intervention planning solely on the diagnosis.

The diversity in manifestation of autism has led over the years to a preference among many clinicians and researchers for the term "autism spectrum disorder" to show that a wide range of manifestations can be expected. One might argue that use of the term ASD itself is a way to refocus on individual characteristics, because it de-emphasizes the traditional discrete diagnostic categories such as autism, pervasive developmental disorder not otherwise specified, and Asperger syndrome. The term ASD has become conventional usage, despite the fact that it has yet to appear in any official diagnostic publication such as the *Diagnostic and Statistical Manual of Mental Disorders* (APA, 1994). An analysis of diagnostic practices using the various criteria that have been applied over the years by Wing and Potter (2002) demonstrated that the change in criteria for autism has been a significant factor in the rise in the numbers of children and adults diagnosed with autism and related disorders. Those who work with children and adults with pragmatic language difficulties and social challenges encounter a wide range of individuals, some of whom fit the classic profile of autism first described by Kanner (1943, 1946). Although others may have support needs in these areas, they may not quite fit the definition of autism or even a related disorder, such as Asperger syndrome (Winner, 2007).

It is not news that in the realm of language impairments, diagnostic labels and etiological categories are never sufficient (or perhaps even desirable—see Kovarsky, Duchan, & Maxwell, 1999) bases for planning intervention. Children and adults with autism, like all people with communication disorders, have unique experiences and characteristics that may predispose them to responding better to one intervention than another. A careful assessment of the whole person and his or her environment is central to formulating support plans that are tailored appropriately for individual circumstances. Family responses and structures, school settings, and factors unique to the individual will influence treatment outcomes. Strategies such as positive behavioral support (Buschbacher & Fox, 2003; Dunlap & Fox, 1999: Koegel, Harrower, & Koegel, 1999) and person-centered planning (Duchan & Black, 2001) are important tools for working with children and families. Using these types of holistic strategies addressing the totality of a child's environment helps solve the conundrum of providing individualized interventions that are nonetheless evidence-based. Certain types of behaviors that can impede the success of children with ASD can be exacerbated or even triggered by the environment. Thus, a child may be well able to function in a supportive environment, but when special needs are not taken into account, the child may appear far less competent than he or she truly is. The intervention literature for children with autism is filled with resources for developing individualized instructional approaches, modifying the physical environment, and developing supportive social structures. Examples include functional behavioral analysis (Maurice, Green, & Luce, 1996), visual supports (Hodgson, 1995), priming (Koegel, Koegel, Frea, & Green-Hopkins, 2003), and training caregivers in strategies for effective interaction (Kashinath, Woods, & Goldstein, 2006; Sussman, 1999). Although evidence exists supporting the effectiveness of most of these, much of the power of such strategies stems from their ability to be adapted to the individual needs of particular children.

## EVIDENCE-BASED PRACTICE CONSIDERATIONS

Although it is undisputed that interventions should be chosen on the basis of the best available evidence, paradoxically, the attempt to validate interventions for a highly variable population may obscure more than it reveals. If only intervention strategies based on randomized controlled trials (Robey & Schultz, 1998) are considered appropriate, then individual differences cannot be fully accommodated in intervention planning. The fact is that even the best evidence derived from a group study may not apply to any particular individual with ASD. Thus, a challenge in devising effective support strategies for ASD arises from the protocols used in much intervention research. The experimental literature itself shows us that individuals with similar characteristics do not show uniform gains in response to treatment protocols. For example, in the famous initial study of the Young Autism Project (Lovaas, 1987; McEachin, Smith, & Lovaas, 1993), 9 children made strong gains (as measured by IQ in the normal range), 7 showed some progress (IQ in the mild range of cognitive impairment), and 2 showed little improvement (IQ in the severe-profound range of cognitive impairment). Thus, clinicians attempting to use evidence-based practices may run up against challenges when selecting treatment protocols. If a particular child is more similar to the nonresponders in a study than the responders, it does not matter whether a study shows a treatment was effective overall. What matters is whether or not it will work for the individual it is intended to benefit. In this way, group designs demonstrate a particular weakness in treatment research. Findings that show statistically significant gains calculated on the basis of group data may obscure the fact that those who gained a lot and those who made no gains at all were lumped together to create the group means. Some intervention researchers advocate single-participant design, where participants serve as their own experimental controls, because in this design the effectiveness of an intervention on an individual level can be demonstrated (Barlow & Hersen, 1984; Odom et al., 2003). However, selecting a treatment on the basis of the response of small numbers of participants in single-participant designs leads to its own difficulties. Even using single-participant designs, a study may show variability of outcome, with some responding to treatment, and others not showing benefit. Depending on the level of detail provided in reports of case studies and single-participant design research, it may or may not be possible to speculate about the individual differences that interacted with treatment to yield the outcomes observed.

Features specific to autism make it particularly troublesome to generalize the results of group studies to individuals. People with ASD may exhibit any of the following, at a wide range of severity levels:

- Cognitive impairment, either in overall intellectual functioning or in specific cognitive subdomains, including executive functioning, understanding of others' mental states (theory of mind), and abstract reasoning (Edelson, 2006; Hale & Tager-Flusberg, 2003; Joseph, McGrath, & Tager-Flusberg, 2005; Joseph & Tager-Flusberg, 2004)
- Heightened or flattened sensory responses (Anzalone & Williamson, 2000; Grandin, 1995; Khalfa et al., 2004)
- Hyper- or hypoarousal (Anzalone & Williamson, 2000)
- Comorbid psychiatric disorders, such as attention deficit and/or hyperactivity disorder, bipolar disorder, obsessive-compulsive disorder, depression,

and anxiety (Leyfer, Folstein, Bacalman, Davis, Dinh, & Morgan, et al., 2006; Tsai, 2005)
- Phonological impairment and/or developmental dyspraxia of speech (Shriberg et al., 2001)
- Language impairment, with some individuals exhibiting a profile similar to individuals with language learning disability and/or specific language impairment (Kjelgaard & Tager-Flusberg, 2001)

Clearly, clinicians must be aware of the potential for any of the above when working with individuals on the spectrum. For some comorbid conditions and behavioral concerns, psychotropic medications may be prescribed, each carrying its own impact on learning and behavioral ability and functioning.

The lengthy list of problems that may coexist with ASD makes it clear that despite a great deal of progress in understanding this disorder, the complexity it exhibits continues to pose a challenge to unraveling commonalities and individual differences alike. There has been a veritable explosion of research in autism over the past decade or so, and the resulting studies, although they help to clarify foundational issues, also present difficulties of interpretation. The amount of scholarly effort devoted to intervention research has steadily increased. In recent years, an emerging consensus has begun to develop defining core principles for best practice (National Research Council, 2001), but major gaps in knowledge remain. Thus, although early intervention has received significant attention (e.g., Bibby, Eikeseth, Martin, Mudford, & Reeves, 2001; Boyd & Corley, 2001; Eikeseth, Smith, Jahr, & Eldevik, 2002; Lovaas, 1987; McEachin et al., 1993; Turner & Stone, 2007), results have yet to crystallize into recommendations that one treatment has the best supporting evidence. Smith (1996) argued that research supporting early intensive behavioral intervention (EIBI) had demonstrated convincing superiority over other interventions. This claim was not fully supported at the time, and it has been weakened by subsequent work showing that EIBI as implemented in the community is not as effective as reports from university-based programs would indicate (Magiati, Charman, & Howlin, 2007; but see also Cohen, Amerine-Dickens, & Smith, 2006). One emerging picture is the role of IQ and language level in predicting treatment outcome for children undergoing early intervention (Ben-Itzchak & Zachor, 2007; Magliati et al., 2007; Joseph, Tager-Flusberg, & Lord, 2002). Children with higher IQs and standardized language scores tend to achieve more gains, whatever the intervention, than children with lower scores. This result might be interpreted to indicate that variability in intervention outcomes is primarily a factor of basic ability. Other factors may also be at work, however. It is unclear that IQ scores, especially in very young children with autism, are completely successful in measuring cognitive functioning (Edelson, 2006). They may instead, or in addition, be indexing such factors as motivation, attentional focus, and social engagement (Koegel, Koegel, & Smith, 1997). If these are the causes of low IQ scores, then intervention targeting these areas might lead to significant gains. It is tantalizing to imagine that cognitive profiling of individuals with ASD might lead to individualized treatment recommendations. However, definitively pinpointing the cause of low scores on standardized tests for any one individual is seldom possible.

The possibility that an individual's ability to function may not be adequately measured by typical protocols leads to another aspect of autism that challenges professionals. Stories have proliferated of children who have made huge changes in a short span of time. Sometimes, these stories refer to children who were apparently developing typically and then suddenly lost language and social skills (Richler et al., 2006). Less well documented (but still frequent enough to tantalize parents) are stories of individuals with severe communication disorders suddenly exhibiting near-miraculous recoveries. Sometimes these are reported following a particular therapy (Stehli, 2004). Although it is difficult to validate these reports of sudden onset of symptoms and sudden recovery, it is important for practitioners to be respectful of parents' perspectives and experiences. The frequency with which such stories occur makes them an important aspect of the world of autism treatment, with families banding together to form foundations focused on curing autism (e.g., Autism Speaks and Cure Autism Now). Some individuals with ASD are offended by the notion of a "cure" (e.g., Aspies for Freedom) and actually oppose the notion that a cure would be a positive thing. This view is less widely shared than the view of many parents that autism is a devastating illness that needs to be treated (see Maurice, 1993, for an eloquent example of this view). Miracle cures and alternative treatments seem to cluster around autism, fueled by the speed of the Internet. Unfortunately, because the diagnosis is itself complex and multifactored and day-to-day variability is part of the autism spectrum, many of these reports will never be verifiable. As any experienced clinician knows, a long time of slow growth and learning may suddenly change, and a child may add many new abilities in a very short time. If that coincides with the introduction of a drug or a novel diet protocol, then the tendency to attribute a causal force to the treatment is understandable. Coincidence and wishful thinking may explain some of the stories of miracle cures, with some clinicians feeling that their years of long hard work helping a child learn do not get the credit they deserve. However, there is some hard evidence that neurological variability may in fact result in fluctuations in functioning. A recent study attempted to validate anecdotal information of transient improved function during an episode of fever (Curran et al., 2007). Curran et al. found that some behavioral improvement may occasionally occur when a child with ASD has a fever. Such reports indicate that there are unknown physical factors leading some children with autism to be unable to tap into the full range of their cognitive resources. It is unknown why higher ability levels or more organized behavior could be exhibited when the neurological conditions caused by fever are present. Such reports speak to within-child variability, a type of individual difference that is just as challenging to account for as between-child differences. As knowledge of neurobiological bases of autism develops, clinicians may receive better guidance on how to optimize treatment timing and protocols relative to biological functioning. For now, it appears that the best we can do is try to be aware that there is the potential for transient changes, up and down, so that we can minimize our own frustration with and burnout related to seemingly mysterious changes in receptivity to intervention.

## INDIVIDUAL DIFFERENCE ISSUES RAISED
## BY NEUROBIOLOGICAL MODELS

Fundamental differences in cognitive resources are a primary cause of variability in response to treatment. Nonetheless, variability still exists among individuals with similar IQ and language profiles. The literature is less informative in elucidating factors that account for why an intervention successful with one person may not be at all effective with another who on the surface appears to have similar strengths and needs. Turning to the literature detailing neurobiological theories of ASD is one way to better understand the actual nature of the learning challenges faced by children with autism. Although controversy exists and the full picture is far from clear, it appears likely that autism involves connections among multiple brain systems (Courchesne & Pierce, 2005; DiCicco-Bloom et al., 2006; Minshew & Williams, 2007). Connections among various regions, such as the frontal lobe and cerebellum, may develop anomalously. In addition, some individuals may have deficits in specific regions. It may be that subtle variations in connectivity, interacting over time with structural differences or defects in the brain, may lead to quite diverse outcomes. The picture is further complicated by the fact that the best current evidence points to ASD as being caused by an interaction of genetic and environmental factors (Ronald, Happé, & Plomin, 2005). Most neurobiological and neuropsychological researchers agree that a unitary cause for autism is not consistent with the manifestations of the disorder and with what is known about its biological basis and development.

Because the environment appears to play a vital role in the biogenesis of ASD, understanding the role of early experience in shaping brain structures is crucial for understanding variability in ASD. Research indicates that children raised in environments where they are deprived of rich social systems and opportunity for independent exploration and problem-solving will have deficits (Mason & Narad, 2005; Perry, Pollard, Blakely, Baker, & Vigilante, 1995). At first glance, comparing children with ASD with those who have experienced abuse and neglect may seem completely off target, and perhaps even offensive. However, the parallel lies not in what the environment does to the child—it is what the child's style of interacting with the environment does to the child. A strong preference for sameness (Kanner, 1943), an aversion to exploring certain textures, and a lack of enjoyment of the social world in infancy may lead a child to develop brain structures well adapted to his or her special concerns (sensory exploration of particular materials, or particular activities that the child finds rewarding, and avoidance of activities found unpleasant). Perhaps such brain differences could lead to special talents (the famous "splinter skills" or "savant" abilities occasionally seen in individuals with ASD), but equally, a neglect of portions of the environment might lead to significant impairments. Social cognition, like all cognition, is based on an organic substrate. However, because the developing brain emerges over time as an interaction between the genetic endowment and the exchange with the environment, a child who neglects social input may not develop the neural connections crucial for full development of social cognition. In a sense, a child with ASD may naturally seek certain experiences, thereby creating a world uniquely suited to his or her cognitive and sensory preferences. If left to his or her own devices and not challenged to seek out less preferred or even possibly aversive experiences, relatively minor early differences may, over the course of development, become major differences, divergent to the extent that they become limiting or disabling to the individual.

A variety of brain structures have been theorized to be implicated in autism, including the cerebellum, the thalamus, and the prefrontal cortex. Although cerebellar involvement is controversial, there is a large body of literature supporting the notion that the cerebellar anomalies play a role in ASD (Allen, 2006). It appears that the cerebellum is involved in more than just motor planning and motor learning, having links to more brain regions than any other single brain structure. It seems to be linked to learning and execution of all types of tasks, and deficits seen in Purkinje cell density suggest that insufficient connection sites are available to handle the input from the various brain regions seeking to connect to the cerebellum. One influential current theory is that the connection between the frontal lobe and the cerebellum is disturbed in ASD (Courchesne & Pierce, 2005). Problems in connectivity lead to issues with processing input, planning, learning, and management of all types of higher level tasks that are dependent on the prefrontal cortex, such as executive functioning and social reasoning. The relative difficulty that children with ASD experience in novel environments may be related to issues in processing novel input and decision making that the frontal lobe and cerebellum handle in a complex system of distributed functioning. Thus, learning may take longer, and more repetitive, structured input may be needed in order to give the system input that it can handle and to ensure that extra time is available to deal with the input. In this model, the rate of presentation of information, predictability of input, number of times that a particular type of experience is repeated, and whether that information is repeated in a form that the system can recognize all might end up being predictor variables for learning outcomes in children with ASD. Whereas a typically developing brain manages to extract regularities from highly diverse input, the brain of a person with autism may be less flexible in recognizing patterns. Such cognitive style preferences may account for the interest that many young children with autism show in highly repetitive activities, such as turning light switches on and off. The presence in older individuals of a strong desire to engage in repeated sequences of questions and answers on a single topic makes sense if the type of processing needed for repetitive exchanges is compared with that required for an open-ended conversation, full of shifting topics and subtle social cues, verbal and nonverbal. This complex landscape of social exchange may defeat people who need more obvious structure in linguistic exchanges in order to succeed, and if patterns are not obvious, they logically seek to create their own.

## SENSORY DIFFERENCES IN ASD

In order to intervene successfully to support all children with ASD to develop to their full potential, it will be crucial to begin to understand more about the impact of neurocognitive preferences on early development. One aspect of neurological development that has received attention is the role of sensory differences (Dennis & Edelman, 2006; Grandin, 1995). Because of the difficulty of documenting these with precision, there is only now emerging a literature in which sensory differences are investigated with rigor. This emerging literature is beginning to confirm that experience of the sensory world may be quite different in children with ASD than in typically developing individuals. Recent work has documented auditory sensitivity (Khalfa et al., 2004) and visual distortions and dysfunctions (Davis, Bockbrader, Murphy, Hetrick, & O'Donnell, 2006). Case reports of tactile sensitivities and proprioceptive disturbances also exist (Grandin, 1995). Patterns of strengths in various realms of sensory attainment have been documented in high-functioning individuals, including some who have savant abilities, such as perfect pitch (Heaton, 2003) or advanced ability to draw three-dimensional objects (Mottron, Belleville, & Ménard, 1999). Some proposals attempt to account for unusual sensory abilities as well as disabilities within a single model (Mottron, Dawson, Soulieres, Hubert, & Burack, 2006). In this view, sensory differences may account for unique aspects of cognitive style that lead to unusual patterns of learning and functioning. Some differences may result in a talent, such as visual pattern recognition leading to hyperlexia, whereas others may have more negative effects, such as a decline in the ability to function in ordinary environments owing to hypersensitivity to background noise.

Because sensory differences appear to be widespread in ASD and the sensory system is obviously key to receiving information from the environment, several treatments for ASD target disturbances of sensation. The theory behind all of these is that sensory differences cause cognitive and behavioral problems. The hope is that improving sensory processing and/or decreasing hypersensitivities will lead to widespread positive change. One of the systems that sensory treatments attempt to affect is communication. Strong claims for treatments of sensory impairments have raised hopes that regulating the sensory system might lead to very large linguistic and cognitive improvements in children and adults with ASD. However, controlled trials (Bettison, 1996; Griffer, 1999; Sinha, Silove, Wheeler, & Williams, 2006) have not supported these claims. Nonetheless, because of the documented issues related to sensory processing, many clinicians continue to work closely with experts in sensory integration, primarily occupational therapists. Goals include increased tolerance for a range of auditory, visual, and tactile stimuli. Both within-child and between-child variability can relate to sensory issues, so understanding a child's sensitivities and working to support his or her ability to cope with the sensory world are cornerstones of a holistic approach to intervention. For example, maladaptive behaviors may serve a sensory function. Thus, assisting a client to either process sensation in a more integrated fashion or replace maladaptive with adaptive sensory activities can be crucial in facilitating more organized behavior. Without attention to these issues, intervention targeting complex social and linguistic competencies may be reduced in its effectiveness. One aspect of individual variability that has been well documented is the resistant nature of repetitive actions that appear to serve a sensory function (National Research Council, 2000). It may be that subtle variations of sensory processing underlie the puzzling variability seen in response to intervention in this disorder.

One outgrowth of increased awareness of sensory differences in autism is the widespread use of visual materials to support learning in children with ASD. Although they are often thought of as primarily sensory in nature, in fact visual supports may have more to do with learning style issues in ASD. This is because the transitory nature of acoustic information poses special challenges for people with ASD, especially children struggling to learn language. Auditory input vanishes as soon as it is complete. Because many children with ASD need much more repetition to learn than typical learners do, auditory input that is not repeated and structured may not register as salient. The fact that visual information stays put and can be studied at the learner's pace lends it a powerful advantage over auditory input. It is for this reason that classrooms around the world have begun using more visual structuring of the environment to promote success in children with ASD (Hodgson, 1995). Simple changes that help many children with autism include the use of visual schedules and other graphic supports, rather than relying on verbal reminders that may go by too quickly to register. These supports are most successful when individualized to the child. A popular example is the use of social stories (Gray, 2000), which are illustrated narratives in simple language constructed specifically to teach children about common situations. These combine visual information with language input tailored to the child's level. Repeated reading of the stories promotes development of language, and the visual reminders reduce cognitive load. Older children may be able to use written language organizers, such as reminder lists and checklists for organizing their study time. All of these materials need to be constructed to specifically target the needs of a particular child. No large-scale studies of the effectiveness of social stories and other graphic supports exist, but a number of small-$n$, single-participant design studies have been undertaken. Findings are generally supportive, but a great deal of variability exists (see, e.g., Scattone, Tingstrom, & Wilczynski, 2006). By definition, a social story or a graphic organizer has to be tailor-made to the child, and thus a deep understanding of the child, the physical environment, and the task demands and social expectations that exist in that environment is a prerequisite to success. Such understanding arises only when a clinician has access to a lot of information about the individual and the people in his or her life. The right social story at the right time may make large changes in a child's ability to cope with a particular challenge. Unfortunately, the variables that influence success of any particular social intervention are so complex that the chances of hitting on the exact right mix of factors to include in a social story (or any complex social pragmatic intervention) may range from very high to very low indeed. From what we now understand about ASD, this makes sense. Whereas the old image of people with autism is of totally mysterious beings who have no rational pattern to their behaviors, the picture that has emerged from research shows that formerly inexplicable behavioral variations, such as repetitive behaviors, do have their own internal logic. However, each person with autism has a unique history, and the coping mechanisms he or she has developed over time will therefore be idiosyncratic to each.

## COGNITIVE-LINGUISTIC DIFFERENCES AND DEVELOPMENT

Although it has been known for some time that variability in outcome is strongly predicted by IQ, more recent work has begun to uncover specific cognitive and linguistic predictors of communicative development in ASD. Smith, Mirenda, and Zaidman-Zait (2007) found that number of words said, verbal imitation skills, pretend play with objects, and gestures to initiate joint attention were all seen in children who showed the most rapid vocabulary growth over time. Thurm, Lord, Lee, & Newschaffer (2007) found in a longitudinal study that nonverbal cognitive ability at age 2 was the strongest predictor of language development at age 5. They also found joint attention and vocal and motor imitation were significant predictors. Although it may not be surprising to learn that children who are speaking more early on tend to show better language development over time, the other predictors are not as obvious. These predictive factors are important for clinicians to consider, especially in planning early intervention. Impaired or absent pretend play is highly correlated with a diagnosis of ASD, to such an extent that elicitation of pretend play is a centerpiece of the Autism Diagnostic Observation Schedule (ADOS) protocol for the assessment of ASD (Lord, Rutter, DiLavore, & Risi, 1999). Careful observation is necessary when looking at children with relatively stronger cognitive functioning, as apparently sophisticated play skills are often seen. However, if play is broken down into pretend versus construction, it becomes apparent that a young child who may have excellent attention span and age-appropriate skill and interest in playing with blocks and pop-up toys has no idea how to play with dolls. The scripted play scenario of a baby's birthday party in the ADOS often elicits blank stares and confusion even in older preschoolers with ASD, whereas very young typically developing toddlers respond with spontaneous delight at the activities of making a birthday cake and singing "Happy Birthday" for the baby. Early interventions that target play may turn out to be imperative for children with ASD. Whether assisted symbolic play was successfully introduced in young children diagnosed with ASD may explain some of the variability in outcome. A variety of programs do emphasize play, including examples using naturalistic, social interactionist principles, such as the Hanen More than Words program (Sussman, 1999) and the Do–Watch–Listen–Say approach (Quill, 2000), as well as the popular DIR Floortime model (Greenspan & Wieder, 2000), where DIR stands for "Developmental, Individual-Difference, Relationship-Based." Structured behavioral approaches also incorporate play, and popular models for EIBI (Maurice, Green, & Luce, 1996) target play skills and use play scenarios both as rewards and to promote generalization of trained skills. Thus, diverse approaches may arrive at similar outcomes when they both target fundamental deficits that respond well to early intervention. In addition, recent work has begun to specifically target teaching symbolic play to young children with autism, with some success (Kasari, Freeman, & Paparella, 2006).

Theorists emphasizing social accounts of language development have long pointed to joint attention as important in early language learning (see, e.g., Carpenter & Tomasello, 2000). Investigations have revealed joint attention as a predictor variable in development of language in children with ASD (Smith et al., 2007; Thurm et al., 2007), and interventions targeting this area have been developed. General social-interactionist, naturalistic paradigms inherently incorporate joint attention, with an emphasis on following the child's lead and providing relevant language targeted to the child's developmental level (e.g., Sussman, 1999). Behavioral paradigms also require children to engage in joint attention, although in most structured programs the focus is on getting the child to attend to foci of attention selected by adults. In addition to these general paradigms, investigators have begun to experimentally validate the use of joint attention interventions specifically (Kasari et al., 2006). The long-term impact of specifically targeting joint attention has yet to be experimentally validated, but the fact that it can be stimulated and increase in spontaneity provides some grounds to hope that increasing joint attention will promote language development and enhanced social functioning in children with ASD.

Imitation, of both verbalizations and gestures, has also been found to predict later language development. Clinicians need to consider carefully how to apply this finding to decision making with individual clients. Certainly, the absence of spontaneous imitation is cause for concern. For children with some limited ability to imitate, it would appear important to elicit, scaffold, and reinforce imitative behaviors as much as possible. Teaching imitation can be difficult where motivation is low. Imitating facial expressions and postures may pose special challenges, as it requires attention to the face, and the eyes, of another. Some research indicates that eye gaze can be more strongly stimulating (and hence perhaps aversive) for some individuals with ASD (Kylliäinen & Hietanen, 2006). Some behavioral approaches to intervention for ASD inherently focus on imitation, in highly structured environments, with external rewards (Lovaas, 1987; Maurice et. al, 1996). These approaches are based on behavioral theories in which child motivation is seen as needing to be instilled via external motivators (such as edible rewards). Imitation of a variety of behaviors is key to these programs, including communicative acts such as gestures and verbalizations. Given the association between imitation and later language development, it may be that some of the successes attributed to behavioral intervention programs may arise in part from the strong emphasis on teaching imitation.

Naturalistic approaches have also targeted imitation. Such approaches emphasize learning in more child-centered, naturalistic environments to ensure high external validity, improve likelihood of generalization, and decrease prompt dependency (see, e.g., Koegel & Koegel, 2006; Smith, Goddard, & Fluck, 2004; Prizant, Wetherby, & Rydell, 2000; Quill, 2000; Sussman, 1999). A recent study directly targeting descriptive gestures using a naturalistic intervention approach found positive results for most of the participants, using a single-participant design (Ingersoll, Lewis, & Kroman, 2007). This research indicates that it is possible to increase spontaneous use of gestures in children with ASD, and thus it would appear at least theoretically possible to ameliorate this particular risk factor. Whether structured behavioral or naturalistic approaches are better for improving gestures has not been investigated to date. Thus, the choice of protocol must be determined by working with families and according to the expertise and clinical judgment of individual clinicians. It is also unknown whether teaching imitation to a child will directly improve communication and language development over time. The research findings showing a correlation may be associated with factors inherent in a child that may not be alterable via intervention. However, many intervention approaches emphasizing imitation have demonstrated successful increases in communication and overall improvements in learning.

Support exists for an approach to intervention that targets development in core deficit areas as potentially offering the key to positive change, as the results from the imitation and joint attention literatures attest. However, caution is needed. There is ample evidence that many individuals on the spectrum struggle with demonstrating theory of mind and perspective taking (e.g., Joseph & Tager-Flusberg, 2004). Because the ability to take the point of view of the listener is key to successful communication, efforts to improve communication by teaching theory of mind have been made (Hale & Tager-Flusberg, 2003). Although improvement in performance on theory of mind tasks was seen, no effect on overall communicative competence resulted from this attempt at direct teaching. Thus, the idea that remediating specific deficit areas may be the means to achieve better outcomes—and thereby perhaps address individual differences in response to intervention—has met with mixed success.

## SUMMARY

It is no exaggeration to say that the strides made in autism research, both basic and clinical, have led to huge advances in our understanding of the disorder. The development of a variety of effective interventions that make real differences in the lives of children and their families is now a fact (Goldstein, 2002; National Research Council, 2001). However, consideration of individual differences leads us to the very limits of current knowledge. In this chapter, I have been able to point to many indicators that predict better or worse outcomes. Early indicators such as lack of imitation, lack of gestures, deficits in joint attention (both soliciting and responding to it), and impaired nonverbal cognition have been shown by many investigators to predict later language outcomes. I have also described a number of important factors that may help explain variability in response to intervention, including sensory processing issues, comorbid illnesses (including psychiatric illnesses), family support and educational support structure differences, child motivation and interest, and the child's distinctive cognitive profile. Factors internal to the child's unique cognitive and sensory system contribute to individual differences. Examples include more or less gaze aversion, hyper- or hypoarousal, greater or lesser comprehension of theory of mind and point of view, stronger or weaker executive functioning, presence or absence of learning disabilities, and the possibility of a specific language impairment separate from the autism diagnosis. Individual coping mechanisms secondary to issues such as sensory processing differences, or comorbid psychiatric disorders such as obsessive-compulsive disorder, are also to be considered when trying to understand why a particular approach may not have worked with a particular child. Fluctuations in the child's social-emotional environment, the starting or stopping of a medication, or other treatment such as a dietary change may cause change in response to intervention strategies. The amount of time spent on a particular unusual interest—for example, a special topic, such as dinosaurs, or a repetitive action, such as turning light switches on and off—is time taken away from learning about other things.

Children are embedded in rich social worlds, and typical learners observe that world closely, imitating the things they see and creatively engaging with the world around them. Most children with autism show some degree of interest in the social world that surrounds them. The issues are the extent of that interest and whether attempts made by caregivers and intervention agents to capture and increase that interest are targeted to a child's unique combination of strengths and weaknesses. The timing of such efforts is clearly significant: early intervention has a large and growing literature to support the potentiality for large gains. Although working with children (and adults) of any age can be beneficial, the magnifying, emergent effects of redirecting a child's system to improved social and communicative development in the early years cannot be duplicated by interventions started in later childhood.

The question of how best to develop an intervention that will help a child with autism engage with the world and learn to his or her best potential cannot be answered definitively with current knowledge. A range of theories exist on what is best for children. One that is often applied to autism is behavioral theory (e.g., Lovaas, 1987), although this theory in the realm of language and communication development has not been in the ascendancy in recent decades. However, it is not necessary to return to a strict behavioral view to profit from some of the successes of this model. A complex range of factors may be significant in understanding how best to positively influence a child's development. Deep understanding requires a careful and minute examination of the experiential world of the children we work with. The close observation of antecedent and consequent events advocated by behavior management specialists is one type of detail-focused approach (Maurice et al., 1996). Family-centered practice (Buschbacher & Fox, 2003; Prelock, Beatson, Bitner, Broder, & Ducker, 2003) is another. Collaborating with other professionals, such as occupational and physical therapists, to better understand sensory and physical challenges faced by our clients is a third. Another means to a deeper understanding of the individuality of our clients is to use ethnographic approaches, such as participant observation (e.g., Simmons-Mackie & Damico, 2001; Kovarsky, Culatta, Franklin, & Theadore, 2001). The purpose of participant observation is to attempt to blur the boundaries between experience and observation. Most observations we complete as clinicians are as onlookers, and close observation is always worth the attempt, but occasional forays into participant observation can leave us with a better appreciation of what a particular experience is like for the experiencer. This requires imagination and creativity, and it needs to be undertaken with caution not to overlay our own beliefs and experiences on those of the person we seek to understand. Nonetheless, attempts to imagine the perspective of a person who sees the world in very different way are worthy efforts. Ethnographic and qualitative assessments may increase the clarity with which we can consider clinical challenges and also the creativity with which we confront them. Clinicians may not have the luxury of sufficient time to spend on detailed observation. One shortcut to assist in conceptualizing the world of individuals with autism is to read some of the ever-growing list of books written by individuals with ASD and their families (e.g., Barron & Barron, 2002; Grandin, 1995). Although it is necessary to be cautious and not over-generalize the particular experiences of the authors of such books, they do offer insight into patterns that influenced the authors' development as individuals. Understanding how they were supported, or not supported, at crucial junctures in their lives may provide clues to the particular circumstances that allowed them to achieve their successes. In addition, this understanding may also show some potentialities perhaps not achieved and provide intriguing clues to directions for future research into optimizing interventions.

Autism is often thought of in terms such as "a mysterious and devastating illness." Whether or not it is an illness is a matter of much debate, with some on the spectrum advocating for their unique qualities as a difference, not a disorder. Temple Grandin (1995) has stated that she would not want to be "cured," as she finds her visual thinking to be a huge advantage, one that she would never want to give up. Whether autism is seen as positive or negative, one thing that can be agreed on is that autism is no longer such a mystery. Many sources of information, from basic and clinical science to personal accounts, are coming together to provide a clearer picture. Much remains to be done, but the days when autism was thought of as a quasimystical disorder, beyond the limits of our understanding, are well and truly gone. One key to increased understanding has been the investigation of individual differences, which has expanded understanding of the nature and scope of the autistic spectrum (Wing & Potter, 2002), providing an impetus for ever-improving research and treatment options. The unique qualities of individuals, their life experiences, and their desires and drives are the ultimate determiners of the course of development and of the response to interventions and supports offered.

## REFERENCES

Allen, G. (2006). Cerebellar contributions to autism spectrum disorders. *Clinical Neuroscience Research, 6*, 195–207.

American Psychiatric Association. (1994). *Diagnostic and statistical manual of mental disorders* (4th ed.). Washington, DC: Author.

Anzalone, M., & Williamson, G. G. (2000). Sensory processing and motor performance in autism spectrum disorders. In A. Wetherby & B. Prizant (Eds.), *Autism: A transactional developmental perspective* (pp. 143–166). Baltimore: Brookes.

Barlow, D., & Hersen, M. (1984). *Single case experimental designs: Strategies for studying behavior change.* New York: Pergamon Press.

Barron, J., & Barron, S. (2002). *There's a boy in here: Emerging from the bonds of autism.* Arlington, TX: Future Horizons.

Ben-Itzchak, E., & Zachor, A. (2007). The effects of intellectual functioning and autism severity on outcome of early behavioral intervention for children with autism. *Research in Developmental Disabilities, 28*(3), 287–303.

Bettison, S. (1996). The long-term effects of auditory training on children with autism. *Journal of Autism and Developmental Disorders, 26,* 361–374.

Bibby, P., Eikeseth, S., Martin, N. T., Mudford, O. C., & Reeves, D. (2001). Progress and outcomes for children with autism receiving parent-managed intensive interventions. *Research in Developmental Disabilities, 22*(6), 425–447.

Boyd, R., & Corley, M. (2001). Outcome survey of early intensive behavioral intervention for young children with autism in a community setting. *Autism, 5*(4), 430–441.

Buschbacher, P. W., & Fox, L. (2003). Understanding and intervening with the challenging behavior of young children with autism spectrum disorder. *Language, Speech, and Hearing Services in Schools, 34*(3), 217–227.

Carpenter, M., & Tomasello, M. (2000). Joint attention, cultural learning, and language acquisition: Implications for children with autism. In A. Wetherby & B. Prizant (Eds.), *Autism: A transactional developmental perspective* (pp. 31–54). Baltimore: Brookes.

Cohen, H., Amerine-Dickens, M., & Smith, T. (2006). Early intensive behavioral treatment: Replication of the UCLA model in a community setting. *Journal of Developmental and Behavioral Pediatrics, 27*(2), S145–S155.

Courchesne, E., & Pierce, K. (2005). Why the frontal cortex in autism might be talking only to itself: Local over-connectivity but long-distance disconnection. *Current Opinion in Neurobiology, 15*(2), 225–230.

Curran, L., Newschaffer, C., Lee, L., Crawford, S., Johnston, M., & Zimmerman, A. W. (2007). Behaviors associated with fever in children with autism spectrum disorders. *Pediatrics, 120*(6), 1386–1392.

Davis, R. A., Bockbrader, M., Murphy, R., Hetrick, W., & O'Donnell, B. F. (2006). Subjective perceptual distortions and visual dysfunction in children with autism. *Journal of Autism and Developmental Disorders, 36*(2), 199–210.

Dennis, R., & Edelman, S. (2006). Sensory and motor considerations in the assessment of children with ASD. In P. Prelock, *Autism spectrum disorders: Issues in assessment and intervention* (pp. 303–344). Austin, TX: Pro-Ed.

DiCicco-Bloom, E., Lord, C., Zwaigenbaum, L., Courchesne, E., Dager, S. R., Schmitz, C., et al. (2006). The developmental neurobiology of autism spectrum disorder. *Journal of Neuroscience, 26*(26), 6897–6906.

Duchan, J., & Black, M. (2001). Progressing toward life goals: A person-centered approach to evaluating therapy. *Topics in Language Disorders, 22*(1), 37–49.

Dunlap, G., & Fox, L. (1999). A demonstration of behavioral support for young children with autism. *Journal of Positive Behavior Interventions, 1*(2), 77–87.

Edelson, M. (2006). Are the majority of children with autism mentally retarded? A systematic review of the evidence. *Focus on Autism and Other Developmental Disabilities, 21*(2), 66–83.

Eikeseth, S., Smith, T., Jahr, E., & Eldevik, S. (2002). Intensive behavioral treatment at school for 4- to 7-year-old children with autism: A 1-year comparison controlled study. *Behavior Modification, 26*(1), 49–68.

Goldstein, H. (2002). Communication intervention for children with autism: A review of treatment efficacy. *Journal of Autism and Developmental Disorders, 32,* 373–396.

Grandin, T. (1995). *Thinking in pictures and other reports from my life with autism*. New York: Doubleday.

Gray, C. (2000). *The new social story book*. Arlington, TX: Future Horizons.

Greenspan, S., & Wieder, S. (2000). A developmental approach to difficulties in relating and communication in autism spectrum disorders and related syndromes. In A. Wetherby & B. Prizant (Eds.), *Autism: A transactional developmental perspective* (pp. 279–306). Baltimore: Brookes.

Griffer, M. (1999). Is sensory integration effective for children with language-learning disorders?: A critical review of the evidence. *Language, Speech, and Hearing Disorders in Schools, 30*, 393–400.

Hale, C. M., & Tager-Flusberg, H. (2003). The influence of language on theory of mind: A training study. *Developmental Science, 6*(3), 346–359.

Heaton, P. (2003). Pitch memory, labeling and disembedding in autism. *Journal of Child Psychology and Psychiatry, 44*(4), 543–551.

Hodgson, L. (1995). Visual strategies for improving communication in autism. Troy, MI: QuirkRoberts.

Ingersoll, B., Lewis, E., & Kroman, E. (2007). Teaching the imitation and spontaneous use of descriptive gestures in young children with autism using a naturalistic behavioral intervention. *Journal of Autism and Developmental Disorders, 37*(8), 1446–1456.

Joseph, R. M., McGrath, & Tager-Flusberg, H. (2005). Executive dysfunction and its relation to language ability in verbal school-age children with autism. *Developmental Neuropsychology, 27*(3), 361–378.

Joseph, R., Tager-Flusberg, H., & Lord, C. (2002). Cognitive profiles and social–communicative functioning in children with autism spectrum disorder. *Journal of Child Psychology & Psychiatry & Allied Disciplines, 43*(6), 807–821.

Joseph, R. M., & Tager-Flusberg, H. (2004). The relationship of theory of mind and executive functions to symptom type and severity in children with autism. *Development and Psychopathology, 16*(1), 137–155.

Kanner, L. (1943). Autistic disturbances of affective contact. *Nervous Child, 2*, 217–250.

Kanner, L. (1946). Irrelevant and metaphorical language in early infantile autism. *American Journal of Psychiatry, 103*, 242–245.

Kasari, C., Freeman, S., & Paparella, T. (2006). Joint attention and symbolic play in young children with autism: A randomized controlled trial. *Journal of Child Psychology and Psychiatry, 47*(6), 611–620.

Kashinath, S., Woods, J., & Goldstein, H. (2006). Enhancing generalized teaching strategy use in daily routines by parents of children with autism. *Journal of Speech, Language, and Hearing Research, 49*, 466–485.

Khalfa, S., Bruneau, N., Roge, B., Georgieff, N., Veuillet, E., Adrien, J., et al. (2004). Increased perception of loudness in autism. *Hearing Research, 198*(1–2), 87–92.

Kjelgaard, M. M., & Tager-Flusberg, H. (2001). An investigation of language impairment in autism: Implications for genetic subgroups. *Language and Cognitive Processes, 16*(2–3), 287–308.

Koegel, L. K., Harrower, J. K., & Koegel, R. L. (1999). Support for children with developmental disabilities in full inclusion classrooms through self-management. *Journal of Positive Behavior Interventions, 1*(1), 26–34.

Koegel, R., & Koegel, L. (2006). *Pivotal response treatments for autism: Communication, social, and academic development*. Baltimore: Brookes.

Koegel, L. K., Koegel, R. L., Frea, W., & Green-Hopkins, I. (2003). Priming as a method of coordinating educational services for students with autism. *Language, Speech, & Hearing Services in Schools, 34*(3), 228–235.

Koegel, L. K., Koegel, R. L., & Smith, A. (1997). Variables related to differences in standardized test outcomes for children with autism. *Journal of Autism and Developmental Disorders, 27*(3), 233–243.

Kovarsky, D., Culatta, B., Franklin, A., & Theadore, G. (2001). "Communicative participation" as a way of facilitating and ascertaining communicative outcomes. *Topics in Language Disorders, 22*(1), 1–20.

Kovarsky, D. Duchan, J. F., Maxwell, M. (1999). *Constructing (in)competence: Disabling evaluations in clinical and social interaction.* Mahwah, NJ: Lawrence Erlbaum Associates.

Kylliäinen, A., & Hietanen, K. (2006). Skin conductance responses to another person's gaze in children with autism. *Journal of Autism and Developmental Disorders, 36*(4), 517–525.

Leyfer, O., Folstein, S., Bacalman, S., Davis, N., Dinh, E., Morgan, J., Tager-Flusberg, H., & Lainhart, J. (2006). Comorbid psychiatric disorders in children with autism: interview development and rates of disorders. *Journal of Autism and Developmental Disorders, 36*(7), 849–861.

Lord, C., Rutter, M., DiLavore, P., & Risi, S. (1999). *Autism Diagnostic Observation Schedule—Generic.* Los Angeles: Western Psychological Services.

Lovaas, O. I. (1987). Behavioral treatment and normal educational and intellectual functioning in young autistic children. *Journal of Consulting and Clinical Psychology, 55*(1), 3–9.

Magiati, I., Charman, T., & Howlin, P. (2007). A two-year prospective follow-up study of community-based early intensive behavioural intervention and specialist nursery provision for children with autism spectrum disorders. *Journal of Child Psychology and Psychiatry, and Allied Disciplines, 48*(8), 803–812.

Mason, P., & Narad, C. (2005). International adoption: A health and developmental perspective. *Seminars in Speech and Language, 26*(1), 1–9.

Maurice, C. (1993). *Let me hear your voice.* New York: Ballantine.

Maurice, C., Green, G., & Luce, S. (1996). *Behavioral intervention for young children with autism.* Austin, TX: Pro-Ed.

McEachin, J., Smith, T., & Lovaas, O. I., (1993). Long-term outcome for children with autism who received early intensive behavioral treatment, *American Journal on Mental Retardation, 97*(4), 359–372.

Minshew, N., & Williams, D. (2007). The new neurobiology of autism: Cortex, connectivity, and neuronal organization. *Archives of Neurology, 64*(7), 945–950.

Mottron, L., Belleville, S., & Ménard, E. (1999). Local bias in autistic subjects as evidenced by graphic tasks: Perceptual hierarchization or working memory deficit? *Journal of Child Psychology and Psychiatry, 40*(5), 743–755.

Mottron, L., Dawson, M., Soulieres, I., Hubert, B., & Burack, J. (2006). Enhanced perceptual functioning in autism: An update, and eight principles of autistic perception. *Journal of Autism and Developmental Disorders, 36*(1), 27–43.

National Research Council. (2001). *Educating children with autism.* Washington, DC: National Academy Press.

Odom, S., Brown, W., Frey, T., Karasu, N., Smith-Canter, L. L., Strain, P. (2003). Evidence-based practices for young children with autism: Contributions for single-subject design research. *Focus on Autism & Other Developmental Disabilities, 18*(3), 166–175.

Perry, B., Pollard, R., Blakley, T., Baker, W., & Vigilante, D. (1995). Childhood trauma, the neurobiology of adaptation, and "use-dependent" development of the brain: How "states" become "traits." *Infant Mental Health, 16,* 271–292.

Prelock, P., Beatson, J., Bitner, B., Broder, C., & Ducker, A. (2003). Interdisciplinary assessment of young children with autism spectrum disorder. *Language, Speech, and Hearing Services in Schools, 35*, 194–202.

Prizant, B., Wetherby, A., & Rydell, P. (2000). Communication intervention issues for young children with autism spectrum disorders. In A. Wetherby & B. Prizant (Eds.), *Autism spectrum disorders: A transactional developmental perspective* (pp. 193–224). Baltimore: Brookes.

Quill, K. (2000). *Do-watch-listen-say: Social and communication intervention for children with autism.* Baltimore: Paul H. Brookes.

Richler, J., Luyster, R., Risi, S., Hsu, W., Dawson, G., Bernier, R., et al. (2006). Is there a 'regressive phenotype' of autism spectrum disorder associated with the measles-mumps-rubella vaccine? A CPEA Study. *Journal of Autism and Developmental Disorders, 36*(3), 299–316.

Robey, R., & Schultz, M. (1998). A model for conducting clinical-outcome research: An adaptation of the standard protocol for use in aphasiology. *Aphasiology, 12*, 787–810.

Ronald, A., Happé, F., & Plomin, R. (2005). The genetic relationship between the social and non-social behaviors characteristic of autism. *Developmental Science, 8*(5), 444–458.

Scattone, D., Tingstrom, D., & Wilczynski, S. (2006). Increasing appropriate social interactions of children with autism spectrum disorders using Social Stories. *Focus on Autism and Other Developmental Disabilities, 21*(4), 211–222.

Shriberg, L., Paul, R., McSweeny, J., Klin, A., Cohen, D., & Volkmar, F. R. (2001). Speech and prosody characteristics of adolescents and adults with high-functioning autism and Asperger syndrome. *Journal of Speech, Language, and Hearing Research, 44*(5), 1097–1115.

Simmons-Mackie, N., & Damico, J. (2001). Intervention outcomes: A clinical application of qualitative methods. *Topics in Language Disorders, 21*(4), 21–36.

Sinha, Y., Silove, N., Wheeler, D., & Williams, K. (2006). Auditory integration training and other sound therapies for autism spectrum disorders: A systematic review. *Archives of disease in childhood, 91*(12), 1018–1022.

Smith, T. (1996). Are other treatments effective? In C. Maurice, G. Green, & S. Luce (Eds.), *Behavioral intervention for young children with autism: A manual for parents* (pp. 45–59). Austin, TX: Pro-Ed.

Smith, C., Goddard, S., & Fluck, M. (2004). A scheme to promote social attention and functional language in young children with communication difficulties and autistic spectrum disorders. *Educational Psychology in Practice, 20*(4), 319–333.

Smith, V., Mirenda, P., & Zaidma Zait, A. (2007). Predictors of expressive vocabulary growth in children with autism. *Journal of Speech, Language, and Hearing Research, 50*(1), 149–160.

Stehli, A. (2004). *Sound of falling snow Stories of recovery from autism and related conditions.* New York: Beaufort Books.

Sussman, F. (1999). *More than words: Helping parents promote communication and social skills in children with autism spectrum disorder.* Toronto, Ontario, Canada: Hanen Centre Publications.

Thurm, A., Lord, C., Lee, L.-C., & Newschaffer, C. (2007). Predictors of language acquisition in preschool children with autism spectrum disorders. *Journal of Autism and Developmental Disorders, 37*, 1721–1734.

Tsai, L. (2005). Medical treatment in autism. In D. Zager (Ed.), *Autism spectrum disorders* (3rd ed., pp. 395–492). Mahwah, NJ: Lawrence Erlbaum Associates.

Turner, L. M., & Stone, L. (2007). Variability in outcome for children with an ASD diagnosis at age 2. *Journal of Child Psychology and Psychiatry*, *48*(8), 793–802.

Wing, L., & Potter, D. (2002). The epidemiology of autism spectrum disorders: Is the prevalence rising? *Mental Retardation and Developmental Disabilities Research Reviews, 8*, 151–161.

Winner, M. G. (2007, November). *Asperger syndrome: Facilitating social thinking across the school day*. Seminar presented at the American Speech-Language-Hearing Association Annual Meeting, Boston, MA.

# 8 Benefiting From Speech Therapy

## The Role of Individual Differences in Treating Children With Speech Sound Disorders

*Amy L. Weiss*

## INTRODUCTION: CONSIDERING CLIENT DIFFERENCES IN SPEECH SOUND DISORDERS

Speech-language pathologists (SLPs) generally consider the normal process of speech sound acquisition completed by age 8 or 9 for young children learning English as their first language (Smit, Hand, Freilinger, Bernthal, & Bird, 1990). This way of thinking, however, can lead to an underestimate of what the typical child is doing developmentally. For example, we know that even three quarters of children demonstrating some degree of speech delay have normalized their speech 3 years earlier, by 6 years of age (Shriberg, 1997; Shriberg, Gruber, & Kwiatkowski, 1994; Shriberg, Kwiatkowski, & Gruber, 1994). The data show that most typically developing children are making great strides in their phonological development during the preschool years, just as they are also demonstrating impressive competencies in semantic, syntactic, morphologic, and pragmatic language development (Hoff, 2009).

Acquisition of the speech sound system means more than that a child can intelligibly produce all of the phones of the adult system they are learning. In addition, the child has developed an orderly system of underlying phonemic contrasts that signify meaning (i.e., phonemes), as well as a rule system that systematically allows for predictable context-based phonetic or phonemic productions that may be called for in the particular dialect that the child is learning to speak. Acquisition also implies that the child knows something about the morphophonemic rules of the language, as illustrated by the three different phonetic realizations of the plural morpheme in English. To be credited with a fully acquired phonological system, the child also recognizes the output constraints of the language (e.g., "pt" can be produced at the ends of English words but not at their beginnings). Thus, learning the sound system of one's language, its phonology, is made up of several component parts, some more abstract than the production of recognizable sounds. (See Edwards & Shriberg, 1983, p. 37, for a useful schematic representation of these components and their relationships.) Note as well that acquisition relates to both the literal (production accuracy) and the abstract (underlying rule systems).

Complicating the picture of typical phonological development is the finding by a number of researchers that there is evidence of variability between children who appear to be learning their sound system in a normal fashion, although general developmental trends are obvious (Leonard, Newhoff, & Mesalem, 1980; McLeod, van Doorn, & Reed, 2001). Given the breadth of the age range considered for typical phonological development, some variability in acquisition rates would have to be assumed. For example, Leonard et al. reported data collected from a pair of identical twins reared in the same household and found nonidentical phonemic repertoires, although similar trends in acquisition were evident (e.g., glides, nasals and plosives were acquired prior to fricatives and affricates). Stoel-Gammon (2007) noted that variability in phonological development can be considered within a child as well as between children. That is, typically developing children up to almost 3 years of age have shown considerable inconsistency (variability) in their productions of consonant–vowel–consonant words (e.g., cap, bite). The within-child variability observed in typically developing children most likely is caused by immaturity of the child's neuromotor system or inconsistently applied phonological rules (Stoel-Gammon, 2007, p. 58). Thus, some variability is characteristic of the child whose phonological system is developing in a typical manner.

As noted by Stoel-Gammon (2007) above, variability in development of the sound system has been attributed not only to differences in the maturity of the child's linguistic system but in the maturity of the motor system as well (see Goffman, 2005, for a review). For example, Kent (1992) suggested that the reason that fricatives are typically learned after stops stems from the relative difficulty of the speech motor control involved in their production. Perhaps not surprisingly, the disparity in movement variability has been shown to be much more pronounced in children diagnosed with specific language impairment, especially for weak syllable production, and in children diagnosed with childhood apraxia of speech (CAS) for production of consistent, recognizable prosodic contours (Goffman, 1999, 2004). This latter point is a good reminder that when considering phonological development, we should evaluate both the child's segmental and suprasegmental achievements.

However, when SLPs, a child's family members, or classroom teachers are alerted to a child's failure to progress along the age-expected path of acquisition, it is usually because of real-world concerns: the child is having a difficult time communicating during activities of daily living. Sometimes the significant others in the child's life will also report that he or she sounds like a much younger child.

Borrowing from a still ecologically valid definition of a speech disorder from Van Riper (1972), when an individual's speech pattern is so different from normal that it frequently draws attention to itself and away from the intended message, a speech sound disorder is present (p. 29). Van Riper included another marker of speech disorder, the causation of the maladjustment of the speaker. For now I will assume that for a speech sound disorder, the latter translates into a reduction of intelligibility that is so severe that it renders the individual unable (or makes the individual believe that he or she is unable) to participate in academic or social endeavors (Felsenfeld, Broen, & McGue, 1994; Fujiki, Brinton, Isaacson, & Summers, 2001).

Note that in Van Riper's (1972) definition, there is no mention of whether the speech sound error pattern can be best described as articulatory or phonologically based. That is, regardless of whether the client's problem has stemmed from deficits of motor output, perceptual deficiency, an underlying organizational immaturity, or perhaps a bit of all three, the essential factor is that when a speaker's ability to communicate is significantly, negatively affected, a speech sound disorder is present. It is for this reason that most SLPs frame their long-term goal in treating an individual with a speech sound disorder as improving that individual's intelligibility, with shorter-term goals focusing on increasing the number of speech sound segments produced correctly or phonological patterns suppressed. Improved intelligibility in conversational activities of daily living provides the best rationale for eventual dismissal from therapy (Kamhi, 2006).

To enhance understanding of assessment and treatment, Shriberg (1997) delineated three populations of speech sound disorders in children for clinical consideration. According to his taxonomy, developmental phonological disorders are made up of two subgroups. The first of these groups, age-wise, is that of children with *speech delay*, a diagnosis appropriate for any child not keeping up with normal developmental milestones by 9 years of age. The second and older group is referred to as those who demonstrate *residual errors*, individuals 9 and older who still have not completed their phonemic inventory. The third and final subgroup is made up of speakers who, regardless of age, demonstrate speech sound errors that are related to concomitant health, educational, or emotional deficits, such as children who may present with Down syndrome, cleft palate, or oppositional defiant disorder. When planning service delivery for individual children representing each one of these groups, SLPs may follow different decision-making patterns. These are often the organic disorders whose etiologies can be traced back to a particular physical or cognitive deficit.

How prevalent are developmental speech sound disorders? Shriberg, Tomblin, and McSweeny (1999) not only reported the prevalence of speech sound disorders among 6-year-olds to be 3.8% but also reported that the likelihood of a speech delay was more prevalent in males than females (4.5% versus 3.1%). Additional estimates of the population of children with speech sound disorders have yielded a median prevalence estimate between 8% and 9% for children in the early school years, ages 5 through 8 (Law et al., 2000; as cited in National Institute on Deafness and Other Communication Disorders, n.d.).

We also know that the problem of speech sound disorders is not a trivial one, especially when considering SLPs who work in school settings. The recently published American Speech-Language-Hearing Association (ASHA)

2008 Schools Survey (ASHA, 2008) of more than 2,500 ASHA-certified SLPs who are primarily employed in school settings demonstrated that, on average, school SLPs are treating children with what the survey's developers termed "articulation/ phonological disorders" more than any other communication disorder category in settings from preschool through secondary school. Specifically, for SLPs working with the preschool population, 93.2% regularly serve clients with this disorder on their caseloads, with an average of more than 18 clients with a diagnosed speech sound disorder served per clinician. As might be expected, these figures increase somewhat for SLPs employed in elementary schools (96.7%, 24.3 clients) and then drop off for those with caseloads in junior high and high schools (86.9%, 8.8 clients), as the expected normalization age is reached and then surpassed. The percentage and average number of clients for SLPs working in secondary school venues may appear to be surprisingly high to some readers. Clients with speech sound disorders represented on the caseloads of SLPs in junior high and high schools may be individuals demonstrating the residual sound errors Shriberg (1997) noted, possibly the "late eight" (Bleile, 2006), or clients with etiological factors such as hearing impairment or orofacial anomalies, or diagnoses such as CAS that are likely to yield persistent (though inconsistent) sound error patterns. Unfortunately, the ASHA survey data as presented make it impossible to differentiate among these possibilities. It may also be the case that many of these older school-age clients have concomitant literacy-learning difficulties. (See Larrivee & Maloney, Chapter 6 in this volume, for more information about the potential linkage between weak phonological processing competencies and problems with literacy success.) Regardless, the considerable proportion of speech sound disorders throughout the age range of school attendance means that SLPs and others who educate young children with speech sound disorders have a vested interest in knowing how to select intervention strategies that are likely to be most efficient and effective for their clients.

## SPEECH SOUND INTERVENTION: WHY DOES THERAPY WORK?

What do we know about the efficacy of interventions for speech sound disorders? One perspective was presented in Gierut's (1998) now decade-old review of the treatment efficacy studies for children with speech sound disorders (circa 1980 through 1995), in which she found that research converged around five outcomes. In an earlier review of that paper (Weiss, 2004), I noted that Gierut had reported that the research of that era supported the SLPs' selection of (a) target sounds or pairs of target sounds that were absent from the child's sound repertoire; (b) sound targets that were typically later-developing, not stimulable, and phonetically more complex; (c) a drill-play treatment mode where feedback is consistently provided, but reinforcement follows only correct productions (see Shriberg & Kwiatkowski, 1982b); (d) both perceptual and production training; and (e) microcomputer software programs in some therapy contexts (Gierut, 1998, pp. S93–S94). What I found most revealing in Gierut's thorough review was that she found a relative lack of emphasis on studying clients' individual differences (e.g., cognitive abilities, temperament, motivation to change) that might influence therapy outcomes (Weiss, 2007). Gierut did explicitly note that this lack of an individual difference focus was a shortcoming of the research she had reviewed. Specifically, she stated that "identification of the sources of individual differences in phonological learning is another fundamental research need" (Gierut, 1998, p. S94). Certainly, Gierut's review is just that, a review of available research at that time, and does not reflect her own personal beliefs about what may influence therapy outcomes for speech sound disorders.

Of interest to me when reading the remaining summaries of efficacy studies for other disorder areas published in the *Journal of Speech, Language, and Hearing Research* (e.g., aphasia, voice) was that the topic of clients' individual differences had been more fully incorporated into investigations that considered success in therapy than was evident for the literature dealing with successful intervention for speech sound disorders. For example, it was often the case that premorbid personality was associated with more or less success in treatment for aphasia (Holland, Fromm, DeRuyter, & Stein, 1996). Although this was only one example, perhaps because of the age of the typical client with a speech sound disorder and a subsequent lack of reliable measures of client motivation or the fact that in speech sound therapy the focus is usually habilitation and not rehabilitation, that individual differences, the personal factors the young client brings to the therapy context, were more difficult to investigate.

Kamhi (2006) recently observed that there is evidence from several reviews (e.g., Bauman-Waengler, 2004; Gierut, 1998; Weston & Bain, 2003) that a number of different therapy strategies, including metaphon, cycles approach, and productive phonological knowledge (PPK), have demonstrated their utility to change children's speech sound systems (p. 272). However, following a careful meta-analysis taking into account evidence-based practice (EBP) criteria, Weston and Bain concluded that despite the number of treatment studies to date, their results provide little information to lead SLPs in specific directions for selecting a best practices treatment paradigm for speech sound disorders. Considering Weston and Bain's conclusion, Kamhi (2006) suggested that the problem for SLPs treating individuals with speech sound disorders may not be a lack of suggestions for ways to approach intervention for speech sound disorders but rather a systematic way to choose among them.

Even more recently, Powell (2008) made the case that SLPs need to account for the following observation: clinical studies that have attempted to apply a standardized treatment methodology to a carefully selected, homogeneous group of individuals with speech sound disorders have yielded nonuniform treatment outcomes across subjects. Despite selection of study participants with similar sets of speech sounds in error and fastidious adherence to a therapy approach, individual differences have been apparent. Powell suggested that this outcome could stem from the fact that there are many different explanations for why a particular child cannot accurately produce the particular speech sounds in a word, ranging from incorrect storage of the word in the mental lexicon to the presence of a structural anomaly. Furthermore, he noted, it is not uncommon for more than one explanation to be at the root of a speech sound production error. We are left to make the following inference: given the number of permutations and combinations of causal factors delineated, it is not easy to determine the best treatment approach on the basis of the appearance of the speech sound error pattern alone. In summary, Powell noted that "in terms of treatment, the published research clearly indicates that one size does *not* fit all" (2008, p. 375; italics in original).

I believe that this is where the importance of investigating individual differences and their role in successful therapy fits in. That is, to accurately evaluate the results of treatment studies for our clients with speech sound disorders, it is necessary that we look at the individual variables (and we can view these as strengths, needs, and/or preferences) that a client brings to the therapy table. It is quite possible that useful information about clients' individual differences underlies the findings already reported in intervention studies, but they have not been highlighted as such. In this chapter, the focus is on what those individual differences are and the role they play when SLPs plan the most appropriate therapy programs for their clients with speech sound disorders.

## INDIVIDUAL DIFFERENCES AND PERSONAL FACTORS RELATED TO THERAPY OUTCOMES

Considering therapy options for any client with a communication disorder should send clinicians to resources for EBP data (Baker & McLeod, 2004; Dollaghan, 2007). By now most SLPs have been exposed to the EBP paradigm that when evaluating an evidence-based approach to treating communication disorders, there are three perspectives to be weighed: data resulting from carefully controlled studies (in a perfect world, that is where treatments have been compared across randomly assigned subject groups), the preferences of the client and the client's family, and the knowledge gained via clinical experiences accrued by the SLP in treating individuals with similar communication problems. Neglecting to incorporate any one of the three components endangers the appropriate application of EBP, but how does the SLP incorporate all of them?

Recently, Gillam and Gillam (2006) made specific suggestions for how clinicians can go about weighing these different components of EBP, especially in situations where the evidence provided by external research does not jibe with the preferences of the client/family and/or the clinician's own perspective or skills. Although Gillam and Gillam were specifically focusing on intervention choices for children with language disorders, there is no reason to assume that their principles would not be worth considering for clients with speech sound disorders. Gillam and Gillam recommended that as part of the evaluation of the external or research evidence available, the clinician consider the goodness of fit between the clients on one's caseload and the participants in the original intervention study. Gillam and Gillam noted that not all studies are equally forthcoming regarding their inclusion of important descriptive data about their participants, including "age, gender, race, ethnicity, socioeconomic status, speech and language abilities, and/or cognitive status" (2006, p. 307). When participants are not fully described, the SLP is less able to determine whether the intervention approach in the study (even if the outcomes of the intervention study are impressive) is applicable to children on his or her caseload. Thus, Gillam and Gillam have acknowledged the important role played by the constellation of personal factors embodied by individual clients and the potential difficulty imposed by studies that obfuscate their retrieval.

As the field of communication disorders has become more sophisticated in its understanding of speech sound disorders, having borrowed from linguistics, psychology, acoustics, and physiology, as well as making its own copious contributions to the literature, several factors under the heading of individual differences or personal factors have been posited as important considerations in the selection of an effective therapy approach or as the rationale for why some treatment approaches appear to be more or less successful with different clients.

## ETIOLOGY

One of the first major attempts to delineate differences between individuals diagnosed with speech sound disorders to aid in the selection of therapy was focused on uncovering the etiology of the problem. Does the client present with an organic or a functional disorder, for example? Determination of the etiology of a speech sound disorder was viewed as critical to providing the most appropriate speech therapy strategies (Shriberg, 1982; Shriberg & Kwiatkowski, 1982a).

In fact, Shriberg and Kwiatkowski (1982a) argued that without a thorough assessment of predisposing factors (e.g., cognitive-linguistic, speech and hearing mechanism, and social-emotional/behavioral) it would be impossible to differentiate one etiology from another. Their perspective was that etiology is an essential matter. If the etiology of a speech sound disorder cannot be determined, it is less likely that the most appropriate therapeutic plan will be chosen. If a specific etiology cannot be determined, then at least the clinician is beholden to gather sufficient data about the client's cognitive-linguistic skills, speech and language mechanism integrity, and social-emotional/behavioral development to ascertain the foundational skill set the client has brought into therapy. Using a 3-point rating scale to measure 90 different variables distributed across the three causal-correlate domains, Shriberg and Kwiatkowski concluded that two thirds of their 43 subjects presented with some evidence of a history of involvement in one or more areas. Specifically, although one third presented with histories suggestive of comprehension problems, 90% showed evidence of expressive language deficiencies. In terms of psychosocial inputs and outputs, 40–60% of the children demonstrated some concerns (e.g., aggression, immaturity, avoidance, sensitivity to new situations). As Shriberg and Kwiatkowski noted, their data were presented in the aggregate to make the case that SLPs should be carefully evaluating these causal-correlates to identify subgroups of children with speech sound disorders that may require different intervention programs (Shriberg & Kwiatkowski, 1982a, p. 239). Reliance on basing therapy-selection decisions on characteristics of speech sound patterns alone, say Shriberg and Kwiatkowski, could result in missing important information about the client's prerequisite abilities that could lead to an ineffective choice of therapy approach. Similarly, Davis (2005) reprised the need to assess multiple factors, such as the client's motor abilities, structural differences, perceptual abilities, neuromotor differences, cognitive-linguistic abilities, and psychosocial abilities, prior to setting goals for individual clients with developmental speech sound disorders.

Furthermore, reliance on a dichotomy of organic versus functional disorders may eliminate some important subdivisions within the classical functional category of "faulty learning" that can best be treated by individualized intervention approaches, according to Shriberg (1982). For example, the speech sound error patterns exhibited by children with histories of chronic serous otitis media accompanied by fluctuating hearing loss may represent a distinct pattern requiring an intervention approach different from that needed by other children with an identical cluster of speech sounds in error (Shriberg et al., 2000; Shriberg, Kent, Karlsson, Nadler, & Brown, 2003).

One relatively obvious example of when background historical information is critical to clinical decision making for treatment of a speech sound disorder would be in the case where a speech sound disorder is caused by (or accompanied by) a moderate-to-severe hearing loss. For a client with this causal-correlate it is likely that unless measures are taken to compensate for the client's reduction in hearing acuity and/or distortion of the auditory signal, a satisfactory therapy outcome will not be achieved. Thus, the provision of amplification is a necessary part of the treatment plan, although it is less likely to be a necessary therapy component if the client with a speech sound disorder presents with normal hearing acuity (see Teagle & Eskridge, Chapter 12). In terms of the importance of determining what speech-language therapy clients bring to the therapy table, I assume that all clinicians recognize the essential need to determine a client's hearing acuity levels before planning therapy without much convincing. My interpretation of the seminal Shriberg and Kwiatkowski (1982a) paper is that in addition to providing a template for assessing the presence and degree of potential causal-correlates to speech sound disorders in service to identifying subgroups of clients who require etiology-appropriate therapy, the authors were also making a very precise case for the importance of determining the individual differences that may exist between clients.

## Is There a Genetic Predisposition for Speech Sound Disorders?

In terms of personal factors that one can bring to the therapy table, there may not be anything as closely related to one's likelihood to be diagnosed with a speech sound disorder as one's genetic makeup. The last 20 years have seen attempts to identify a speech sound disorders phenotype.

Lewis, Ekelman, and Aram (1989) examined a group of 20 children who had been diagnosed with severe phonological disorders along with their siblings and compared them with a same-sized group of children with typically developing speech sound systems and their siblings on measures of motor ability, language, and reading, as well as phonological competencies. The investigators found that the children with disordered phonology demonstrated a significant positive correlation with their siblings on measures of phonological ability. The children in the control group and their siblings did not. In addition, family histories revealed that the children with speech sound disorders had many more family members with language disorders, dyslexia, and other speech disorders than did the histories of the control families, suggesting that for some children with severe phonological disorders, a familial link might be present.

Building on the notion of familial linkage, Shriberg et al. (2005) more recently studied a group of 72 preschoolers who had functional speech sound disorders. That is, no etiology had been determined. Their intent was to identify the subcategory of children with genetically linked speech sound disorders. When the children were segregated into groups by the number of relatives they had with speech or language disorders, Shriberg et al. found that those who had what the authors termed a *higher genetic load* for a speech sound disorder, defined as having two or more family members with speech or language disorder, were significantly more likely to show a similar speech pattern. Specifically, Shriberg et al. noted that children with a higher genetic load for speech sound disorder were more likely to produce sound omission errors on typically later-developing sounds but less likely to produce distortion errors.

Lewis et al. (2006) concluded from a review of the available studies investigating speech sound disorders through familial aggregation, studying sets of twins, and molecular genetics that there is probably not one genetic explanation for speech sound disorders. Rather, "an individual's susceptibility for speech sound disorders may be due to a single gene effect … or to multiple underlying genetic and environmental etiologies" (p. 1304). Lewis et al. further stressed that the interaction of the genetic factors that may place children at risk for developing speech sound disorders and those factors that counteract these and play a protective function is not well understood. In all cases, Lewis et al. noted that genetic influences are mediated by environmental ones. For example, when Campbell et al. (2003) calculated odds ratios for six risk factors (i.e., male gender, low socioeconomic status, low education level, African American race, persistent otitis media, and presence of a developmental communication disorder in a first-degree relative) to see whether 3-year-olds with speech delays were more likely to be identified with any of these factors, they found that both mother's education level and male gender yielded elevated ratios that were clinically significant (p. 353). Familial history of a communication disorder and low socioeconomic status also showed elevated risk ratios but not quite to the extent that gender and mother's education did. Lewis et al. concluded that additional genetic studies will be most helpful in delineating the essential phenotypic characteristics of speech sound disorders to assist SLPs in accurately identifying speech sound disorders early on, as well as understanding the relationships between speech sound disorders, reading disorders, and the diagnosis of specific language impairment.

## ARTICULATION OR PHONOLOGY?

Related to etiology is determination of the best way to characterize the speech sound pattern. Within the subgroups of speech sound disorders described by

Shriberg (1997) (e.g., speech delay, residual errors, and special populations), another clinical delineation is commonly made by SLPs who want to answer the question of whether the error pattern produced by the client can be best represented as an articulation or a phonological disorder. As noted by Bernthal, Bankson, and Flipsen (2009), the term *articulation disorder* has classically referred to production-based disorders, while the term *phonological disorder* refers to speech sound disorders that are rule-governed (p. 2). They go on to note that "it may be difficult to determine which of these concepts is most appropriate in describing a particular client's error pattern" (Bernthal et al., 2009, p. 2). This is an important comment because SLPs try to determine the best descriptor for their clients' speech sound disorders often because they assume that the selection of the therapy approach most appropriate for their client depends on that determination. For example, production-based error patterns commonly found in residual errors will most likely respond to intervention that provides motor practice and subsequent feedback. On the other hand, phonological disorders require focus on the organization of the sound system that can be provided by the use of a minimal pairs approach or a cycles goal attack strategy, for example (Hodson & Paden, 1991).

## ARE OTHER LINGUISTIC DEFICITS PRESENT?

A related factor typically considered when deciding upon a therapy approach for a particular child's speech sound disorder is whether the phonological deficits are accompanied by deficits in other language areas. We know that more than half of the children diagnosed with speech sound disorders do demonstrate language involvement (Paul & Shriberg, 1982; Shriberg & Kwiatkowski, 1982a), and this being the case, we are faced with the clinical question of which type of intervention, one focused on the speech sound system or on development of morphosyntax, would be more efficacious.

In a study that investigated the benefits of providing grammatical intervention to 25 children who were diagnosed with deficits in both phonology and morphosyntax, Fey et al. (1994) found no significant increase in their participants' phonological skills. However, when the converse was attempted (Tyler & Sandoval, 1994), that is, when intervention was focused on the specific phonemes (e.g., /s/, /z/) that accounted for their subjects' inability to accurately convey grammatical morphemes, there was a resulting increase in correct production of those grammatical morphemes composed of the target phonemes. More recently, Tyler, Lewis, Haskill, and Tolbert (2003) reported the results of an ambitious study that focused on the progress of 40 children between the ages of 3 and 6 diagnosed with both speech and language disorders. They simultaneously looked at both the effects of different service delivery models (e.g., cycles, vertical) and, embedded therein, the conveyance of therapy provided for speech, language, or both. Tyler et al. (2003) reported that their participants fared best when they were provided with therapy that addressed both grammatical and phonological goals. In addition, Tyler et al. (2003) concluded that the choice of therapy targets for children with phonological and morphosyntactic deficits probably rests with the SLP's ability to determine how interdependent the two sets of goals are (p. 73). That is, if the grammatical morpheme errors are closely associated with the specific speech sounds missing from a young client's repertoire, it stands to reason that targeting those particular sounds will more likely generalize to the use of those phonemes in service to the grammatical morphemes in question (Tyler, 2005). In fact, Tyler (2008) most recently published an organizational framework for delineating how clinicians can make evidence-based decisions about selection of an intervention approach for a specific child with a speech sound disorder. She used as her first major dichotomy the clinician's choice of focusing directly on speech or on language, thus focusing indirectly on speech.

## Beyond Etiology

The suggestion to consider variables beyond etiology is a recurring theme. When Gildersleeve-Neumann (2007) discussed what she called "precursors to motor learning" in a recent article about treatment of CAS, she noted that "client motivation, family situation, the child's attitude toward treatment, and individual factors such as developmental delay or attention deficit can all have an effect on learning" (p. 30). She also admonished SLPs to recognize that for successful treatment, a client must not only be invested in the therapy but believe that the intervention will work (p. 30). The latter, she argued, may be the most important factor to ensure a positive therapeutic outcome (Gildersleeve-Neumann, 2007, p. 30).

Kwiatkowski and Shriberg (1993) attempted to give clients' motivation to change their speech its due. They acknowledged that there is a lengthy history of research that has attempted to determine why children do not all progress in therapy at the same rate or meet with the same degree of success in the therapy process for speech sound disorders (Bernthal et al., 2009; Newman, Creaghead, & Secord, 1985). This failure to provide statistical evidence for predictive variables of success (e.g., age, gender, etiology, phonological patterns in error) led these investigators to address what they viewed as a neglected variable in the study of individual differences, motivation. To accomplish this, Kwiatkowski and Shriberg proposed a two-factor framework for learning that featured the interaction between both capability (i.e., linguistic variables and risk factors potentially influencing therapy success) and focus (i.e., the motivational events and effort displayed by the client). In addition to capability and focus, two additional, important features of this variable mix involved the ability of the client to mobilize the information that stimulability and self-monitoring could lend to the learning process. The authors suggested that delineating two separate features of capability and focus reflect the real-world experiences of clinicians who have had the experience of clients who may be motivated to change their speech-sound patterns but do not have the skills (capabilities) to make those changes. Conversely, other clients present with the basic skills to effect changes in speech sound patterns but are not motivated to make those changes.

In their retrospective study (Kwiatkowski & Shriberg, 1993) of 164 children with speech sound disorders, capability and focus variables were coded. Although the capability variable (measured as consonant inventory) was the most powerful single predictor of a positive therapy outcome, the majority of children who made maximal progress in intervention were those who were coded as *good* in terms of both capability and focus variables. Kwiatkowski and Shriberg (1993) cautioned that there were some participants who had also been scored as *good* for both the capability and focus variables yet achieved minimal progress in therapy. This led the investigators to conclude that "predictive models of speech change that include only linguistic capability and risk variables—however well developed linguistically or statistically—will not be sufficient to predict the progress of individual children" (p. 15).

## Selecting Therapy Targets

One of the variables frequently investigated in terms of its relationship to effectiveness of speech sound therapy has been the clinician's approach to selection of the speech sound targets incorporated into therapy. Although this may appear to be a clinician-centered variable and not qualify as a personal factor, I would argue that selection of targets is often based on an individual client's phonological repertoire. That is, what we are really considering is the individual client's degree of understanding and use of his or her own phonological system, and selection thus qualifies as an individual difference.

Usually, the clinical question is stated as follows: Which sounds, when targeted in therapy, are most likely to generalize the organization of the child's sound system to sounds not specifically targeted in therapy? The issue is how to best facilitate generalization. Gierut and colleagues (Elbert & Gierut, 1995; Gierut, 2001; Gierut, Elbert, & Dinnsen, 1987; Gierut, Morrisette, Hughes, & Rowland, 1996) have promoted an approach to target selection rooted in the concept of PPK. PPK is, at its core, a hierarchy that delineates the extent to which a sound produced in error is considered to be part of the child's underlying speech sound organization. That is, individual error sounds in a young client's speech pattern may represent relative levels of PPK. For example, some sounds may be absent from the child's repertoire; others may be inconsistently produced correctly in all word positions or always produced correctly in one or two word positions. These differences are explained as illustrating more or less phonological knowledge. The question for SLPs has been to decide how to utilize the variable of PPK when selecting sound targets. Specifically, should SLPs start therapy with sound targets that represent more PPK in the child's repertoire, or conversely with those representing less PPK? Said another way, is it more efficacious to begin therapy by targeting sounds that are closer to acquisition in the fullest sense of the word or sounds that have the least incorporation to the child's sound system?

The outcomes of a series of studies using multiple baseline designs have led Gierut and colleagues to conclude that the initially counterintuitive tack of starting with the sounds representing least PPK renders more success (Gierut, 2005; Gierut, Elbert, & Dinnsen, 1987; Gierut, Morrisette, Hughes, & Rowland, 1996). The investigators have explained their findings by suggesting that when a sound absent from the client's repertoire (lowest possible PPK) is targeted, the basics of the sound's relationship to the organization of the client's phonological system have to be addressed through therapy. For example, when targeting error sounds that fall on the lower end of the PPK continuum, it is necessary to convey to the child how this new sound contrasts with others in a meaningful way to yield a phonemic distinction. Focusing the child on the essential principles of the sound system's organization is more likely to generate a "spread of effect" to other sounds not specifically targeted that the child has already "figured out" to a greater extent. Because the specific therapy mode is not prescribed as much as the method for selecting the target sounds, Gierut (2005) refers to selecting targets as focusing on the *what* of therapy, rather than the *how*. Notice, however, that this selection methodology relates to an individual child's level of PPK; there is no predetermined selection criterion based on normative data that may or may not be a good fit for the child.

Using PPK to select targets for intervention has received considerable attention because it runs counter to traditional therapy approaches that have suggested prioritizing sound targets that are closer to acquisition or at least sounds that are viewed as developmentally appropriate. In fact, in a study of 48 children randomly assigned to receive therapy on sound targets representing either *most knowledge/ earliest developing* (ME) or *least knowledge/latest developing* (LL), Rvachew & Novak (2001) found significant differences between their two groups of subjects, but not in the direction that would have been predicted by Gierut et al. (1996).

Specifically, Rvachew and Novak (2001) investigated how generalization, progress in therapy, and the client's indication of satisfaction with therapy were impacted by selecting therapy targets that represented ME versus LL targets (p. 612). Their results showed that children receiving therapy on the LL targets (i.e., nondevelopmental sounds) demonstrated less systemic generalization within their phonological repertoire than children assigned to the ME group. Furthermore,children who received therapy focusing on the ME targets also showed greater progress to a statistically significant degree than those children assigned to the LL group. Both findings are contradictions of Gierut et al.'s (1996) findings. Last, Rvachew and Novak did not find differences between the groups of children in terms of their enjoyment with the speech therapy. Their takeaway message was for SLPs to be confident in targeting error sounds that are earlier developing and for which a child has shown greater PPK. However, just as Kwiatkowski and Shriberg (1993) had seen progress in sound learning in some children with characteristics they found ran counter to progress in most children, Rvachew and Novak also observed children from the LL group who made more progress in therapy than children in the ME group. Clearly, selection of target phonemes remains an issue about which there is some disagreement and on which further study is needed.

## Stimulability

The concept of stimulability can be viewed as a subtopic under the rubric of the knowledge of the phonological system that the child has attained. That is, if a child is able to correctly imitate another's production of an error sound, we can say that that child is stimulable for that sound's production and has some knowledge, both motor and linguistic, about that sound (Rvachew, Rafaat, & Martin, 1999). According to Miccio and colleagues (Miccio, 2005; Miccio, Elbert, & Forrest, 1999; Powell & Miccio, 1996), stimulable sounds are more ready for incorporation into the client's production repertoire than are nonstimulable sounds. In fact, some SLPs purposely do not prioritize a child's stimulable sounds for therapy because these are the sounds the child is most likely to acquire without the benefit of therapy. One of the benefits of targeting stimulable sounds, however, is that because of their typically rapid acquisition, success may breed additional success in terms of compliance with a therapy regimen for a young child. On the down side, as suggested by Gierut et al. (1996), stimulable sounds represent more phonological knowledge in a child's phonological system, and thus the spread of effect from them to nonstimulable sounds is less remarkable than if nonstimulable sounds were targeted in therapy. It is for this reason that some clinical investigators have recommended targeting the stimulability of nonstimulable sounds as its own clinical goal (Miccio, 2007; Powell, 1996). Note that in Kwiatkowski and Shriberg's (1993) capability-focus model, stimulability also played an important role. Specifically Kwiatkowski and Shriberg suggested that "capability defines the potential for demonstrating stimulability or self-monitoring; access to this potential presumably requires some threshold level of Focus" (p. 11).

## Does the Client Take Responsibility for Sound Change?

Two recent anecdotal reports about young children with speech sound disorders illustrate the role that taking responsibility for sound change can potentially make. As described here, the two children demonstrated perspective-taking abilities that, when infused with their individual temperaments, translated to different responses to therapy.

Weiss (2004) described a young child named Sid who had been treated for several semesters in a university clinic for a severe phonological disorder that rendered his speech virtually unintelligible. One semester after multiple expressions of concern that his speech was less mature than his younger sister's during client–clinician discussion, Sid abruptly made incredible progress by increasing his intelligibility in connected speech to the point where dismissal was considered. What had rendered this change? It was the clinician's contention that Sid's awareness of his problems communicating and the personal identity he assumed he adopted as a result (i.e., talking like a baby) were incompatible with how he wanted to view himself and that this disparity motivated him to make changes to his speech pattern. Weiss's explanation is consistent with personal construct therapy (Hayhow, 1987; Stewart & Leahy, Chapter 10), an approach to facilitating change that has been used more widely with clients who stutter.

In a description of his daughter Franne's history of therapy for multiple speech sound errors, Kamhi (2000) suggested that Franne's ability to perceive the disconnect between practicing her speech sounds and being able to communicate served as a roadblock to her progress. That is, Franne was aware that using speech to practice did not have the same underlying goal as using speech to meaningfully communicate. Thus, she refused to practice her sounds at home, where communicating was her intended use of her speech and not the receipt of feedback from her parents regarding the accuracy of her productions (Kamhi, 2000). This recounting of Franne's refusal to practice may give SLPs some pause when requesting families to institute a home program to facilitate carryover.

Franne's negative response to the carryover phase of therapy and Sid's positive response to recognition that he could be an agent for change in the progress of his intervention may both represent features of these children's temperaments. Temperament refers to a genetically determined, persistent set of features that, according to Strelau (1998), can be identified early in a child's development. Some examples of temperamental features include level of anxiety or degree of extroversion or introversion. Thus, Franne's "stubborn nature" (her father's description in Kahmi, 2000, p. 183) and Sid's stick-to-itiveness (Weiss's description in Weiss, 2004) in the face of their individual frustrations with the failure to permit meaningful communication in Franne's case and with being viewed as an immature speaker in Sid's, seem to have spurred each child to respond in a predictable way based on temperamental characteristics. One of the temperamental features that experienced SLPs probably routinely attend to and utilize when making session-by-session alterations to clinical programs is an individual child's ability to cope with frustration or taking risks when challenged. Although I know of no large-scale study of children's risk taking related to speech therapy, there are anecdotal reports of children who appear relatively unfazed by challenge and others who approach attempts at generalizing sounds with trepidation (Weiss, 2007).

Historically, attempts to find correlations between children's personality traits and progress in speech therapy have not met with consistently positive results (Bloch & Goodstein, 1971; Reid, 1947; Winitz, 1969), although Hawk (1948) suggested that measuring the personalities of our clients with speech disorders should yield useful clinical information. Interestingly, there is at least one study that reported a statistically significant relationship between parents' personality profiles and the presence of functional speech sound disorders in their children (Wood, 1946). Shriberg and Kwiatkowski (1994) provided the most compelling evidence for SLPs' consideration of personality/temperament features in their profiling of children with developmental phonological disorders. Shriberg and Kwiatkowski reported that more than half of their 178 participants had been characterized as either being "somewhat too sensitive" or "overly sensitive" (p. 1115), a finding that led Shriberg and Kwiatkowski to state that "for intervention questions ... such information clearly confirms the need to account for psychosocial variables in the overall plan of treatment" (p. 1115). As these examples illustrate, temperament factors are ignored only at the peril of jeopardizing success when SLPs try to maximize therapeutic efficacy for children with speech sound disorders.

## CONCLUSIONS

It is clear from the literature reviewed that clinical investigators are generally aware that a one-size-fits-all approach to selecting treatment for speech sound disorders, as Powell (2008) noted, ignores the diversity of potential for change represented by the individual children who make up our clinical caseloads.

If it is true that you can lead a horse to water but cannot make him (or her) drink, then it is likewise also true that you cannot force your clients to correctly produce a speech sound, you can only provide the tools for them to do so. Ultimately, the client decides whether or not new sounds will be incorporated into his or her sound system. Our job is to serve as consistent, knowledgeable guide, supporter, and in some cases, cheering section. And, one of the best ways we can fulfill those roles is by accurately determining what our starting point truly is when we begin the therapy process by knowing who our client is. As I hope this chapter has demonstrated, this cannot be accomplished without a more comprehensive evaluation than of that young client's phonetic and phonemic inventories. Knowledge of our clients' capability and focus, as Kwiatkowski and Shriberg (1993) explained, along with careful observation of how an individual client can be best taught are both critical aspects of the science and art of therapy decision making.

## REFERENCES

American Speech-Language-Hearing Association. (2008). *2008 schools survey summary report: Number and type of responses*. Rockville, MD: Author.

Baker, E., & McLeod, S. (2004). Evidence-based management of phonological impairment in children. *Child Language Teaching and Therapy, 20*, 261–285.

Bauman-Waengler, I. (2004). *Articulatory and phonological impairments: A clinical focus* (2nd ed.). Boston: Allyn & Bacon.

Bernthal, J., & Bankson, N., & Flipsen, P., Jr. (2009). *Articulation and phonological disorders: Speech sound disorders in children* (6th ed.). Boston: Allyn & Bacon.

Bleile, K. (2006). *The late eight*. San Diego: Plural Publishing Inc.

Bloch, E., & Goodstein, L. (1971). Functional speech disorders and personality: A decade of research. *Journal of Speech and Hearing Disorders, 36*, 295–314.

Campbell, T., Dollaghan, C., Rockette, H., Paradise, J., Feldman, H., Shriberg, L., et al. (2003). Risk factors for speech delay of unknown origin in 3-year-old children. *Child Development, 74*, 346–357.

Davis, B. (2005). Goal and target selection for developmental speech disorders. In A. Kamhi & K. Pollock (Eds.), *Phonological disorders in children: Clinical decision making in assessment and intervention* (pp. 89–100). Baltimore: Paul H. Brookes Publishing Co.

Edwards, M., & Shriberg, L. (1983). *Phonology: Applications in communicative disorders*. San Diego, CA: College-Hill Press.

Felsenfeld, S., Broen, P., & McGue, M. (1994). A 28-year follow-up of adults with a history of moderate phonological disorder: Educational and occupational results. *Journal of Speech and Hearing Research, 37*, 1341–1353.

Fey, M., Cleave, P., Ravida, A., Long, S., Dejmal, A., & Easton, D. (1994). Effects of grammar facilitation on the phonological performance of children with speech and language impairments. *Journal of Speech and Hearing Research, 37*, 594–607.

Fujiki, M., Brinton, B., Isaacson, T., & Summers, C. (2001). Social behaviors of children with language impairment on the playground: A pilot study. *Language, Speech, and Hearing Services in Schools, 32*, 101–113.

Gierut, J. (1998). Treatment efficacy: Functional phonological disorders in children. *Journal of Speech, Language, and Hearing Research, 41*, S85–S100.

Gierut, J. (2001). Complexity in phonological treatment: Clinical factors. *Language, Speech, and Hearing Services in Schools, 32*, 229–241.

Gierut, J. (2005). Phonological intervention: The how or the what? In A. Kamhi & K. Pollock (Eds.), *Phonological disorders in children: Clinical decision making in assessment and intervention* (pp. 201–210). Baltimore: Paul H. Brookes Publishing Co., Inc.

Gierut, J., Elbert, M., & Dinnsen, D. (1987). A functional analysis of phonological knowledge and generalization learning in misarticulating children. *Journal of Speech and Hearing Research, 30*, 462–479.

Gierut, J., Morrisette, M., Hughes, M., & Rowland, S. (1996). Phonological treatment efficacy and developmental norms. *Language, Speech, and Hearing Services in Schools, 27*, 215–230.

Gildersleeve-Neumann, C. (2007). Treatment for childhood apraxia of speech: A description of integral stimulation and motor learning. *The ASHA Leader, 12*, 10–13, 30.

Gillam, S., & Gillam, R. (2006). Making evidence-based decisions about child-language intervention in schools. *Language, Speech, and Hearing Services in Schools, 37*, 304–315.

Goffman, L. (1999). Prosodic influences on speech production in children with specific language impairment: Kinematic, acoustic, and transcription evidence. *Journal of Speech, Language, and Hearing Research, 42*, 1499–1517.

Goffman, L. (2004). Kinematic differentiation of prosodic categories in normal and disordered language development. *Journal of Speech, Language, and Hearing Research, 47*, 1088–1102.

Goffman, L. (2005). Assessment and clarification: An integrative model of language and motor contributions to phonological development. In A. Kamhi & K. Pollock (Eds.), *Phonological disorders in children: Clinical decision making in assessment and intervention* (pp. 51–64). Baltimore: Paul H. Brookes Publishing Co.

Hawk, S. (1948). Personality measurement in speech correction. *Journal of Speech and Hearing Disorders, 13*, 307–312.

Hayhow, R. (1987). Personal construct therapy with children who stutter and their families. In C. Levy (Ed.), *Stuttering therapies: Practical approaches* (pp. 1–18). London: Croom Helm.

Hodson, B., & Paden, E. (1991). *Targeting intelligible speech* (2nd ed.). Austin, TX: Pro-Ed.

Hoff, E. (2009). *Language development* (4th ed.). Belmont, CA: Wadsworth/Cengage Learning.

Holland, A., Fromm, D., DeRuyter, F., & Stein, M. (1996). Treatment efficacy: Aphasia. *Journal of Speech, Language, and Hearing Research, 39*, S27–S36.

Kamhi, A. (2000). Practice makes perfect: The incompatibility of practicing speech and meaningful communication. *Language, Speech and Hearing Services in Schools, 31*, 182–185.

Kamhi, A. (2006). Treatment decisions for children with speech-sound disorders. *Language, Speech, and Hearing Services in Schools, 37*, 271–279.

Kent, R. (1992). The biology of phonological development. In C. Ferguson, L. Menn, & C. Stoel-Gammon (Eds.), *Phonological development: Models, research, implications* (pp. 65–90). Timonium, MD: York Press.

Kwiatkowski, J., & Shriberg, L. (1993). Speech normalization in developmental phonological disorders: A retrospective study of capability-focus theory. *Language, Speech, and Hearing Services in Schools, 24*, 10–18.

Leonard, L., Newhoff, M., & Mesalem, L. (1980). Individual differences in early child phonology. *Applied Psycholinguistics, 1*, 7–30.

Lewis, B., Ekelman, B., & Aram, D. (1989). A familial study of severe phonological disorders. *Journal of Speech, Language, and Hearing Research, 32*, 713–724.

Lewis, B., Shriberg, L., Freebairn, L., Hansen, A., Stein, C., Taylor, H., & Iyengar, S. (2006). The genetic bases of speech sound disorders: Evidence from spoken and written language. *Journal of Speech, Language, and Hearing Research, 49*, 1294–1312.

McLeod, S., van Doorn, J., & Reed, V. (2001). Consonant cluster development in two year olds: General trends and individual difference. *Journal of Speech, Language, and Hearing Research, 44*, 1144–1171.

Miccio, A. (2005). A treatment program for enhancing stimulability. In A. Kamhi and K. Pollock (Eds.), *Phonological disorders in children: Clinical decision making in assessment and intervention* (pp. 163–174). Baltimore: Paul H. Brookes Publishing Co.

Miccio, A., Elbert, M., & Forrest, K. (1999). The relationship between stimulability and phonological acquisition in children with normally developing and disordered phonologies. *American Journal of Speech-Language Pathology, 8*, 347–363.

National Institute on Deafness and Other Communication Disorders. (n.d.). *Statistics on voice, speech, and language*. Retrieved August 22, 2008, from http://www.nidcd.nih.gov/health/statistics/vsl.asp#2

Newman, P., Creaghead, N., & Secord, W. (1985). *Assessment and remediation of articulatory and phonological disorders*. Columbus, OH: Charles E. Merrill Publishing Company.

Paul, R., & Shriberg, L. (1982). Associations between phonology and syntax in speech-delayed children. *Journal of Speech and Hearing Research, 25*, 536–547.

Powell, T. (1996). Stimulability considerations in the treatment of a child with a persistent disorder of speech sound production. *Journal of Communication Disorders, 29*, 315–333.

Powell, T. (2008). The use of nonspeech oral motor treatments for developmental speech sound production disorders: Interventions and interactions. *Language, Speech, and Hearing Services in Schools, 39*, 374–379.

Powell, T., & Miccio, A. (1996). Stimulability: A useful clinical tool. *Journal of Communication Disorders, 29*, 237–254.

Reid, G. (1947). The etiology and nature of functional articulatory defects in elementary school children. *Journal of Speech and Hearing Disorders, 12*, 143–150.

Rvachew, S., & Nowak, M. (2001). The effect of target-selection strategy on phonological learning. *Journal of Speech, Language, and Hearing Research, 44*, 610–623.

Rvachew, S., Rafaat, S., & Martin, M. (1999). Stimulability, speech perception skills, and the treatment of phonological disorders. *American Journal of Speech-Language Pathology, 8*, 33–43.

Shriberg, L. (1982). Toward classification of developmental phonological disorders. In N. Lass (Ed.), *Speech and language: Advances in basic research and practice* (pp. 2–18). New York: Academic Press.

Shriberg, L. (1997). Developmental phonological disorders: One or many? In B. Hodson & M. L. Edwards (Eds.), *Perspectives in applied phonology* (pp. 105–131). Gaithersburg, MD: Aspen Publishers, Inc.

Shriberg, L., Flipsen, P., Thielke, H., Kwiatkowski, J., Kertoy, M., Nellis, R., et al. (2000). Risk for speech disorder associated with early recurrent otitis media with effusion: Two retrospective studies. *Journal of Speech, Language, and Hearing Research, 43*, 79–99.

Shriberg, L., Gruber, F., & Kwiatkowski, J. (1994). Developmental phonological disorders III: Long-term speech-sound normalization. *Journal of Speech and Hearing Research, 37*, 1151–1177.

Shriberg, L., Kent, R., Karlsson, H., Nadler, C., & Brown, R. (2003). A diagnostic marker for speech delay associated with otitis media with effusion: Backing of obstruents. *Clinical Linguistics and Phonetics, 17*, 529–547.

Shriberg, L., & Kwiatkowski, J. (1982a). Phonological disorders I: A diagnostic classification system. *Journal of Speech and Hearing Disorders, 47*, 226–241.

Shriberg, L., & Kwiatkowski, J. (1982b). Phonological disorders II: A conceptual framework for management. *Journal of Speech and Hearing Disorders, 47,* 242–256.

Shriberg, L., & Kwiatkowski, J. (1994). Developmental phonological disorders I: A clinical profile. *Journal of Speech and Hearing Research, 37,* 1100–1126.

Shriberg, L., Kwiatkowski, J., Gruber, F. (1994). Developmental phonological disorders II: Short-term speech-sound normalization. *Journal of Speech and Hearing Research, 37,* 1127–1150.

Shriberg, L., Lewis, B., Tomblin, J., McSweeny, J., Karlsson, H., & Scheer, A. (2005). Toward diagnostic and phenotypic markers for genetically transmitted speech delay. *Journal of Speech, Language, and Hearing Research, 48,* 834–852.

Shriberg, L., Tomblin, J., and McSweeny, J. (1999). Prevalence of speech delay in 6-year-old children and comorbidity with language impairment. *Journal of Speech, Language, and Hearing Research, 42,* 1461–1481.

Smit, A., Hand, L., Freilinger, J., Bernthal, J., & Bird, A. (1990). The Iowa articulation norms project and its Nebraska replication. *Journal of Speech and Hearing Disorders, 55,* 779–798.

Stoel-Gammon, C. (2007). Variability in speech acquisition. In S. McLeod (Ed.), *The international guide to speech acquisition* (pp. 55–60). Clifton Park, NY: Thomson Delmar Learning.

Strelau, J. (1998). *Temperament: A psychological perspective.* New York: Plenum Press.

Tyler, A. (2008). What works: Evidence-based intervention for children with speech sound disorders. *Seminars in Speech and Language, 29*(4), 320–330.

Tyler, A. (2005). Promoting generalization: Selecting, scheduling, and integrating goals. In A. Kamhi & K. Pollock (Eds.), *Phonological disorders in children: Clinical decision making in assessment and intervention* (pp. 67–75). Baltimore: Paul H. Brookes Publishing Co.

Tyler, A., Lewis, K., Haskill, A., & Tolbert, L. (2003). Outcomes of different speech and language goal attack strategies. *Journal of Speech, Language, and Hearing Research, 46,* 1077–1094.

Tyler, A., & Sandoval, K. (1994). Preschoolers with phonological and language disorders: Treating different linguistic domains. *Language, Speech, and Hearing Services in Schools, 25,* 215–234.

Van Riper, C. (1972). *Speech correction: Principles and methods* (5th ed.). Englewood Cliffs, NJ: Prentice-Hall, Inc.

Weiss, A. (2004). The child as agent for change in therapy for phonological disorders. *Child Language Teaching and Therapy, 20,* 221–244.

Weiss, A. (2007). Personal factors and their influence on speech acquisition. In S. McLeod (Ed.). *The international guide to speech acquisition* (pp. 91–95). Clifton Park, NY: Thomson Delmar Learning.

Weston, A., & Bain, B. (2003, November). *Current v. evidence-based practice in phonological intervention: A dilemma.* Poster session presented to the Annual Convention of the American Speech-Language-Hearing Association, Chicago.

Winitz, H. (1969). *Articulatory acquisition and behavior.* New York: Appleton-Century-Crofts, Inc.

Wood, K. (1946). Parental maladjustment and functional articulatory defects in children. *Journal of Speech and Hearing Disorders, 11,* 255–275.

# 9 Consideration of Individual Differences in Speech Development, Outcome, and Management
## *Children With Cleft Lip and Palate*

*Kathy L. Chapman and Mary A. Hardin-Jones*

## INTRODUCTION

Children with isolated cleft lip and palate[1] are often described as a heterogeneous group. Although many have normal speech and language development, it is estimated that more than 50% of these children require intervention for speech and language delays at some point (Hardin-Jones & Jones, 2005; Peterson-Falzone, Hardin-Jones, and Karnell, 2009). Much that has been written about individual differences for children with speech sound disorders (see Weiss, Chapter 8, this volume) is likely applicable to children with cleft palate. At the same time, because of the nature of clefting and the resulting effect on speech production, there are factors that are unique to this population. As with a number of areas in the field of communication disorders, there is a lack of well-designed intervention studies. In addition, those that are available have rarely provided information about individual participant characteristics and how those characteristics affected outcome. The literature on this subject, along with the larger body of work examining speech and language development of these children, will guide us as we explore the individual child characteristics that influence our intervention planning and the successful outcomes. In this chapter, we provide (a) a brief overview of speech and language development of children with cleft palate, with an emphasis on individual differences in speech acquisition; (b) a discussion of the individual

---

[1] This chapter focuses on children with cleft palate with/without cleft lip. Therefore, the term cleft palate will be used throughout to refer to this group of children.

differences that are unique and not so unique to this population that will likely influence management decisions and outcome; and (c) a review of the speech intervention literature for children with cleft palate, highlighting (when possible) individual client characteristics that may have influenced study findings.

## INDIVIDUAL DIFFERENCES IN SPEECH DEVELOPMENT OF CHILDREN WITH CLEFT PALATE

Over the past 50 years, numerous studies have examined the speech skills of children with cleft palate. Almost without exception, group studies comparing children with cleft palate and their noncleft peers at any age from infancy to adolescence report that children with cleft palate are behind age expectations for speech development (see Peterson-Falzone et al., 2009, for a review). At the same time, there are many children with cleft palate who seem to catch up in terms of speech development soon after palatal repair and exhibit normal speech development from a young age (Hardin-Jones & Chapman, 2008; Jones, Chapman, & Hardin-Jones, 2003). As most large-scale research studies are interested in describing group differences, it is not clear exactly how many children with cleft palate exhibit normal speech at all stages of development and how many achieve it following intervention. However, a few studies have documented either the percentage of children who received or were referred for intervention (Broen, Moller, Devers, & Doyle, 1996; Dalston, 1990; Hardin-Jones & Jones, 2005; Sell et al., 2001) or the percentage of children who exhibited normal speech sound development at the time of examination. In these latter studies, some of the children achieved normal speech after a period of intervention (Chapman, 2004a, 2008, 2009). Regardless, reports of the percentage of children who never required intervention during the preschool years ranged from 16% (Sell et al., 2001) to approximately 50% (Broen et al., 1996). That number decreased to 25% by 14–15 years of age (Dalston, 1990). Also, the number of children reportedly exhibiting normal speech sound development was 38–40% at age 3 (Chapman, 2004a; Chapman et al., 2008) and 46% at ages 5–6 (Chapman, 2009).

### PRESPEECH DEVELOPMENT

Although the age at time of primary palatal surgery continues to decrease in the United States, most babies undergo palate repair at approximately 10–12 months of age (mean age of 11 months; Hueberner & Marsh, 2002). Although this is earlier than was typical in the past, babies are still beginning the process of language learning with a mechanism that is inadequate for speech. Not surprisingly, studies of the early prespeech development of babies with cleft palate (during the 1st year of life and prior to primary palatal repair) have found babies with cleft palate to be delayed compared with noncleft babies on most measures of early vocal development (Chapman, 1991; Chapman, Hardin-Jones, Schulte, & Halter, 2001; Scherer, Williams, & Proctor-Williams, 2008). Although variability characterizes both groups of babies at this stage of development, there is less individual variation for the babies with cleft palate for production of stop consonants.[2] In a longitudinal, multicenter study of speech and language development of young children with cleft palate, our findings indicated that whereas most noncleft babies produced a range of stops varying in place of articulation and voicing, there was considerable variability across babies in the individual stops that were produced. In contrast, fewer stops were produced by the babies with cleft palate, and when they were produced, they included bilabial (and voiced), velar, or glottal stops. Although the means for size of consonant inventories and production of canonical syllables were smaller for the babies with cleft palate, the amount of variability within the two groups was similar (Chapman et al., 2001). In the first case, the mean size of consonant inventory for the babies with cleft palate was half of what was seen for the noncleft babies (5 versus 10, respectively); however, three babies produced 8 different consonants (equal to the smallest number of consonants produced by any of the noncleft babies), and two babies produced only 2 different sounds. Similarly, in terms of canonical babbling, variability was observed not only in the makeup of these syllables (see above) but in the number of canonical syllables produced. Across the sample of 30 babies, the canonical babbling ratios ranged from 0 (i.e., no canonical syllables) to 0.62 (i.e., 62% of syllables were canonical). So, in spite of the fact that these babies were similar in that all had an unrepaired cleft of the hard and soft palate, the impact of clefting on early speech development was quite variable.

One of the most interesting aspects of individual differences noted in the 9-month-olds tested in this study was related to production of stop consonants. Even though all babies had unrepaired clefts, some of them produced oral stops and others did not. This ability to produce oral stops at 9 months (and prior to palatal surgery) was related to speech production abilities at 21 months (Chapman, Hardin-Jones & Halter, 2003). However, the relationship between speech skills in the early postsurgery period and later performance appeared even stronger, as oral stop production postsurgery was related to speech and lexical skills at 21 months (Chapman et al., 2003).

Interestingly, although children with cleft palate continue to show individual variability in their production of stop consonants over time, the relationship between stop production and later speech and language performance is not as straightforward at it appears on the basis of the findings of Chapman et al. (2003). While a majority of babies with good oral stop production beginning in the presurgery period have good speech outcomes, this is not true for all children with cleft palate. Chapman (2004a) was interested in determining whether the findings of Chapman et al. (2003) would be replicated if speech outcomes were examined at 39 months rather than 21 months. No significant correlations were noted between the speech measures presurgery or postsurgery and speech outcomes at 39 months. Surprisingly, negative correlations were observed between two speech

---

[2] Although stop consonants occur frequently in the babbling of typically developing babies, the absence of oral stops in the babbling of babies with cleft palate is attributed to the inability to generate the intraoral air pressure needed for their production.

measures presurgery and language outcome measures, but positive correlations were noted between oral stop production postsurgery and the language outcome measures. Examination of the individual child data suggested that some of the babies who were good babblers presurgery exhibited velopharyngeal inadequacy (VPI) postsurgery, which, not surprisingly, resulted in poor speech outcomes at 39 months. In addition, a few babies with very poor performance presurgery had normal speech production skills at 39 months following a period of speech-language intervention.

In spite of these findings, for individual children, oral stop production in the postsurgery period is a good predictor of the need for intervention. In a retrospective study of the impact of early intervention for toddlers with cleft palate, not only was stop production an important referral criteria, but it was a fairly stable predictor of those children who would continue to do well (i.e., were not referred for intervention) as late as 3 years of age (Hardin-Jones & Chapman, 2008). Interestingly, although the presence and acquisition of stops in the postsurgery period is a good indicator of which individual children will have a good speech outcome, the absence or slow acquisition of stops in the same period is not as accurate in predicting a poor speech outcome. For example, in a study by Jones et al. (2003), there was never an example of a toddler who showed substantial gains in size of consonant inventory and production of stops approximately 5 months postsurgery who demonstrated a poor speech outcome at age 3. In contrast, there were several toddlers who showed little change in the first 5 months postsurgery but who were judged to have normal speech and resonance at age 3, following a period of intervention.

In order to describe the individual variation in the speech development of children with cleft palate over time, we combined the data from Chapman et al. (2003) and Chapman (2004a) and standardized the children's scores on the speech and language measures across the four assessment points. By comparing within and across the 15 children, we were able to describe individual paths of development from presurgery to 39 months of age. Furthermore, as we now have information on their final resonance outcomes, we consider velopharyngeal status in our descriptions of the four profiles.

## BOX 9.1 VARIABLE PATHS OF DEVELOPMENT

First, the children were divided into two groups based on their velopharyngeal status (adequate velopharyngeal function [AVPF], velopharyngeal inadequacy [VPI]). In the first group, approximately one half of the children exhibited speech within normal limits at 39 months, and the rest exhibited delayed speech. Of those with AVPF, two were never referred or enrolled in intervention. An examination of their progress over time suggested that they were a bit below their peers with cleft palate presurgery, but after primary palatal repair at approximately 12 months, they began to show steady improvement across the study period. This pattern of change was similar for another child who also exhibited normal speech and language at 39 months, but he had the benefit of early intervention starting when he was only 1 year of age. Both of these patterns are different from that exhibited by two other boys with AVPF and normal speech development at 39 months. These boys exhibited performance below their peers presurgery, but did not begin to show consistent and significant improvement in speech postsurgery or by 21 months. However, at 39 months and following a period of intervention, both boys were within normal limits for speech and language. The final three children had AVPF but delayed speech at 39 months. Interestingly, two of the three showed inconsistent but better than average performance (compared with peers with cleft palate) postsurgery and at 21 months, but by 39 months they were delayed in speech development. The final child, after good performance presurgery, began to show delays postsurgery that continued until 39 months in spite of the fact that he was enrolled in intervention at 17 months.

The children in the VPI group also followed varied paths of development. One of these children stands out as unusual because in spite of the fact that he exhibited moderate hypernasality, he was producing all sounds expected for his age at 39 months. An examination of his speech and language performance until that time indicated that he performed below his peers on all measures presurgery, postsurgery, and at 21 months of age. This profile is especially interesting as he was not enrolled in intervention at any time over the period of the study.

As mentioned above, several of the children in this study had good speech production abilities in the presurgery period. In fact, four of the children with VPI scored at least 1 standard deviation above the mean for the children with cleft palate on at least one of the speech outcome measures presurgery. Interestingly, the four varied in how quickly they began to perform below their peers with cleft palate. One began to show a decline in performance postsurgery, two did not really show a decline until 21 months, and the final child exhibited good speech and language skills until 39 months of age. The two exhibited more mixed profiles, as their performance was not uniformly poor across ages and measures. Interestingly, although these last two children had been referred for intervention, only one was enrolled in intervention at 39 months.

## Speech Development Postsurgery

The expectation is that primary palatal surgery (including closure of the hard and soft palate) will provide the child with an adequate mechanism for normal speech development. Although this is true for a majority of children with cleft palate, approximately 20% of children will require additional surgery at some point in time to establish adequate velopharyngeal function (Peterson-Falzone et al., 2009). Regardless of velopharyngeal status following primary surgery, a majority also require speech-language intervention (Hardin-Jones & Jones, 2005), which highlights the difficulty that many children with cleft palate experience in learning the sound system of their language. Our studies examining speech development post-palatal closure have suggested that as a group, toddlers with cleft palate were delayed compared with noncleft peers for size of consonant inventory and production of oral stops, with the exception of /p/, at 17 (Jones et al., 2003) and 21 (Chapman et al., 2003) months of age. At this later age, liquids were also less frequently correct in the speech of the toddlers with cleft palate. The differences between the performance of the two groups would likely have been greater except that few fricatives and affricates are produced by typically developing toddlers at this young age.

Some of the most interesting findings characterizing the speech development of toddlers with cleft palate were not the group findings but data that focused on individual children's acquisition of phonology in the 2nd year of life. For example, Jones et al. (2003) provided data comparing consonant inventories of 14 children with cleft palate and their individually matched peers at 17 months and approximately 5 months postsurgery. These comparisons highlighted the differences in development for toddlers with cleft palate postsurgery as the number of consonants that were added to each child's inventory ranged from as few as one to as many as nine different sounds. In addition, 5 of the 14 toddlers with cleft palate seemed to be catching up in terms of speech development, as their consonant inventories were equal to or larger than those of their matched peers.

In a different study, Estrem and Broen (1989) examined the lexical selectivity of five toddlers with cleft palate during the single word period (children ranged in age from 16.5 to 24 months of age). Group data suggested that compared to noncleft toddlers, these toodlers attempted more words with initial nasals, vowels, approximates, and sounds produced at the extreme places of articulation (i.e., labial and glottal) of vocal tract. However, individual child data suggested that only three of the five children followed this pattern. Another child followed a different pattern and actually attempted more words containing word initial stops and fricatives and multisyllabic words. She also had a "production template for multisyllabic words": a repeated CVCV sequence containing a pharyngeal stop and a vowel (p. 19). The last child also attempted more words containing initial stops, but the stops were preceded by homorganic nasals (e.g., *ball* became *mba*) (p. 20). As might be expected, the latter two were the least accurate in terms of matches with the target. In addition to documenting lexical selectivity in children with cleft palate, these data showed individual differences in learning styles among these five children. The first three appeared to be following a style where they chose words with sounds that were within their phonological capabilities. This pattern is similar (although not identical) to that originally described by Ferguson (1979) as "the cautious system-builder" (p. 196). In contrast, the last two toddlers were willing to try words containing sounds that were not as easily produced and appeared to be more willing to be less intelligible as a result. In both cases, they employed idiosyncratic patterns that may have been related to palatal clefting.

One of the most obvious examples of individual differences in the speech sound development of typically developing children (e.g., Goad & Ingram, 1987; Leonard, Newhoff, & Masalem, 1980; McLeod, van Doorn, & Reed, 2001; Vihman, Ferguson, & Elbert 1986; Vihman & Greenlee, 1987), as well as children with developmental phonological disorders (see Shriberg, Gruber, & Kwiatkowski, 1994), is variability across children in age of mastery for the various sounds. Similar variability can be seen in the consonant inventories of children with cleft palate in the 1st year of life (Chapman et al., 2001; Scherer et al., 2008) and at 2 (Chapman & Hardin, 1992) and 3 (Chapman, 2004a; Scherer, Williams, & Proctor-Williams, 2008) years of age. Some of the variability noted in the data for 2- and 3-year-olds is likely related to the fact that each of these samples included children with normal speech development, children with delayed speech development, and children with delayed speech development and VPI. However, even when we examined the stable consonant usage of our 3-year-old children with cleft palate who were functioning within normal limits for speech development, there were differences across children in sounds that were mastered (i.e., were produced with at least 70% accuracy), as seen in Table 9.1.

## OLDER CHILDREN

As has been documented in the literature for typically developing children and children with developmental phonological disorders (see Shriberg et al., 1994 for a review), speech production skills improve with age. In fact, studies of age of acquisition for children learning English suggest that all sounds are acquired by

---

**TABLE 9.1**
**Individual Differences in Sound Production at 39 Months: Stable Consonants**

| Stable Consonant | Percentage of Children |
|---|---|
| b, p, m, n, w, j, h | 100% |
| k, g, f, s | >80% |
| ʃ | >70% |
| v, tʃ | 50% |
| d, ŋ, r | >20% |
| t, l, z, θ, ð, ʒ, dʒ | <20% |

8 to 9 years of age (Smit, Hand, Freilinger, Bernthal, & Bird, 1990). Research on speech normalization of children with developmental speech sound disorders who were enrolled in intervention as preschoolers suggests that many of these children normalize by age 6 (Shriberg, Kwiatkowski, & Gruber, 1994), with most of the remaining showing normalization by 8½ years of age (Shriberg, Gruber, et al., 1994). Unfortunately, comparable longitudinal speech data are not available for children with cleft palate. The collection of such data is complicated by a number of factors, the most obvious being that children with cleft palate form a highly heterogeneous group, and normalization occurs over a longer period of time. Also, the study sample may be biased toward inclusion of individuals with poorer speech, as those with good speech are less likely to be followed by craniofacial teams over time. Finally, the older the children at the time when speech skills are examined, the less likely it is that the findings can be generalized to children who are the same age but born more recently than the comparison cohort (Peterson-Falzone et al., 2001). These later-born children have the benefit of advances in management that typically result in better speech outcome (e.g., Counihan, 1960; Peterson-Falzone et al., 2001; Riski, 1995; Van Demark, Morris, & VandeHaar, 1979). With these cautions in mind, examination of longitudinal data reported over several treatment centers and over many years (Van Demark et al.; Karnell & Van Demark, 1986; Lohmander & Persson, 2008; Riski & DeLong, 1984) suggests that although significant improvement in speech development is occurring at younger ages, children with cleft palate do not perform as well as age-matched peers at 7 (Lohmander & Persson, 2008), 8 (Riski & DeLong, 1984); 16 (Karnell & Van Demark, 1986), or even 18 (e.g., Van Demark et al., 1979) years of age. At these later ages, although some of the variability in performance may still be related to velopharyngeal function, dentition and malocclusion (and their management) play a more significant role (see below). Again, these reports do not mention the number of children with normal speech development. However, several companion papers by Bardach, Morris, and colleagues (Bardach et al., 1984, 1990, 1992; Morris et al., 1993) described speech outcomes for adolescents with different cleft types. They reported normal speech in 57% of the group with bilateral cleft lip and palate but did not provide this type of information for adolescents with other cleft types. For those who continued to have speech problems, we know that speech sound distortions were a common finding.

## INDIVIDUAL DIFFERENCES: INFLUENCES ON CLINICAL DECISION MAKING AND SUCCESSFUL OUTCOME

Prior to sitting down at the computer to write this chapter, the first thing we did was list individual differences that might influence clinical decision making and/or successful outcomes for children with cleft palate. During the course of that exercise, what struck us was how often, as we identified the potential sources of variation, the discussion led us to recall a particular child (and sometimes a family) whom we had seen clinically or who had participated in our research studies. Although the children were similar in that they had been born with a cleft palate, they were different in so many other ways. Each of these children brought something unique to our understanding of speech development and disorders of children with cleft palate. This suggested to us how important each individual child's unique personal characteristics are to his or her success. Weiss (2004; Chapter 8, this volume) has provided excellent discussions of how these personal characteristics influence intervention outcomes for children with speech sound disorders, as well as how we as clinicians should think about these variables in intervention planning. The same concepts are applicable to children with cleft palate who exhibit speech sound delays.

## ROLE OF VELOPHARYNGEAL FUNCTION IN THE MANAGEMENT OF CHILDREN WITH CLEFT PALATE

Velopharyngeal function is one of the most important factors influencing intervention planning and successful speech outcome for children with cleft palate. It can influence rate of speech development, selection of therapy goals, and rate of improvement achieved by children in therapy. Although definitive assessment of velopharyngeal function (e.g., imaging study) is not typically carried out for most children until 3–4 years of age, perceptual evidence of VPI, including hypernasality and audible nasal emission, may be evident as early as a child's first words. Another possible early indicator of VPI following surgical repair of the palate is the absence of oral stops in the child's consonant inventory. As described above, some children with repaired cleft palate avoid production of oral stops. In some cases, they may attempt only words with nonpressure consonants (e.g., vowels, nasals, or approximates), or they may attempt words with pressure consonants but produce nasal substitutions, glottal substitutions, or other consonants that do not require velopharyngeal closure (e.g. /h/). These latter substitutions exacerbate the perception of nasality and lead to an impression of gross VPI (Peterson-Falzone et al., 2009). Until the child begins attempting production of oral stop consonants, it is not possible to evaluate the functional potential of the velopharyngeal mechanism. This latter point is critical to any study of velopharyngeal function. Since velopharyngeal closure is required for the production of pressure consonants (e.g., stops, fricatives, and affricates), these types of consonants must be present in a child's speech in order to study the functional potential of the velopharyngeal mechanism (Peterson-Falzone et al., 2009). If they are not present, establishing correct placement for these sounds (ignoring nasal emission and/or hypernasality) is a treatment priority (Peterson-Falzone, Trost-Cardamone, Karnell, & Hardin-Jones, 2006).

Differential diagnosis of VPI is critical for establishing appropriate management decisions. Although nasal emission is typically associated with VPI, at times nasal emission will be present without hypernasality and will be evident only on select consonants. In such cases, the pattern of nasal emission can provide important information about the nature of the problem. *Phoneme-specific nasal emission*, which is a learned behavior, typically involves nasal emission on one or more of the sibilants /s, z, ʃ/ (sometimes /tʃ, dʒ/). Nasal emission evident only on /p, b, t, d, s, z/ may be indicative of an *anterior palatal fistula*, whereas nasal emission on only

/k, g/ is typically associated with a *posterior palatal fistula* (Trost-Cardamone, 1990; Peterson-Falzone et al., 2009). Of course, phoneme-specific nasal emission and nasal emission due to VPI would be managed differently. In the case of phoneme-specific nasal emission, therapy would be recommended to eliminate the learned behavior. For nasal emission secondary to VPI, therapy would not be recommended.

Some speech-language pathologists (SLPs) who have had little experience in the area of cleft palate often assume (or may have been taught) that speech therapy should not be recommended for children with VPI because their errors are the result of structural inadequacy and therefore cannot be modified with behavioral interventions. Although that is true under some circumstances, for a majority of children with suspected VPI, speech therapy is indicated prior to any referral for an objective assessment of velopharyngeal function. Whether or not speech therapy is indicated for a child with suspected VPI will depend on each child's individual profile. The two cases described in Box 9.2 provide guidelines for when a child suspected of VPI would be referred for intervention versus when the child would be referred for an objective evaluation of velopharyngeal function.

## BOX 9.2   CASE STUDIES 1 AND 2

### CASE 1: R.F.
#### Description
R.F. was born with a unilateral cleft of the lip and palate. His palate was closed at 12 months 13 days. Pressure equalizing (PE) tubes were placed for the first time at lip surgery (4 months). He had at least six bouts of otitis media (OM) over a 3-year period (based on parent report and review of physician records) and had passed all audiological evaluations performed at regular craniofacial team visits. No palatal fistulae were present. R.F. had not been enrolled in therapy. Results of a speech and language assessment at 39 months revealed the following:

- Correct production of all age-appropriate sounds, although audible nasal emission was noted on production of fricatives
- No compensatory articulations
- Moderate hypernasality during conversational speech
- Receptive and expressive language skills within normal limits as measured by the Preschool Language Scale
- Mean length of utterance (MLU) and number of different words were low normal

#### Recommendation
R.F. was referred for an objective evaluation of velopharyngeal function.

### Rationale

The hypernasality and nasal emission in R.F.'s speech could not be modified with speech therapy.

### CASE 2: B.P.

#### Description

B.P. was born with a bilateral cleft of the lip and palate. His palate was closed at 13 months 19 days. PE tubes were placed at 6 months. B.P. had 16 documented cases of OM by 39 months of age (based on parent report and review of physician records) and had passed all audiological assessments at regular craniofacial team visits. No palatal fistulae were present. B.P. had been enrolled in therapy beginning at 27 months. Results of a speech and language assessment at 39 months revealed the following:

- A severe speech sound delay characterized by (a) a small inventory of stable consonants (i.e., only five sounds, /m, n, w, j, h/, were produced with greater than 70% accuracy), (b) glottal stop substitutions, and (c) nasal substitutions.
- Moderate hypernasality during conversational speech.
- Receptive and expressive language skills within normal limits as measured by the Preschool Language Scale.
- MLU was more than 1 standard deviation below the mean for his age, but the number of different words was low normal.

#### Recommendations

B.P. continue to receive speech and language therapy focusing on elimination of glottal stops and correct placement of age appropriate stops and fricatives.

#### Rationale

Speech therapy is effective in eliminating compensatory articulations and nasal substitutions, as well as in establishing correct placement for production of age-appropriate oral stops and fricatives. Correct placement for pressure consonants must be established prior to referral for an objective evaluation of velopharyngeal function.

## NATURE OF THE SPEECH PROBLEMS OF CHILDREN WITH CLEFT PALATE

### Articulation Versus Phonological

There is some debate about how the speech problems of children with cleft palate should be described. Traditionally, the speech problems of children with cleft palate have been considered organic and directly related to the structural deficits associated with clefting (i.e., articulation problems). More recently, however, some have suggested that the difficulties these children experience in speech production and even speech perception may also be phonological in nature (Chapman, 1993, 2008; Fey, 1992; Grunwell & Russell, 1988; Russell & Grunwell, 1993; Whitehill, Francis, & Ching, 2003). According to Fey, the speech development of young children with cleft palate illustrates how articulation and phonology are interrelated: "the child who cannot articulate the sounds of the language being learned will, necessarily, develop a phonology that differs in important ways from the adult phonology" (p. 228). The phonological rules they use, like those of all young children learning the sound system of their language, are the result of the limitations of the developing speech production mechanism and the impact of these limitations on certain sound classes. Fey and others have argued that a child with cleft palate may fail to produce certain sound contrasts (e.g., nasal–oral) because of structural limitations associated with clefting. These early patterns may not automatically disappear just because velopharyngeal function is restored but become part of the developing phonological system (e.g., Fey; Chapman, 1993; Grunwell & Russell, 1988; Russell & Grunwell, 1993).

We agree with the suggestions by Shriberg and Kwiatkowski (1982) and Weiss (Chapter 8, this volume) that is it important to determine the etiology of the speech sound delay for the purposes of planning intervention. At the same time, it should not be assumed that just because a child has a repaired cleft palate, his or her speech errors are only articulation based. Although many children with cleft palate may exhibit misarticulations secondary to VPI, fistulae, or dental deviations, there are probably almost equal numbers of children without these structural limitations (and some with these problems) who exhibit phonological-based errors. Each child's speech production system should be examined, taking into consideration information related to clefting (cleft type, age, type of surgery, etc.) and also knowledge about how articulation and phonology interact in speech sound learning. Such an approach will lead to intervention planning tailored to the individual child rather than to a particular diagnostic label.

## Compensatory Articulations

*Compensatory articulations* (CAs) are possibly the most talked about speech characteristic of children with cleft palate. CAs are sounds produced with constrictions inferior to the velopharyngeal port (e.g., glottal stops, pharyngeal fricatives) that are substituted for oral consonants (e.g., /b/ and /s/). These atypical patterns are thought to be a consequence of VPI and are considered to be difficult to eliminate, even with intervention. As is the case with all error patterns seen in this population, they are used by some children but not all. There is some indication that the number of children producing CAs is decreasing, and this observation is probably related to decreasing age at time of palatal surgery (Hardin-Jones & Jones, 2005). Furthermore, children vary in the actual CAs they produce, as well as in how consistently they are used as substitutions for more anterior consonants. In the past, clinicians thought that because these patterns were a consequence of VPI, they should not be targeted in therapy until after management of VPI. More recently, however, it has been suggested that surgical management be postponed until these errors are eliminated because as they are replaced with oral productions, velopharyngeal movement increases (Golding-Kushner, 1981; Henningsson & Isberg, 1986; Ysunza, Pamplona, & Toledo, 1992) and intelligibility improves (see Peterson-Falzone et al., 2009). Because CAs are considered deviant productions that are learned in response to a structural inadequacy, traditionally, articulation or motor-phonetic approaches have been employed in therapy (see Peterson-Falzone et al., 2006, for a description of these procedures). Interestingly, however, Pamplona, Ysunza, and Espinoza (1999) found that a phonological approach was faster than an articulation approach in eliminating CAs in children with CAs and VPI. These findings should be replicated, however, before abandoning the more traditional approaches entirely. More data are needed not only comparing the relative effectiveness of these approaches but analyzing the patterns of CA usage for a large number of children with cleft palate (Chapman, 2004b).

## PALATAL FISTULA

A palatal fistula (hole) typically reflects a failure in healing following surgical repair of the palate. Patency, size, and location are all important factors that will determine the extent to which a palatal fistula will influence speech for an individual child. Because the nasal and oral surfaces of the palate may be closed as separate layers during surgery, a fistula that is present on the oral surface of the palate is not necessarily patent (open) through the nasal surface. When a patent fistula is present, air can pass from the oral cavity through the fistula and result in either inaudible or audible nasal emission. We are not concerned about nasal emission that is not audible to the listener. Depending upon the size and shape of the fistula, however, the severity of audible nasal emission can severely distort pressure consonants and lead to an impression of VPI. As indicated above, however, the patterns of nasal emission associated with VPI and palatal fistula are different. VPI tends to impact most if not all pressure consonants, whereas fistulae tend to influence only those consonants produced with a constriction directly anterior to them. Therefore, audible nasal emission associated with anterior palatal fistulae (at the incisive foramen) would be evident on alveolar and labial obstruents, whereas that associated with posterior fistulae (at site of soft and hard palate juncture) would be evident only on velar stops (Peterson-Falzone et al., 2006, 2009). As with nasal emission due to VPI, nasal emission related to a palatal fistula cannot be modified with speech therapy.

Patent palatal fistulae can also influence a child's articulation. One CA pattern produced by children with repaired cleft palate is the middorsum palatal stop. This particular misarticulation has been observed as a substitution for alveolar and velar stops, and sounds equally like a /t/ and /k/ or a /d/ and /g/. Some clinicians have speculated that the presence of middorsum palatal stops in children with an anterior or central palatal fistula may represent the child's attempt to cover the fistula with the tongue and prevent nasal emission (Golding-Kushner, 2001; Hoch,

Golding-Kushner, Siegel-Sadewitz, and & Shprintzen, 1986; Peterson-Falzone et al., 2009). Whenever possible, a fistula should be obturated (either prosthetically or surgically) before attempting to modify place of articulation for these errors. When obturation cannot be accomplished in a timely fashion, Golding-Kushner noted that the fistula can be used as a placement target (e.g., "Put your tongue in front of the hole"; p. 110).

A child with repaired cleft palate who demonstrates inaudible nasal emission related to a palatal fistula should be carefully monitored during the early mixed dentition stage (i.e., 7–8 years of age). Palatal expansion performed prior to bone grafting of an alveolar cleft at that age can result in enlargement of the fistula and subsequent audible nasal emission.

## DENTAL/OCCLUSAL STATUS

Dental problems and malocclusions, including rotated anterior teeth, missing teeth, maxillary arch collapse, and crossbite, are common in children with cleft lip and palate. The combined impact of these problems coupled with changes to the oral cavity that occurs with orthodontic and orthognathic (surgery involving the jaw) management place these children at increased risk for oral distortions of sibilant fricatives and affricates. This type of error frequently accounts for the majority of articulation errors seen in older children and adolescents with cleft palate (Van Demark et al., 1979; Peterson-Falzone et al., 2009). However, as Peterson-Falzone et al. (2009) pointed out,

> It is not possible to fully account for the ability of speakers to adapt to or compensate for dental-occlusal anomalies, nor is it possible to predict the perceptual results when two or more problems interact.... The clinician must remember that although many individuals with clefts may demonstrate oral distortions that appear related to their dental-occlusal status, others may demonstrate perceptually adequate speech even when severe dental-occlusal problems are present. (p. 238)

When speech sound distortions are present and are severe enough to warrant intervention, trial therapy is typically initiated to determine whether the child can benefit from placement cues and sound shaping strategies in articulation therapy. If the child cannot modify the errors, then therapy is typically deferred until orthodontic or orthognathic surgery is complete.

The severity of dentition/occlusion in children with cleft palate is probably correlated to some degree with cleft type. The majority of group comparisons that have been conducted suggest that children with clefts involving the lip and palate are at greater risk for hypernasality and poorer articulation than children with isolated cleft palate (Brunnegard & Lohmander, 2007; Fletcher, 1978; Haapanen, 1994; Hardin-Jones & Jones, 2005; Riski & Delong, 1984). The extensive tissue deficiency associated with complete clefts of the lip and palate may account for differences noted in resonance, whereas the numerous dental/occlusal problems associated with the alveolar cleft (e.g., maxillary collapse, missing teeth, protrusion of the premaxilla) may explain the poorer articulation observed in these children.

## Language Status

Although data are not available regarding the co-occurrence of speech and language delay in children with cleft palate, most believe they are at risk for language delays. However, a review of studies examining the language skills of these children revealed a lack of consensus across studies, likely related to large individual variation across children and small sample sizes. There is also some suggestion that language delays in this population may be directly or indirectly related to speech delays (e.g., Broen, Devers, Doyle, Prouty, & Moller, 1998; Chapman, 2008; Chapman, Tecco Graham, Gooch, & Visconti, 1998; Frederickson, Chapman, & Hardin-Jones, 2006). Regardless, language status is an important variable influencing intervention planning and outcome for children with cleft palate.

Many toddlers with cleft palate who are enrolled in early intervention programs will present with delays in lexical development, as vocabulary deficits have been reported by a number of investigators (Broen et al., 1998; Chapman et al., 2003; Scherer & D'Antonio, 1995). In addition, although 6 of the 15 toddlers profiled here were performing below their peers without cleft palate on measures of lexical development at 21 months (Chapman et al., 2003), the remaining were either similar to or performing in advance of their peers without cleft palate.

As with any young child showing delays in both speech and language, it is not always easy to determine whether the child will benefit most from intervention focused on language, intervention focused on speech, or intervention targeting both areas. The results of research examining this question for children with speech and language delays without cleft palate have been inconclusive (see Tyler, 2005, for a review). However, work by Scherer, D'Antonio, et al. (2008) suggested that intervention focused on lexical development for toddlers with cleft palate resulted in improvements in vocabulary and speech production. However, because speech delays may be driving the lexical delays in this population (see Chapman, 2008), the approach described by Scherer and colleagues should be contrasted with an intervention program focusing on speech, while also measuring gains in both speech and lexical development to determine which is more efficacious. Although some children responded more positively than others to the intervention described in the Scherer, D'Antonio et al. (2008) study, age, severity of other impairments, and possibly velopharyngeal status were the only child factors cited as influencing a child's individual response to intervention. It is likely that the degree of impairment in speech versus language may have also had an impact on the child's progress in therapy.

Although not written specifically for young children with cleft palate, the recommendations of Stoel-Gammon and Stone (1991) have direct applicability to intervention planning for those young children with cleft palate showing delays in both speech and language. According to these authors, it is important to determine whether (a) the delays are equal in speech and language, (b) speech is more delayed than language, or (c) atypical errors are present in the child's speech. If assessment results suggest that speech and language competencies are "commensurate," a language-focused approach that provides the child with opportunities to produce new sounds within the context of lexical training may be most appropriate (Stoel-Gammon & Stone, 1991). For example, early vocabulary development might focus on acquisition of words containing bilabial stops that are not yet established in the child's sound system (for a description, see Scherer, 1999; Scherer, D'Antonio, et al., 2008). Alternatively, for toddlers whose speech development is slower than their language development, whether or not therapy is recommended may vary because of the age of the child, severity of the delay, and whether or not atypical patterns are present. For example, if the child is young, recently had primary palatal surgery, and is delayed but has begun to show improvements in speech development (especially acquisition of oral stops), this child might be monitored and reevaluated at 3-month intervals. In contrast, if the child exhibits atypical patterns (i.e., glottal productions, frequent use of vowel or nasal substitutions, etc.) regardless of language status, therapy focusing on elimination of these productions should be initiated (Stoel-Gammon & Stone, 1991).

As children with cleft palate grow older, they are less likely to exhibit delays in receptive or expressive language (see Chapman, 2008, for a review). However, research suggests they are at risk for deficits in conversational skills (Chapman et al., 1998; Frederickson et al., 2006) and prereading skills (Chapman, 2009), both of which seem to be related to severity of their speech delay. The idea that children with cleft palate might talk less frequently in an attempt to compensate for reduced speech intelligibility is not new (e.g., Faircloth & Faircloth, 1972; Morris, 1968; Scherer & D'Antonio, 1995). Using the conversational model proposed by Fey (1986), we attempted to examine this proposal (Chapman et al., 1998; Frederickson et al., 2006). Although a majority of children with cleft palate were found to be active conversationalists (i.e., assertive and responsive; Fey, 1986), approximately one fourth to one half of preschoolers fit the profile of a passive conversationalists (i.e., responsive but unassertive in conversation; Fey, 1986), and a few children were categorized as verbal noncommunicators (i.e., assertive but unresponsive in conversation; Fey, 1986) (Chapman et al., 1998; Frederickson et al., 2006). Because it appears that children may adopt a passive conversational style to compensate for poor intelligibility, improving intelligibility (through either intensive speech therapy or physical management) should be a priority. At the same time, because of the effect that either of these conversational styles might have on other areas of functioning (i.e., development of peer relationships, etc.), activities to increase conversational assertiveness and/or responsiveness should be incorporated into all therapy sessions (see Brinton & Fujiki, 1994, for suggestions). If they are not, we may find children being dismissed from intervention with intelligible speech but poor conversational skills that continue to impact not only on language but on social aspects of functioning as well (Chapman & Hardin, 1990).

Finally, children with cleft palate who still exhibit poor speech production skills at 5–6 years of age are also at risk for delays in prereading skills

(Chapman, 2009). This is not surprising considering the work by Richman and colleagues on reading performance of school-age children with cleft palate (Richman & Eliason, 1984; Richman, Eliason, & Lindgren, 1988; Richman & Ryan, 2003; Richman, Wilgenbusch, & Hall, 2005) and the large body of literature documenting the high incidence of reading problems in children with speech and language delays without cleft palate (Catts, Fey, Tomblin, & Zhang, 2002; Catts & Kamhi, 2005). Again, although there was large individual variation among the children with cleft palate on the early reading tasks, the preliteracy skills of children with cleft palate should be monitored, especially in the area of alphabet knowledge (Chapman, 2009). Ideally, children with cleft palate who exhibit moderate to severe delays in speech beyond the preschool years would be candidates for intensive intervention, not only to improve intelligibility but to prevent delays in the acquisition of early reading skills. Paul (2007) has provided suggestions for how such activities could be incorporated into therapy for speech sound disorders.

## HEARING/OTOLOGIC STATUS

Otitis media is common in children with cleft palate. This continues to be true in spite of aggressive management and monitoring of both hearing and otologic status of these children. Although clinical intuition suggests that speech and language delays observed in this population may be related to otitis media, there is little supportive experimental data. Nevertheless, many children with cleft palate who require speech-language services have past or present ear disease and associated hearing loss that should be considered in treatment planning. Middle ear status and hearing should be carefully monitored during therapy so that appropriate medical referral and/or accommodations are made for reduced hearing and other consequences of middle ear disease. (See Chapter 8 by Weiss and Chapter 12 by Teagle & Eskridge in this volume for more discussion of the influence of otitis media and hearing loss on speech development.)

## QUALITY OF INTERVENTION

Public law mandates that early intervention programs and public schools provide appropriate speech-language pathology services to all children who meet eligibility criteria for these services. As Golding-Kushner (2001) pointed out, however, children with delays may not always meet the criteria for state-funded services. Even those who receive therapy do not always receive appropriate intervention. Although some type of service is typically available to children in large urban areas, intervention can be difficult for parents to access when they live in rural communities. When assessing the services available for a child, it is important to establish not only that the services are available to the child but that the family has the actual ability to access them. Working parents may not always be able to take off from work to transport their child to therapy—particularly if the therapy is out of town.

The schedule (frequency) of intervention may be a more important consideration for some children than others. Although we often link severity of the problem with frequency of intervention, the type of error that a child exhibits is often ignored when therapy schedules are established. Two children who demonstrate the same number of errors on a single word articulation test often look quite different when the type of error is examined. Atypical sound substitutions (e.g., glottal stops, nasal substitutions, and initial consonant deletions) have a much greater impact on speech intelligibility than sound substitutions involving developmental phonological processes (e.g., final consonant deletion, velar fronting, and stopping). Although children who demonstrate atypical sound substitutions and poor speech intelligibility should qualify for more frequent therapy than those with less severe problems, a one-size-fits-all approach to scheduling is often adopted because it is easier to maintain with large caseloads. In addition to the type of error, the nature of the problem should also be considered when determining the frequency of services to provide. Numerous clinicians have reported that children with phoneme-specific nasal emission respond better to shorter, intensive therapy than to therapy delivered on a more conventional schedule (e.g., 30 minutes twice a week) (Peterson-Falzone et al., 2009, 2006). We have found that to be true in our clinical practice, as illustrated in the case of Ally, described in Box 9.3.

---

### BOX 9.3   CASE STUDY 3: ALLY

Ally was a 7-year-old girl who had been followed by a regional cleft palate team since infancy. She demonstrated mild hypernasality (not clinically significant) and phoneme-specific nasal emission on /s/. Intensive speech therapy to eliminate the latter problem was recommended at each team visit from the time Ally was 3 until her 7th-year examination. During this time, she was seen for group therapy in the public schools twice a week for 30 minutes. Her speech-language pathologist reported no improvement and repeatedly recommended surgical management each year. Ally was scheduled for intensive therapy at the hospital and seen for 4 hours a day for 3 days. An oral /s/ (referred to as a "long t" to avoid the nasal emission associated with /s/) was established using conventional shaping procedures (e.g., tttttttss) on the first day of therapy. As is true of so many children who demonstrate this behavior, progress was very rapid once Ally heard herself produce an oral /s/ and realized that she could easily produce the sound. By the end of the 3-day treatment period, Ally was correctly producing word initial and word final /s/ in sentences with 95% accuracy. Carryover into conversational speech was also evident. This short, intensive period of intervention was far more productive than the previous 4 years of therapy because correct production of the target sound was established very quickly and a large number of tokens were repeated in a short period of time to stabilize the production.

Hardin-Jones and Chapman (2008) compared speech and language measures for a group of toddlers with cleft palate who received early intervention to a group who had been referred but did not receive intervention. Both groups demonstrated comparable phonetic and lexical performance at the time intervention was recommended. On follow-up at 27 months of age, little difference was evident between the two groups. The authors speculated that lack of improvement could have been impacted by the selection of inappropriate goals. Increasing oral motor awareness and strength was identified as a treatment goal for the majority of children even though all toddlers were producing bilabial consonants and the majority were also producing alveolars and velars. Hardin-Jones and Chapman (2008) questioned the rationale of such a treatment goal, stating that "because all of the toddlers demonstrated the ability to produce oral constrictions for stops and other age-appropriate consonants, it is unclear what the intended outcome of the oral motor exercises was supposed to be" (p. 94).

## PARENTS AS ACTIVE PARTICIPANTS

Most SLPs would agree that parental involvement in the treatment process is a critical factor that has the potential to impact both the effectiveness and efficiency of intervention (e.g., Bowen & Cupples, 2004; Golding-Kushner, 2001; Hardin-Jones & Chapman, 2008; Scherer, D'Antonio, & McGahey, 2008). Pamplona and associates (Pamplona, Ysunza, González, Ramírez, & Patiño, 2000; Pamplona, Ysunza, & Uriostegui, 1996) investigated the role of active parent participation on treatment outcomes for children with cleft palate. They reported that children with active maternal participation demonstrated greater linguistic improvement than their counterparts. Their findings were not surprising since one might logically expect parents who are involved in the therapy process to be more likely to address therapy goals at home. This involvement should facilitate the speed with which these skills are generalized outside of the clinical setting.

Although lack of parent involvement would not preclude a child from being enrolled in therapy, parents should be actively engaged in treatment sessions whenever possible. As Golding-Kushner (2001) pointed out, active participation of parents "enables them to receive ongoing training and demonstrates their involvement to the child," as well as ensuring "an easier transition for the child to respond to the parent in a therapist role when the clinician is not present" (p. 60).

## LEARNING STYLES

Phonological learning styles have been identified in the early stage of phonological development for typically developing children (see Shore, 1995, for a review) and in the early lexical selection strategies of young children with cleft palate (Estrem & Broen, 1989). In addition, differences in learning styles may also explain why children with cleft palate respond differently to VPI. Many children who demonstrate VPI following initial repair of the palatal cleft demonstrate obligatory hypernasality and audible nasal emission but make no effort to prevent the nasal loss of air. Other children develop strategies to limit the perceptual impact of VPI. One such strategy that results in CAs (i.e., glottal stops and pharyngeal fricatives) reduces nasalization by substituting sounds with constrictions inferior to the velopharyngeal port for consonants with a place of articulation within the oral cavity. Another gesture that is believed to be compensatory in nature is the *nasal grimace*. Although not highly effective in minimizing the perception of nasalization, the nasal grimace reflects an attempt to stop airflow anteriorly that could not be stopped posteriorly at the velopharyngeal port. *Camouflage* is another strategy developed by some children that involves an attempt to minimize the perceptual impact of VPI by using a breathy voice or substituting /h/ for pressure consonants (Hutters & Bronsted, 1987).

As discussed above (under *Nature of the Speech Problems of Children With Cleft Palate*), even though these strategies may develop in response to VPI, they should be eliminated (or substantially reduced) with speech therapy prior to surgical management of VPI.

Children with cleft palate, like those without clefts, do not always learn best through the auditory modality. CA patterns that have persisted for many years and become entrenched into the child's phonological system, for example, may require the addition of more extensive feedback than is typically provided in most treatment sessions. When available, biofeedback tools that provide visual feedback, such as electropalatography, nasometry, and nasopharyngoscopy, can be used to augment therapy for those children who do not benefit from conventional articulation therapy methods.

## MATURATION

Maturation will have a large impact on the outcomes of treatment for children with cleft palate. The most definitive assessment of velopharyngeal function requires some type of imaging study. Although a young child might demonstrate perceptual evidence of VPI, those under the age of 3½ or 4 are often too young or immature to cooperate for such an assessment. SLPs who work with these children are often frustrated by the fact that a cleft palate team will not proceed with a recommendation for surgery for a very young child, even when speech is severely nasalized and suggests VPI. Why defer surgery? Although nasalization of speech may indicate that the velopharyngeal port is not closing appropriately during speech, we have no way of knowing *why* closure is not being obtained until the mechanism is visualized during speech production tasks. For example, is the palate mobile, but too short to contact the posterior pharyngeal wall? Do the lateral pharyngeal walls move? The answers to these and related questions often dictate the type of operation that is used to treat the problem as well as the size of tissue flaps that are used. For many children with repaired cleft palate who demonstrate VPI, sound omissions and substitutions have a greater impact on speech intelligibility than does resonance. It is considered preferable to address these phonological errors in therapy and defer surgical management until the child is old enough and mature enough to cooperate for an imaging study.

Maturation will also influence decisions whether to use biofeedback in treatment. Although the Nasometer could be used in nasalance reduction therapy with preschoolers to provide visual feedback, nasopharyngoscopic feedback would not be feasible for this age group since they are unlikely to tolerate having an endoscope in their nose during this type of therapy.

## AGE

Age plays an important role in both surgical and behavioral management of children with cleft palate. Although surgical management for VPI is often delayed for very young children who may be too immature to cooperate for an imaging study, demonstrate pervasive glottal/pharyngeal substitutions, and/or do not yet have pressure consonants in their repertoire, most clinicians try to make a definitive diagnosis between 4–5 years of age. The goal is not only to ensure that the child has an adequate mechanism before he or she goes to school but also to ensure that surgical management has been accomplished before old patterns of behavior become entrenched. Data reported in several clinical reports have demonstrated that pharyngeal flap surgery is more successful in young children than in older adolescents and adults (e.g., Van Demark and Hardin, 1986).[3]

Clinicians have also reported that CA patterns (and other errors) are more easily eradicated in younger patients than older patients (Peterson-Falzone et al., 2009).

## MOTIVATION

Motivation is a mitigating factor that should not be overlooked in treatment outcomes for children with cleft palate. Because these children may demonstrate speech sound errors related to multiple factors (e.g., developmental delay, inappropriate learning, dental/occlusal status, and VPI), many will receive intervention throughout the preschool and school-age years. It is not difficult to understand how the persistence of intervention over time can lead to a lack of enthusiasm and discouragement, particularly if progress obtained during a treatment period is slow and/or not maintained over time. There may be times when treatment is not advisable, even when the goal of normal speech has not yet been attained. For example, a child may have eliminated all developmental substitution errors but continue to demonstrate severe oral distortion of sibilants. If the child is not stimulable for correct production, therapy should be deferred until dental management has been completed and the potential for improvement exists. As Hardin (1991) pointed out, "There is little to be gained and much to lose by keeping a patient in therapy when progress is not being made" (p. 14).

---

[3] The most common surgical management for children with VPI is pharyngeal flap surgery. This procedure involves attaching a superiorly based flap of tissue that has been excised from the posterior pharyngeal wall to the soft palate. Two small holes are left open on either side of the flap to permit air to pass into the nose for nasal consonants and nasal breathing. Mesial movement of the lateral pharyngeal walls against the flap serves to close the holes and prevent nasal air loss during production of obstruent consonants.

In their treatment study of 13 children with repaired cleft palate, Van Demark and Hardin (1985) reported that one highly motivated child who demonstrated glottal stops and pharyngeal fricatives pretreatment demonstrated remarkable improvement during their therapy program. He eliminated all CAs by the end of the program and was stabilizing his new patterns at the conversational level when the program ended. On 9-month follow-up, the child had regressed, and CAs were once again evident. He had only been seen for maintenance therapy twice a month in the public schools, and that time apparently was insufficient to stabilize the new articulatory patterns. Unfortunately, this once-motivated child was highly discouraged on follow-up and refused further intervention.

## INTERVENTION RESEARCH: CHILDREN WITH CLEFT PALATE

Research examining the effectiveness of behavioral intervention for children with cleft palate is "limited in both quantity and design" (Peterson-Falzone et al., 2009, p. 322). Early studies were descriptive, rarely included comparison groups or experimental controls, and offered little insight into the individual child charac- teristics that may have influenced the success of intervention. Not surprisingly, SLPs have relied heavily on the armchair philosophy of experienced clinicians throughout the years and adopted time-honored strategies that have gained popu- larity through familiarity if not actual evidentiary support. In recent years, treat- ment studies have been strengthened by the inclusion of experimental designs employing randomization. However, to date, several recent studies have employed random assignment. As we increase our efforts to validate the treatment we pro- vide, it is incumbent upon the SLP to integrate knowledge obtained through research with the expertise obtained through clinical experience to maintain a strong evidence-based practice.

### CONVENTIONAL INTERVENTION APPROACHES

Since many of the special articulation problems of children with repaired cleft palate reflect errors in place of articulation (e.g., CAs), traditional articulation approaches to remediation have typically been recommended. Although a number of authors have described outcomes of articulation therapy for single cases (Hall & Tomblin, 1975) and larger groups (Van Demark & Hardin, 1986), only a handful of studies have compared the effectiveness of different treatment approaches for these children. Pamplona et al. (1999) randomly assigned 29 children with repaired cleft palate who demonstrated CAs (and VPI) to two intervention groups: one group received articulation therapy and the other received phonological intervention. They reported that the therapy time required to eliminate the CAs was significantly reduced when a phonological approach was used. In a follow-up report, Pamplona, Ysunza, and Ramirez (2004) described outcomes for 30 children with cleft palate with CAs (and VPI) who were randomly assigned to receive phonological intervention (Group 1) or naturalistic intervention (Group 2). These investigators reported no difference in therapy time needed to eliminate the

CAs with either approach. A closer examination of this report suggested that the child participants were similar for many variables that typically influence choice of intervention approach and success in intervention, including cleft type, age, language skills (all were within normal limits), error patterns (all produced CAs), hearing, parent participation, and velopharyngeal function (all exhibited VPI), and finally, no children presented with palatal fistulae. In spite of the similarities across children, the actual therapy time required for each child was quite variable. For example, in the latter study (Pamplona et al., 2004), the average time in therapy was 14 and 16 months for the two treatment groups, respectively, but individual children received anywhere from 6 to 22 months of therapy in Groups 1 and from 4 to 27 months of therapy in Group 2. In the former study (Pamplona et al., 1999), the time in therapy was shorter for children receiving the phonologic approach, and the standard deviation was substantially smaller (4 versus 10). Also, the children were enrolled in therapy for 6–22 months in the phonologic group and for 14–42 months in the articulation group. Of course, the children likely varied in severity of their speech problems, which may have accounted for differences in length of therapy. Examination of other child characteristics and error patterns may have provided information about why some children required less time in intervention and whether one approach was more effective for individual children. However, these details were not provided, so these questions remain unanswerable.

Scherer and colleagues conducted a series of intervention studies involving toddlers with cleft palate. In Scherer's 1999 report, she examined outcomes of a vocabulary intervention program for three toddlers using a multiple baseline design and reported that the intervention increased word use and phonological performance for each of the participants. In two subsequent studies (Brothers & Scherer, 2002; Scherer, 2003), researchers compared outcomes of parent-implemented interventions for four toddlers. Consonant inventory for toddlers who received a conventional, focused stimulation language intervention was compared with that of toddlers who received a focused stimulation intervention supplemented by increased aspiration on word-initial stop consonants. According to the investigators, both interventions were equally effective in expanding the toddler's consonant inventories. In the final report in this series, Scherer, D'Antonio, et al. (2008) compared vocabulary diversity for two groups of children: 10 children with repaired cleft palate who received parent-directed, naturalistic vocabulary intervention and 10 language-matched, noncleft children who did not receive therapy. They reported that although the cleft group increased vocabulary diversity, their performance level did not reach that of the comparison group. The children participating in the language-based approaches employed by Scherer were all similar in that they were delayed in speech and language, but other variables were not controlled and certainly may have influenced which children made more or less progress in intervention.

Clinical investigators have also examined the response of children with cleft palate to different models of intervention and reported greater gains with short-term, intensive therapy than therapy provided for shorter periods over a longer period of time (Albery & Enderby, 1984; Van Demark & Hardin, 1986). Van Demark and Hardin studied 13 children enrolled in a 6-week, intensive summer residential program and reported that although the children made significant gains in articulation during the program, no significant difference was evident between posttreatment articulation scores and scores obtained 9 months later following public school therapy. Although this latter finding was probably related in part to frequency of intervention (the children received only 30–35 hours of intervention during the school year), Van Demark and Hardin noted that immaturity and poor motivation probably contributed to the lack of improvement seen in at least three children. In contrast, Pamplona and colleagues (2005) reported no difference in the speech outcomes for children enrolled in intensive therapy compared with therapy delivered on a more conventional time frame. The former group received 4 hours of therapy 5 days a week for 3 weeks, whereas the control group received small-group intervention for 1 hour twice a week for 1 year. However, the participants in the conventional group received almost twice as many hours of therapy (104) as the children in the intensive therapy group (60 hours), suggesting that there might be an advantage for the intensive therapy group (Pamplona et al., 2005).

Although articulation and phonological-based therapies cannot eliminate hypernasality and audible nasal emission when they are directly related to VPI, such intervention can improve function of the mechanism when glottal/pharyngeal substitutions and phoneme-specific nasal emission are eliminated. Henningsson and Isberg (1986) demonstrated with radiographic evidence that patients achieve better velopharyngeal function when they produce oral stops than when they produce glottal stops. Ysunza et al. (1992) reported videonasopharyngoscopic and multiview videofluoroscopic outcomes of velopharyneal function for 31 children who received articulation therapy to eliminate CAs. Results of imaging studies obtained prior to and following elimination of CA errors demonstrated an increase in velopharyngeal motion and a reduction in the size of the velopharyngeal gap for each of the children in this study.

Some authors have reported that children who demonstrate adequate velopharyngeal closure make faster progress in therapy than children with VPI (Van Demark, 1974). Although VPI certainly does not facilitate efforts to establish correct articulation, numerous reports have also demonstrated that children with cleft palate can improve their articulation even when VPI is present (Chisum, Shelton, Arndt, & Elbert, 1969; Pamplona et al., 2005; Van Demark, 1974; Van Demark & Hardin, 1986). It is important to point out that although a child may improve their articulation with therapy, this behavioral intervention does not impact velopharyngeal gap size (Shelton, Chisum, Youngstrom, Arndt, & Elbert, 1969).

Research conducted by Pamplona and colleagues (Pamplona, Ysunza, González, et al., 2000; Pamplona, Ysunza, et al., 1996) has also underscored the importance of parent participation in the therapy process for children with cleft palate. Using random group assignment, the authors compared outcomes for children who received intervention with an SLP with those obtained by children who received intervention with an SLP and parent. The authors reported greater linguistic improvement for children whose mothers accompanied them to the sessions. They also observed that the mothers who participated in the treatment sessions altered their patterns of interaction with their child.

Collectively, these clinical research findings suggest that factors such as status of the velopharyngeal mechanism, dentition, and motivation probably play a large role in degree and rate of improvement that a child with a cleft palate experiences in speech-language intervention. As is true for noncleft children, therapy outcomes are enhanced when parents get involved in the intervention process and address the goals of intervention with their child on a routine basis.

## Palatal Exercises

One of the earliest approaches used to improve velopharyngeal function in children with cleft palate included palatal exercises (blowing, sucking, etc.). Early studies were interested in examining the effectiveness of blowing, sucking, and swallowing exercises on velopharyngeal function. This interest was based on the assumption that velopharyngeal closure obtained during one of these tasks could be transferred to speech. Kanter (1948) noted in an anecdotal fashion that although palatal exercises based on blowing were a stock procedure in intervention at the time, little spontaneous carry-over of improved palatal function was evident in spontaneous speech. Research conducted by others more than 20 years later substantiated Kanter's early observations. Changes in velopharyngeal gap size (Massengill, Quinn, Pickrell, & Levinson, 1968; Powers & Starr, 1974) and clinical judgments of nasality (Powers & Starr, 1974) have not been substantiated following the use of blowing exercises. Consequently, SLPs who specialize in treatment of children with cleft palate abandoned palatal exercises many years ago. Unfortunately, it appears that many clinicians have rediscovered oral motor exercises in recent years and are choosing to integrate them into their clinical practice (Lof, 2008). This resurgence is attributed, at least in part, to the many companies that promote their use. SLPs should remember that although profits typically motivate company priorities, strong ethical practice should always drive ours. There is neither logical nor empirical evidence to support the use of blowing activities in strengthening the velopharyngeal musculature for children with velopharyngeal valving disorders or children with developmental articulation problems. For a complete discussion on the problems associated with nonspeech oral motor treatments, the reader is referred to the Clinical Forum in the July 2008 issue (volume 39) of the *Language, Speech, and Hearing Services in Schools* journal (Lass & Pannbacker, 2008; Lof & Watson, 2008; Powell, 2008a, 2008b; Ruscello, 2008).

One experimental exercise regimen that may hold some promise for strengthening the velopharyngeal musculature is continuous positive airway pressure (CPAP) therapy. First described by Kuehn in 1991, CPAP therapy involves the use of a common CPAP device that delivers continuous positive air pressure to a patient via a nasal mask. Air pressure generated by the CPAP device can be used to specifically exercise the muscles of the soft palate because these muscles will have to work against the positive air pressure generated by the device in order to close the velopharyngeal port. Kuehn and colleagues (1991, 2002) reported that although some patients have reduced their hypernasality with CPAP therapy, others have not responded to the treatment at all, and in fact, some actually experienced an increase in hypernasality following treatment. Kuehn and colleagues hypothesized that patient compliance may have contributed to differential effects noted for different participants and centers. Because of the rigorous practice schedule and modifications required in the CPAP-based intervention over time, it is easy to see that the success or failure of this approach may depend on the motivation of the participant (and the participant's parents). Although Kuehn and colleagues did not discuss other client variables that may have contributed to the outcomes described above, they did suggest that future research should attempt to identify the ideal candidate for this approach (Kuehn et al., 2002). Logically, one would anticipate that the ideal candidate for this procedure would be the child with a mobile velum and a small velopharyngeal gap.

## BIOFEEDBACK

Although biofeedback tools are often recommended to improve velopharyngeal function and/or reduce hypernasality, relatively few studies have been conducted to examine the effectiveness of these tools for children with cleft palate. Two commonly employed assessment tools that have been used in biofeedback therapy are the Nasometer and nasopharyngoscopy. The Nasometer is a clinical tool that measures the relative amount of nasal acoustic energy present as a patient speaks and provides that information to the user in the form of a nasalance score. Although it is used primarily as an assessment instrument, the *Nasometer* provides a visual trace of the information that can be displayed in real time for a patient. Fletcher (1972, 1978) demonstrated that providing children and adolescents with nasalance feedback resulted in decreases in nasalance scores for a majority of participants. Fletcher, Adams, and McCutcheon (1989) speculated that individuals with scores greater than 35% would not likely achieve normal resonance without secondary physical management, such as a pharyngeal flap. Peterson-Falzone, Hardin-Jones, and Karnell (2001) concluded that good candidates for a nasalance reduction program would probably be patients with mild, inconsistent hypernasality.

Several investigators have examined the use of nasopharyngoscopy as a feedback tool for patients with velopharyngeal dysfunction. An endoscope is passed transnasally, and the patient is encouraged to monitor movements of his or her velopharyngeal structures during connected speech on a video monitor. Clinical outcomes associated with several early investigations (Miyazaki, Matsuya, Yamaoka, & Nishio, 1974 [as cited in Peterson-Falzone et al., 2001]; Nishio, Yamaoka, Matsuya, & Miyazaki, 1976; Yamaoka, Mastuya, Miyazaki, Nishio, & Ibuki, 1983) indicated that some patients who demonstrated the ability to achieve velopharyngeal closure on nonspeech tasks could be taught to achieve closure during select speech tasks (e.g., production of plosives and fricatives, sustained vowels). It was not always clear, however, whether the improvement noted was maintained over time when biofeedback was withdrawn or whether the degree of improvement resulted in fewer surgical cases. Nasopharyngoscopic feedback has also been used as an adjunct to speech therapy when eliminating phoneme-specific nasal emission (Brunner, Stellzig-Eisenhauer, Pröschel, Verres, & Komposch, 2005; Witzel, Tobe, & Sayler, 1988) and when eliminating inconsistent, residual nasalization following pharyngeal flap surgery (Witzel, Tobe, & Sayler, 1989; Ysunza, Pamplona, Femat, Meyer, & Garcia-Velasco, 1997).

Nasopharyngoscopic feedback is still considered an experimental procedure and has not yet been adopted as a routine clinical tool. We do not yet know which patients will benefit the most from this procedure, but as pointed out by Peterson-Falzone et al. (2001), those who achieve velopharyngeal closure during blowing and some pressure consonants appear to be the patients who will most likely benefit from this type of intervention. Witzel et al. (1989) pointed out that the visual information provided by the procedure may be particularly advantageous for the older patient whose speech patterns are "long-standing and ingrained" (p. 134).

## CONCLUSIONS

Since we began working with children with cleft palate as master's degree students in the 1970s, we have seen many changes in the management of these children. Age at time of primary palatal surgery has decreased, new surgical techniques such as the Furlow-double opposing Z-plasty have been developed, nasendoscopy is routinely used for objective evaluation of velopharyngeal function, children are receiving earlier and more aggressive management for middle ear problems, and speech and language intervention is available to children at much younger ages, to name a few. As a result of these advances in cleft care, VPI rates appear to have decreased, and fewer children develop CAs and severe speech problems than in the past (Hardin-Jones & Jones, 2005). At the same time, after studying the speech outcome of 212 preschoolers with cleft palate, Hardin-Jones and Jones (2005) concluded, "There are actually limited data available to support the notion that children managed today are more likely to demonstrate normal speech than are children managed 20 years ago....It is important to recognize that many of these children continue to require therapy for articulation/phonological problems" (p. 11).

As SLPs, we may not be able to decrease the number of children with cleft palate needing therapy. However, we can improve our clinical decision making and quality of the services we provide so that if intervention is needed, it is short term and not long term, and speech normalization occurs by age 5.

Finally, intervention studies need to be conducted so that we can determine whether the approaches that are currently advocated (derived primarily from expert opinion rather than well-designed and controlled intervention studies) are actually the most effective approaches for children with cleft palate. However, when designing and interpreting the results of these studies, we must not lose sight of the personal characteristics that each child brings to the intervention process that affect successful outcomes.

## REFERENCES

Albery, L., & Enderby, P. (1984). Intensive speech therapy for cleft palate children. *British Journal of Disorders of Communication, 19,* 115–124.

Bardach, J., Morris, H. L., Olin, W. H., Gray, S. D., Jones, D. L., Kelly, K. M., et al. (1990). The Iowa-Hamburg Project: Late results of multidisciplinary management at the Iowa Cleft Palate Center. In J. Bardach & H. L. Morris (Eds.), *Multidisciplinary management of cleft lip and palate.* Philadelphia: W. B. Saunders Co.

Bardach, J., Morris, H. L., Olin, W. H., Gray, S. D., Jones, D. L., Kelly, K. M., et al. (1992). Results of multidisciplinary management of bilateral cleft lip and palate at the Iowa Cleft Palate Center. *Plastic Reconstructive Surgery, 89,* 419–432.

Bardach, J., Morris, H. L., Olin, W., McDermott-Murray, J., Mooney, M., & Bardach, E. (1984). Late results of multidisciplinary management of unilateral cleft lip and palate. *Annals of Plastic Surgery, 12,* 235–242.

Bowen, C., & Cupples, L. (2004). The role of families in optimizing phonological therapy outcomes. *Child Language Teaching and Therapy, 20,* 245–260.

Brinton, B., & Fujiki, M. (1994). Ways to teach conversation. In J. Duchan, L. E. Hewitt, & R. M. Sonnenmeier (Eds.), *Pragmatics from theory to practice* (pp. 59–71). Englewood Cliffs, NJ: Prentice Hall.

Broen, P. A., Devers, M. C., Doyle, S. S., Prouty, J. M., & Moller, K. T. (1998). Acquisition of linguistic and cognitive skills by children with cleft palate. *Journal of Speech, Language, and Hearing Research, 41,* 676–687.

Broen, P., Moller, K., Devers, M., & Doyle, S. (1996, April). *Accuracy of speech production of 30 month old children with cleft palate.* Paper presented at the annual meeting of the American Cleft Palate-Craniofacial Association, San Diego, CA.

Brothers, M., & Scherer, N. (2002, November). *Parent-implemented treatment for young children with cleft lip and palate.* Poster presented at the annual meeting of the American Speech-Language-Hearing Association, Atlanta, GA.

Brunnegard, K., & Lohmander, A. (2007). A cross-sectional study of speech in 10-year-old children with cleft palate: Results and issues of rater reliability. *Cleft Palate-Craniofacial Journal 44,* 33–44.

Brunner, M., Stellzig-Eisenhauer, A., Pröschel, U., Verres, R., & Komposch, G.(2005). The effect of nasopharyngoscopic biofeedback in patients with cleft palate and velopharyngeal dysfunction. *Cleft Palate-Craniofacial Journal, 42,* 649–657.

Catts, H. W., Fey, M. E., Tomblin, J. B., & Zhang, X. (2002). A longitudinal investigation of reading outcomes in children with language impairments. *Journal of Speech, Language, and Hearing Research, 45,* 1142–1157.

Catts, H. W., & Kamhi, A. (2005). *Language and reading disabilities.* Boston: Pearson, Allyn & Bacon.

Chapman, K. L. (1991). Vocalizations of toddlers with cleft lip and palate. *Cleft Palate-Craniofacial Journal, 28,* 172–178.

Chapman, K. L. (1993). Phonologic processes in children with cleft palate. *Cleft Palate-Craniofacial Journal, 30,* 64–72.

Chapman, K. L. (2004a). Is presurgery and early postsurgery performance related to speech and language outcomes at 3 years of age for children with cleft palate? *Clinical Linguistics & Phonetics, 18,* 235–257.

Chapman, K. L. (2004b, November). *The interaction of phonological and articulation disorders in children with cleft palate.* Paper presented at the annual meeting of the American Speech-Language-Hearing Association, Philadelphia, PA.

Chapman, K. L. (2008). Speech and language of children with cleft palate: Interactions and influences. In K. T. Moller & L. E. Glaze (Eds.), *Cleft Palate: Interdisciplinary issues and treatment—For clinicians by clinicians.* Austin: Pro-Ed Publications.

Chapman, K. L. (2009). The relationship between reading skills and speech and language performance of children with cleft lip and palate. *Cleft Palate-Craniofacial Journal.* Manuscript submitted for publication.

Chapman, K. L., & Hardin, M. A. (1990). Communicative competence in children with cleft palate. In J. Bardach & H. Morris (Eds.), *Multidisciplinary management of cleft lip and palate* (pp. 721–726). Philadelphia: W. B. Saunders Co.

Chapman, K. L., & Hardin, M. A. (1992). Phonetic and phonological skills of two year olds with cleft palate. *Cleft Palate-Craniofacial Journal, 29,* 435–443.

Chapman, K. L., Hardin-Jones, M. A., Goldstein, J. A., Halter, K. A., Havlik, R. J., & Schulte, J. (2008). Timing of palatal surgery and speech outcome. *Cleft Palate Craniofacial Journal, 45,* 297–308.

Chapman, K. L., Hardin-Jones, M. A., & Halter, K. (2003). The relationship between early speech and later speech and language performance for children with cleft palate. *Clinical Linguistics & Phonetics, 17,* 173–197.

Chapman, K. L., Hardin-Jones, M. A., Schulte, J., & Halter, K. (2001). Vocal development of 9- month-old babies with cleft palate. *Journal of Speech, Language, and Hearing Research, 44,* 1268–1283.

Chapman, K. L., Tecco Graham, K., Gooch, J., & Visconti, C. (1998). Conversational skills of preschool and school-aged children with cleft lip and palate. *Cleft Palate-Craniofacial Journal, 35,* 503–516.

Chisum, L., Shelton, R. L., Arndt, W. B., & Elbert, M. (1969). The relationship between remedial speech instruction activities and articulation change. *Cleft Palate Journal, 6,* 57–64.

Counihan, D. T. (1960). Articulation skills of adolescents and adults with cleft palate. *Journal of Speech and Hearing Disorders, 25,* 181–187.

Dalston, R. M. (1990). Communication skills of children with cleft lip and palate: A status report. In J. Bardach & H. Morris (Eds.), *Multidisciplinary management of cleft lip and palate* (pp. 746–757). Philadelphia: W. B. Saunders Co.

Estrem, T., & Broen, P. A. (1989). Early speech production of children with cleft palate. *Journal of Speech and Hearing Research, 32,* 12–23.

Faircloth, S. R., & Faircloth, M. A. (1972). Delayed language and linguistic variation. In K. R. Bzoch (Ed.), *Communicative disorders related to cleft lip and palate* (pp. 130–135). Boston: Little, Brown & Company.

Ferguson, C. A. (1979). Phonology as an individual access system: Some data from language acquisition. In C. J. Fillmore, D. Kempler, & W. S-Y. Wang (Eds.), *Individual differences in language ability and language behavior* (pp. 189–201). New York: Academic Press.

Fey, M. (1986). *Language intervention with young children.* San Diego, CA: College-Hill Press.

Fey, M. E. (1992). Clinical forum: Articulation and phonology treatment. Articulation and phonology: Inextricable constructs in speech pathology. *Language, Speech and Hearing Services in Schools, 23,* 225–232.

Fletcher, S. G. (1972). Contingencies for bioelectric modification of nasality. *Journal of Speech and Hearing Disorders, 37,* 329–346.

Fletcher, S. G. (1978). *Diagnosing speech disorders from cleft palate.* New York: Grune and Stratton.

Fletcher, S. G., Adams, L. E., & McCutcheon, M. J. (1989). Cleft palate speech assessment through oral-nasal acoustic measures. In K. R. Bzoch (Ed.), *Communicative disorders related to cleft lip and palate* (pp. 246–257). Boston: Little, Brown.

Frederickson, M., Chapman, K. L., & Hardin-Jones, M. (2006). Conversation skills of children with cleft palate: A replication and extension. *Cleft Palate-Craniofacial Journal, 43,* 179–188.

Goad, H., & Ingram, D. (1987). Individual variation and its relevance to a theory of phonological acquisition. *Journal of Child Language, 14,* 419–432.

Golding-Kushner, K. J. (1981). *Articulation and velopharyngeal insufficiency: A rationale for pre-surgical speech therapy.* Paper presented at the Fourth International Congress on Cleft Palate and Related Craniofacial Anomalies, Acapulco, Mexico.

Golding-Kushner, K. J. (2001). *Therapy techniques for cleft palate speech and related disorders.* San Diego, CA: Singular Publishing Group, Inc.

Grunwell, P., & Russell, J. (1988). Phonological development in children with cleft lip and palate. *Clinical Linguistics & Phonetics, 2,* 75–95.

Haapanen, M. L. (1994). Cleft type and speech proficiency. *Folia Phoniatrica Logopedics, 46,* 57–63.

Hall, P. K., & Tomblin, J. B. (1975). Case study: Therapy procedures and remediation of a nasal lisp. *Language, Speech, and Hearing Services in Schools, 6,* 29–32.

Hardin, M. A. (1991). Cleft palate: Intervention. *Clinics in Communication Disorders, 1,* 12–18.

Hardin-Jones, M., & Chapman, K. L. (2008). Early intervention: A retrospective look at outcome. *Language, Speech, and Hearing Services in Schools, 39,* 89–96.

Hardin-Jones, M. A., & Jones, D. L. (2005). Speech production of preschoolers with cleft palate. *Cleft Palate-Craniofacial Journal, 42,* 7–13.

Henningsson, E. G., & Isberg, A. M. (1986). Velopharyngeal movement patterns in patients alternating between oral and glottal articulation: A clinical and cineradiographical study. *Cleft Palate Journal, 23,* 1–9.

Hoch, L., Golding-Kushner, K., Siegel-Sadewitz, V. L., & Shprintzen, R. J. (1986). Speech therapy. *Seminars in Speech and Language, 7,* 313–326.

Hueberner, D. V., & Marsh, J. L. (2002, May). *Management for cleft lip and palate:* The first 18 months. Paper presented at the annual meeting of the American Cleft Palate-Craniofacial Association, Seattle, WA.

Hutters, B., & Brondsted, K. (1987). Strategies in cleft palate speech—With special reference to Danish. *Cleft Palate, 24,* 126–136.

Jones, C. E., Chapman, K. L., & Hardin-Jones, M. A. (2003). Speech development of children with cleft palate before and after palatal surgery. *Cleft Palate-Craniofacial Journal, 40,* 19–31.

Kanter, C. E. (1948). The rationale of blowing exercise for patients with repaired cleft palates. *Journal of Speech Disorders, 12,* 281–286.

Karnell, M. P., & Van Demark, D. R. (1986). Longitudinal speech performance in patients with cleft palate: Comparisons based on secondary management. *Cleft Palate Journal, 23,* 278–288.

Kuehn, D. P. (1991). New therapy for treating hypernasal speech using continuous positive airway pressure (CPAP). *Plastic and Reconstructive Surgery, 88,* 959–966.

Kuehn, D. P., Imrey, P. B., Tomesm L., Jones, D. L., O'Gara, M. M., Seaver, E. J., et al. (2002). Efficacy of continuous positive airway pressure (CPAP) in the treatment of hypernasality. *Cleft Palate-Craniofacial Journal, 39,* 267–276.

Lass, N. J., & Pannbacker, M. (2008). The application of evidence-based practice to non-speech oral motor treatments. *Language, Speech, and Hearing Services in Schools, 39,* 408–421.

Lof, G. L., & Watson, M. M. (2008). A nationwide survey of nonspeech oral motor exercise use: Implications for evidence-based practice. *Language, Speech, and Hearing Services in Schools, 39,* 392–407.

Leonard, L., Newhoff, M., & Masalem, L. (1980). Individual differences in early childhood phonology. *Applied Psycholinguistics, 1,* 7–30.

Lohmander, A., & Persson, C. (2008). A longitudinal study of speech production in Swedish children with unilateral cleft lip and palate and two-stage palatal repair. *Cleft Palate-Craniofacial Journal, 45,* 32–41.

Massengill, R., Quinn, G. W., Pickrell, K. L., Levinson, C. (1968). Therapeutic exercise and velopharyngeal gap. *Cleft Palate Journal, 5,* 46–55.

McLeod, S., van Doorn, J., Reed, V. A. (2001). Consonant cluster development in two-year-olds: General trends and individual differences. *Journal of Speech, Language, and Hearing Research, 44,* 1144–1171.

Miyazaki, T., Matsuya, T., Yamaoka, M., & Nishio, J. (1974, April). *A nasopharyngeal fiberscope.* Film presented at the annual meeting of the American Cleft Palate Association, Boston, MA.

Morris, H. L. (1968). Etiological bases for speech problems. In D. D. Spriestersbach & D. Sherman (Eds.), *Cleft palate and communication* (pp. 119–168). New York: Academic Press.

Morris, H. L., Bardach, J., Ardinger, H., Jones, D., Kelly, K. M., Olin, W. H., & Wheeler, J. (1993). Multidisciplinary treatment results for patients with isolated cleft palate. *Plastic and Reconstructive Surgery, 92,* 842–851.

Nishio, J., Yamaoka, M., Matsuya, T., & Miyazaki, T. (1976). How to exercise the velopharyngeal movement by the velopharyngeal fiberscope. *Japanese Journal of Oral Surgery, 20, 450. Abstracted in Cleft Palate Journal, 13,* 310.

Pamplona, M. C., Ysunza, A., & Espinosa, J. (1999). A comparative trial of two modalities of speech intervention for compensatory articulation in cleft palate children: Phonologic approach versus articulatory approach. *International Journal of Pediatric Otorhinolaryngology, 49,* 21–26.

Pamplona, M. C., Ysunza, A., González, M., Ramírez, E., & Patiño, C. (2000). Linguistic development in cleft palate patients with and without compensatory articulation disorder. *International Journal of Pediatric Otorhinolaryngology, 54,* 81–91.

Pamplona, M. C., Ysunza, A., Patino, C., Ramirez, E., Drucker, M., & Mazon, J. J. (2005). Speech summer camp for treating articulation disorders in cleft palate patients. *International Journal of Pediatric Otorhinolaryngology, 69,* 351–359.

Pamplona, M. C., Ysunza, A., & Ramirez, E. (2004). Naturalistic intervention in cleft palate children. *International Journal of Pediatric Otorhinolaryngology, 68,* 75–81.

Pamplona, M. C., Ysunza, A., Uriostegui, C. (1996). Linguistic interaction: The active role of parents in speech therapy for cleft palate patients. *International Journal of Pediatric Otorhinolaryngology, 37,* 17–27.

Paul, R. (2007). *Language disorders from infancy through adolescence* (3rd ed.). Philadelphia: Mosby.

Peterson-Falzone, S. J., Hardin-Jones, M. A., & Karnell, M. (2001). *Cleft palate speech* (3rd ed.). St. Louis, MO: Mosby Inc.

Peterson-Falzone, S. J., Hardin-Jones, M. A., & Karnell, M. (2009). *Cleft palate speech* (4th ed.). St. Louis, MO: Mosby Inc.

Peterson-Falzone, S. J., Trost-Cardamone, J. E., Karnell, M. P., & Hardin-Jones, M. A. (2006). *Treating cleft palate speech.* St. Louis, MO: Mosby Inc.

Powell, T. W. (2008a). Epilogue: An integrated evaluation of nonspeech oral motor treatments. *Language, Speech, and Hearing Services in Schools, 39,* 422–427.

Powell, T. W. (2008b). Prologue: The use of nonspeech oral motor treatments for developmental speech sound production disorders: Interventions and interactions. *Language, Speech, and Hearing Services in Schools, 39,* 374–379.

Powers, G. L., & Starr, C. D. (1974). The effects of muscle exercises on velopharyngeal gap and nasality. *Cleft Palate Journal, 11,* 28–35.

Richman, L. C., & Eliason, M. (1984). Type of reading disability related to cleft type and neuropsychological patterns. *Cleft Palate Journal, 21,* 1–6.

Richman, L. C., Eliason M. J., & Lindgren, S. D. (1988). Reading disability in children with clefts. *Cleft Palate Journal 25,* 21–25.

Richman, L. C., & Ryan, S. M. (2003). Do the reading disabilities of children with cleft fit into current models of developmental dyslexia? *Cleft Palate-Craniofacial Journal, 40,* 154–157.

Richman, L. C., Wilgenbusch, T., & Hall, T. (2005). Spontaneous verbal labelling: Visual memory and reading ability in children with cleft. *Cleft Palate-Craniofacial Journal, 42,* 565–569.

Riski, J. E. (1995). Speech assessment of adolescents. *Cleft Palate-Craniofacial Journal, 32,* 109–113.

Riski, J. E., & DeLong, E. (1984). Articulation development in children with cleft lip/palate. *Cleft Palate Journal, 21,* 57–64.

Ruscello, D. M. (2008). Nonspeech oral motor treatment issues related to children with developmental speech sound disorders. *Language, Speech, and Hearing Services in Schools, 39,* 380–391.

Russell, J., & Grunwell, P. (1993). *Speech development in children with cleft lip and palate.* In P. Grunwell (Ed.), Analysing cleft palate speech (pp. 19–47). London: Whurr Publishers.

Scherer, N. J. (1999). The speech and language status of toddlers with cleft lip and/or palate following early vocabulary intervention. *American Journal of Speech-Language Pathology, 8,* 81–93.

Scherer, N. J. (2003, November). *Parent-implemented early vocabulary intervention for toddlers with cleft.* Paper presented at the annual meeting of the American Speech-Language-Hearing Association, Chicago, IL.

Scherer, N. J., & D'Antonio, L. L. (1995). Parent questionnaire for screening early language development in children with cleft palate. *Cleft Palate-Craniofacial Journal, 32,* 7–13.

Scherer, N. J., D'Antonio, L. L., & McGahey, H. (2008). Early intervention for speech impairment in children with cleft palate. *Cleft Palate-Craniofacial Journal, 45,* 18–31.

Scherer, N. J., Williams, A. L., & Proctor-Williams, K. (2008). Early and later vocalization in children with and without cleft palate. *International Journal of Pediatric Otorhinolaryngology, 72,* 827–40.

Sell, D., Grunwell, P., Mildinhall, S., Murphy, T., Cornish, T. A., Bearn, D., Shaw, W. C., Murray, J. J., Williams, A. C., & Sandy, J. R. (2001). Cleft lip and palate care in the United Kingdom: The clinical standards advisory group (CSAG) study. Part 3: Speech outcomes. *Cleft Palate-Craniofacial Journal, 38,* 30–37.

Shelton, R. L., Chisum, L., Youngstrom, K. A., Arndt, W. B., & Elbert, M. (1969). Effect of articulation therapy on palatopharyngeal closure, movement of the pharyngeal wall, and tongue posture. *Cleft Palate Journal, 6,* 440–448.

Shore, C. (1995). *Individual differences in language development.* London: Sage Publications.

Shriberg, L. D., Gruber, A. F., & Kwiatkowski, J. (1994). Developmental phonological disorders III: Long-term speech-sound normalization. *Journal of Speech and Hearing Research, 37,* 1151–1177.

Shriberg, L. D., & Kwiatkowski, J. (1982). Phonological disorders I: A diagnostic classification system. *Journal of Speech and Hearing Disorders, 47*, 226–241.

Shriberg, L. D., Kwiatkowski, J., & Gruber, A. F. (1994). Developmental phonological disorders II: Short-term speech-sound normalization. *Journal of Speech and Hearing Research, 37*, 1127–1150.

Smit, A. B., Hand, L., Freilinger, J. J., Bernthal, J. E., & Bird, A. (1990). The Iowa Articulation Norms Project and its Nebraska replication. *Journal of Speech and Hearing Research, 55*, 779–798.

Stoel-Gammon, C., & Stone, J. R. (1991). Assessing phonology in young children. *Clinical Communication Disorders, 1*, 25–39.

Trost-Cardamone, J. E. (1990). The development of speech: Cleft palate misarticulations. In D. E. Kernahan & S. W. Rosenstein (Eds.), *Cleft lip and palate: A system of management.* Baltimore: Williams & Wilkins.

Van Demark, D. R. (1974). Some results of intensive speech therapy for children with cleft palate. *Cleft Palate Journal, 11*, 41–49.

Van Demark, D. R., & Hardin, M. A. (1985). Longitudinal evaluation of articulation and velopharyngeal competence of patients with pharyngeal flaps. *Cleft Palate Journal, 22*, 163–172.

Van Demark, D. R., & Hardin, M. A. (1986). Effectiveness of intensive articulation therapy for children with cleft palate. *Cleft Palate Journal, 23*, 215–224.

Van Demark, D. R., Morris, H. L., & VandeHaar, C. (1979). Patterns of articulation abilities in speakers with cleft palate. *Cleft Palate Journal, 16*, 230–239.

Vihman, M. M., Ferguson, C. A., & Elbert, M. (1986). Phonological development from babbling to speech: Common tendencies and individual differences. *Applied Psycholinguistics, 7*, 3–40.

Vihman, M. M., & Greenlee, M. (1987). Individual differences in phonological development: Ages one and three years. *Journal of Speech and Hearing Research, 30*, 503–521.

Weiss, A. L. (2004). The child as agent for change in therapy for phonological disorders. *Child Language Teaching and Therapy, 20*, 221–244.

Whitehill, T. L., Francis, A. L., & Ching, C. K.-Y. (2003). Perception of place of articulation by children with cleft palate and posterior placement. *Journal of Speech, Language, and Hearing Research, 46*, 451–461.

Witzel, M. A., Tobe, J., & Salyer, K. (1988). The use of nasopharyngoscopy biofeedback therapy in the correction of inconsistent velopharyngeal closure. *International Journal of Pediatric Otorhinolaryngology, 15*, 137–142.

Witzel, M. A., Tobe, J., & Salyer, K. E. (1989). The use of videonasopharyngoscopy for biofeedback therapy in adults after pharyngeal flap surgery. *Cleft Palate Journal, 26*, 129–134.

Yamaoka, M., Mastuya, T., Miyazaki, T., Nishio, J., & Ibuki, K. (1983). Visual training for velopharyngeal closure in cleft palate patients: A fiberscopic procedure (preliminary report). *Journal of Maxillofacial Surgery 11*, 191–193.

Ysunza, A., Pamplona, M. C., Femat, T., Mayer, I., & Garcia-Velasco, M. (1997). Videonasopharyngoscopy as an instrument for visual feedback during speech in cleft palate patients. *International Journal of Pediatric Otorhinolaryngology, 41*, 291–298.

Ysunza, A., Pamplona, C., Toledo, E. (1992). Change in velopharyngeal valving after speech therapy in cleft palate patients. A videonasopharyngoscopic and multi-view videofluoroscopic study. *International Journal of Pediatric Otorhinolaryngology, 24*, 45–54.

# 10 Uniqueness and Individuality in Stuttering Therapy

*Trudy Stewart and Margaret M. Leahy*

Behind each face there is a unique world that no one else can see. This is the mystery of individuality. The shape of each soul is different. No one else feels your life the way you do. No one else sees or hears the world as you do....Given the uniqueness of each of us, it should not be surprising that one of the greatest challenges is to inhabit your own individuality and to discover which life-form best expresses it.

**O'Donoghue (2007), p. 147**

## INTRODUCTION

Therapy can be described as a unique encounter; one that is different for each of the individuals engaged in it and that is different each time it is experienced. Therapy for adults who stutter is also unique, both in its form and in its experience. There are three essential elements in the management of stuttering in adults that together make up this unique event: the clinician, the therapy, and the client who stutters. This triad can be used to explore dynamics in the intervention that can affect therapy outcomes. This chapter will discuss the triad with reference to the individual nature of clinical practice, which Rolfe (2006) describes as consisting of "interactions between unique individuals, with unique experiences and it always takes place in unique situations" (p. 39).

## THE CLIENT

The adult who stutters comes to therapy with extensive life experience with speaking as well as stuttering, high expectations, and aspirations toward solving a problem that has proved intractable. This client has his or her own unique agenda. Through engaging in the process of therapy, the client aspires to achieve answers to the enigma of his or her personal problems with stuttering. Ultimately, being rid of the burden of stuttering is a motivating force. In almost all instances, there are many questions that need to be aired by the client, as well as many uniquely personal experiences and stories regarding stuttering to be shared with the clinician.

The client has abilities as well as difficulties, degrees of insight and knowledge about stuttering and about therapy. Fundamental to this client's contributions in a therapeutic interaction are the constructs he or she brings and uses in the engagement with a clinician, and these will be discussed later in this chapter.

In considering this first element in our triad, we are aware that we write from our perspective as clinicians, relying on our empathetic skills and our personal experiences with clients to allow us to see how our triad is changed by these variables. We might hypothesize that how the client presents and the client's narrative, willingness to engage in the therapy process, and constructions of self and the dynamic with the therapist all have a bearing on the outcome.

## PRESENTATION

How an individual describes his or her difficulties to a clinician provides the clinician with an important window on what the client believes the issues to be. Some adults who stutter see the limitations of dysfluent speech purely in terms of their immediate daily lives, aware only of the difficulties that stuttering presents in specific settings, such as public transportation, restaurants, or shops. Other clients are aware of the implications of, for example, avoidance behaviors on their lives, the effect on their confidence in speaking situations, and the fundamental consequence on their ability to construe themselves as being in control.

Aside from the specific kinds of problems described, how individuals narrate their stories is also of interest. Narratives can reflect a range of emotions and beliefs that people have come to after years of living in certain ways. It is important for clinicians to reflect not only on the content of what is said but attend to the underlying message conveyed by the mode of delivery.

## CLINICAL EXAMPLE

When working on the completion of a checklist documenting covert or emotional components of his stutter, Martin began talking about the relationship he had with his parents and his troubled childhood. He became upset but obviously felt it was important to explore and describe the link he had made between these past troubles and his stutter. It was very difficult and emotionally intense for him to recount his experiences, but this effort reflected his determination to begin the process of coming to terms with events and his desire to be open with the clinician.

## ABILITY TO ENGAGE IN A THERAPEUTIC PROCESS

It is important to consider the point at which an individual embarks upon therapy. It may come after months of searching and considering options or it may be precipitated by a single significant event. A useful model for looking at this "entry point" is Prochaska and DiClemente's transtheoretical model of change (1982):

1. Precontemplation: This is a time when change is not considered because it may be thought of as too difficult.

2. Contemplation: This is when the person considers the advantages and disadvantages of change.
3. Preparation: Here, various processes are put into place as a precursor for the next stage.
4. Action: Change is under way.
5. Maintenance: The person uses strategies to ensure that skills and behaviors learned in the previous stage are consistently present over time.

In our experience, most clients present themselves at the point of action when beginning therapy. However, if a clinic has a long waiting list for initial appointments, a clinician can miss the opportunity to engage with the client at this important moment. Waiting for several weeks may mean an individual returns to the phase of contemplation, and the clinician will have to begin the process of motivating and moving the client back into action.

Occasionally, other factors are at work that prevent clients from engaging in therapy. There are individuals whose past experiences have led them to believe they do not have the ability to change. Their stories may include previous therapy, the results of which have been difficult to maintain, or relationships where they have felt the victim of others' change and/or been unable to initiate change autonomously. They may feel that in other aspects of their lives, as well as in their stuttering, they are not the agents of their own change and can best be described as having an external locus of control. (An *external locus of control* is the sense that events run their course regardless of individuals' attempts to influence the direction of the outcome, whereas an *internal locus of control* contributes to feelings of being able to effect change on the environment and events [Craig, Franklin, & Andrews, 1984].)

In instances where clients have feelings of not being in control, not being effective, it is important for them to have an experience that demonstrates a small area of change early in the therapy process. This should be an area of little importance to them, a nonspeech behavior such as a change in routine (e.g., going to work by a different route), making a different choice (e.g., eating different food for lunch), or having a different experience (e.g., going away for the day). In this way, people loosen a way of thinking about themselves because they have seen themselves behaving differently. They can now attach greater meaning to their behavior as people who change because of this experience.

## WORKING WITH MEANING

Many clinicians recognize that in order for therapy to be meaningful and have long-term benefits for clients, it must be congruent with their constructions about a range of issues. If the therapy is at odds with the individual's beliefs about how a speech and language clinician should behave, what therapy should be like, or what fluency should sound like, for example, then the result will not be integrated into the person's construction system. There are several examples in the literature and in our personal experiences of individual clients who demonstrated excellent skill in the fluency techniques in the clinic. However, on excursions to the outside, the individual was observed not to use the techniques and experienced marked dysfluent speech as a result. It appears that the individual chose to stutter rather than be fluent in a controlled way. Clinicians may puzzle over why a client prefers to stutter when all the therapeutic efforts are directed toward creating a fluent type of speech. However, if the techniques are not seen by clients as part of who they believe themselves to be, the use of control techniques will remain artificial. The techniques will function no better than a coat that is taken down in the worst of weathers and found to fit poorly and have worn fabric due to neglect. Therefore, a clinician must primarily be interested in gaining an understanding of what is meaningful to a client. In this way the clinician is able to adapt the therapeutic process to fit with this understanding.

To develop the most effective clinical program, a clinician needs to take into account the client's learning style, including response to medium (i.e., visual, auditory, etc.), and need for theoretical rationale. However, it is important to consider the type of therapy and the way it is presented to the client. In our experience, some clients need to be introduced to the therapeutic model and given an opportunity to adjust their stance to it, in other words to socialize to the model. For example, some individuals assume they will participate in therapy that uses the medical model as a framework. Thus, they expect clinicians to provide answers for their problems and tell them what changes they need to make. Many clinicians currently prefer to work in a more didactic way and allow clients to experiment with several options before deciding for themselves which one to adopt. A client coming to therapy expecting a speech and language clinician to be the expert may be uncomfortable at first with an alternative way of working. In addition to some explanation, this client may need time to consider the meaning of this practice for him or her.

Another issue to consider is what triggers change in a client's system. Working on behavior change may successfully allow clients to experience differences in the way they operate in his daily life. Frequently, small changes that may or may not be related to stuttering can be all that is required to create meaning for some clients.

## CLINICAL EXAMPLE

Jim realized he did not have to rush to answer the bus driver's question about his required destination. Giving himself just a second or two to regulate his breathing and gain eye contact with the driver had a significant effect on his feelings of control and composure. When this behavior change is successful, it can in turn begin a realization that changes are possible and develop confidence in the process.

Some clients, however, need different experiences for the change process to begin. They may respond to requests for trying changes in behavior with a "yes but" response (e.g., "Yes, but it was a different driver today"; "Yes, but I didn't really keep eye contact for very long and lost it again when I said my fare"). In these cases, the focus needs to be on the client's understanding of his or her construction system. The clinician will need to present a hypothesis to the client relating the client's behavior to a possible attitude or belief. For example, "I wonder if you are unable to spend those extra seconds composing yourself before speaking to the driver because you experience that time as silence. Perhaps you equate silence with blocking, so you would rather not experience the silence because it is like stuttering, and you are unable to tolerate stuttering." If the client is accepting of this hypothesis presented by the clinician, he or she may be willing to experiment with tolerating silence, which could lead to developing tolerance of silent blocks in the client's own speech.

## THE CLINICIAN

The clinician is a person who has interest in and curiosity about communication and experience in evaluating communication abilities and disabilities. The clinician engages in therapy to understand and help alleviate the client's presenting problems, aiming to develop the client's potential communication effectiveness. The clinician has been educated to develop the knowledge, skills, and attitudes of a professional speech and language pathologist and strives to provide the best possible service available in terms of efficiency and effectiveness. The clinician has an ethical responsibility to be the best possible therapist in clinical situation. Although the clinician shares professional knowledge and has skills and attitudes similar to other members of the profession, he or she brings unique personal traits and life experience to the therapy situation. How the clinician construes fluency, stuttering, his or her own role in therapy, and the client's role are all individual differences to be considered.

The role the clinician plays in affecting positive outcomes has long been recognized in other fields, as well as speech and language pathology. Bernstein Ratner (2006, p. 260), discussing the clinician's specific participation, states that "in some meta-analysis of therapy outcomes, therapists seem to matter more than therapies in achieving outcomes." Our clinical experience would complement this view. We are aware of some speech and language clinicians achieving better outcomes with the same program than others who are equally experienced. It is interesting to consider the factors that we believe have contributed to these more individualized results. Certainly some specific skills can be identified. For example, to engage in evidence-based practice (EBP), Canadian Cochrane Network and Centre (2003) recommended five steps for clinicians:

1. Ask a clear, focused question.
2. Find the best evidence.
3. Critically appraise the evidence and determine whether it can be used with the client.
4. Integrate the evidence with clinical judgment and client values and circumstance.
5. Evaluate performance.

In order to successfully engage in an EBP process, there are certain prerequisites for a speech and language clinician.

1. The clinician must have the ability to adopt a hypothesis-testing approach. Some clinicians operate from more short-term considerations, where management is based on sessional objectives. In this instance, the focus is on *how* the client's symptoms appear and the development of tasks that will ameliorate the condition. This is in contrast to those clinicians who are able to assimilate information presented by a client's narrative, along with formal and informal assessments, and devise a statement relating to *why* the client is presenting in a particular way.
2. The clinician needs to have access to evidence to assess others' experiences with different treatment approaches. Remarkably, there are specialists who are not sufficiently supported and therefore have limited continuing professional development opportunities, poor library or referencing facilities, and restricted peer support.
3. The clinician needs to have well-developed critical evaluation skills in order to appraise the available evidence. He or she needs to not only understand the concepts presented in the literature but to be able to apply these to particular clients and their situations where appropriate.
4. The clinician must be able to discuss the product of assessing clients' circumstances and be able to recommend management options in such a way that is meaningful to the clients and motivates them to engage in a therapeutic process when this is an outcome that matches their needs.
5. The clinician should have the ability to record and reflect on the dynamics in the therapeutic process (i.e., monitoring change in the client and an awareness of what is working, what is effective in therapy).

An obvious conclusion that one might draw from consideration of the clinician's competencies is that more experienced clinicians can be more effective. In our opinion, these skills are not necessarily the prerogative of advanced practitioners with years of experience. In fact, they can be observed in some less experienced individuals. Where these particular competencies are limited or absent, they can be developed, given appropriate support and supervision from experienced practitioners. Indeed, it is incumbent on advanced practitioners to provide this help to ensure the succession of appropriate levels of competency in the speech-language pathology profession.

Now let us consider how the clinician interacts with the other elements in our triad.

## Clinician and Therapy

A client-centered model is recommended as good practice when working with adults who stutter. In clinical sessions this would be observed as a nonexpert stance, allowing clients to take the lead. Focusing on client narrative also supports this perspective. That is, each client brings something individual to the therapy context and can teach the clinician how to best accommodate the treatment process to the client's needs. Some clinicians might find themselves at odds with this practice and prefer a more directive, behavioral approach to a client's problem. In such an instance, were a clinician to try and adopt a client-centered stance in the face of a different preference, the result would be less than convincing to the client and consequently less effective.

## Clinician and Client

Individuals, regardless of profession, background, or competency, are better at forming successful, cooperative relationships with some individuals than others. More specifically, some individuals can find "empathetic spots" and areas of commonality with some other people more easily than with others. This feature of human relationships can also be applied to therapeutic interactions; clinicians will relate better to some clients than others. The more skilled clinician may be able to operate with a degree of success in the face of reduced commonality but would be aware of progress in less than ideal circumstances and may have to work harder as a consequence.

The clinician–client dynamic and its reflection in positive therapeutic outcomes was clearly illustrated in recent work in the field of discourse analysis (see Duchan & Leahy, 2008). One of the major contributors to the field of stuttering during the 20th century was Charles Van Riper (1904–1995), who developed the stuttering modification approach to therapy. An example of this approach was video recorded in the Action Therapy tapes (Van Riper, 1977). Although Van Riper had the reputation of sometimes being unduly harsh as a therapist, he generally achieved good results. His session on desensitization, which is part of the Action Therapy tapes, is with an 18-year-old student, referred to in the following extract as client C. This session has been analyzed (Leahy, 2008), and parts of the analysis are worthy of consideration in this context.

The desensitization session with C. opens with a sequence, where the therapist (V.R.) acknowledges C. and refers to the previous week's task.

1. V.R.: Well C., here we are again eh a moment ago I felt your pulse and
2. it was racing em but you've had a hard week
3. C.: Yes
4. V.R.: Having to identify your stuttering
5. I guess and I'd like to know if the thing has happened to you
6. that usually happens to many stutterers after they begin
7. to explore their stuttering to catalogue it to examine it to take a look at
8. it to feel it a lot of emotion usually rises up, any in you?
9. C.: Yes I find it very hard to I I find it really hard to elauelauelauelauelau
10. look at my stuttering em it just I feel like in the past week I've been (+t)
11. stuttering a lot more more severely
12. V.R.: And I did that to you didn't I? eh the dirty dog
13. C.: (laughs)

V.R.'s focus on task is immediate, following a cursory reference to C.'s racing pulse. In this brief introduction, V.R. has established his professional stance, created in a medical reference in feeling C.'s pulse. By referring to what "usually happens to many stutterers" (line 6), V.R. emphasizes his expertise and experience, and he later uses a metaphoric reference for increasing emotion. C. agrees (line 9), stuttering severely, refers to the difficulty he has had in looking at his stutter. V.R. acknowledges his response, displaying some self-depreciating humor as he does so (line 12). In the sequence, V.R.'s initial frame of medical and specialist expertise in stuttering establishes his formal, authoritative role, socially distant from the client. However, V.R. shifts his footing by using humor, minimizing the social distance, presenting a warmer and more understanding persona than that of the expert. The use of humor helps build solidarity and affiliation, and it can mitigate embarrassment and solicit cooperation (Simmons-Mackie & Schultz, 2003). In this instance, it serves both the former and latter functions. Along with his use of humor, the responsibility for how C. has been during the previous week has been assumed by V.R. in the remark (line 12), indicating his sense of control. However, the remark also demonstrates that V.R. has uttered words that C. could not: "the dirty dog" referring to himself, in a self-depreciating way. This shows how V.R. was able to align with the client, saying words that the client could not, using humor to build up the rapport, and ensure that the client was motivated and "on side." The distinct roles employed by Van Riper—the socially distant expert-in-control along with the warm, humorous, caring person—represent what has been termed "tough love" in other contexts: where the harsh or stern quality expressed masks the genuine concern that motivates the harsh words or behavior.

At later stages in the session, Van Riper demonstrates his authority, as well as showing empathy, in anticipating the client's responses to questions about his feelings. He also uses metaphors to demonstrate clearly his understanding of the pain experienced by people who stutter. Although elements of the interaction show a harsh and critical quality, this is balanced to an extent by Van Riper's ability to empathize, to align with the client, and thus to encourage positive client responses. (See Leahy, 2008, for further discussion on the interaction style of Van Riper.) The close inspection provided by analysis of clinical discourse helps us gain a good understanding of why Van Riper's therapy was successful: Even though therapy incorporated a harsh quality that could predominate the interaction, Van Riper's warmth, humor, and alignment with the client shine through, ultimately helping the client to become a more confident communicator.

## THE THERAPY

### THERAPY FOR STUTTERING

Therapy for stuttering has historical roots in attempts to understand fluency, dysfluency, and motor speech. Since the 1960s, understanding of psychological aspects of stuttering has developed and has incorporated interpretations (Van Riper,

1971, 1973; Sheehan 1984), including the impact of the stutter, and applications of particular approaches to change (e.g., Fransella's 1972 application of Personal construct psychology [Kelly, 1991] to stuttering [Leahy, 2002; Stewart & Birdsall, 2001]). The therapeutic management of stuttering involves direct attention to all that is involved in speaking and to the bigger picture where speech occurs, encapsulating psychosocial interaction perspectives. Currently, the therapeutic approach may be viewed as being drawn from cognitive, behavioral, and psychological techniques (or a combination of some or all of these) and incorporates techniques to improve fluency control alongside work on varying the stuttering behavior itself.

Five general principles of therapy are generally accepted as good practice.

1. Identification: "A method by which a person learns about all the different components of his stammer. It enables him to take the pieces apart, examine them and put them back together as one might reassemble an engine. This process enables the individual to develop a fuller understanding of his stammering and perhaps increase his awareness of features that had hitherto been apparent only to his listeners. In addition … it allows the person to confront his difficulties directly, perhaps after a lifetime of running away from them or trying to hide specific features from himself and others." (Turnbull & Stewart, 1999, p. 51)

2. Desensitization: Basically, work in this area aims to change the way clients construe their stuttering and help individuals see it as something they do rather than something they are. Van Riper (1973) targets three areas in his approach to desensitization: confrontation of the disorder, core behavior (which raises a client's tolerance for "fixations and oscillations"), and resisting communicative stress and listener penalty.

3. Avoidance reduction: This area is generally associated with the work of Joseph Sheehan (1975, 1979). Therapy, for Sheehan, consisted solely of work on avoidance and required two kinds of acceptance: "Firstly he (the stutterer) must develop sufficient acceptance of himself as a stutterer to stop concealing the problem from himself and others—long enough to undertake a systematic, weakening of the handicapping behaviours via principles of learning. Second, he must accept the goal of less than perfect fluency, for no one has that" (Sheehan, 1979, p. 178).

4. Fluency modification: This includes work on breathing and relaxation, rate control, easy onset, block modification, and so forth.

5. Maintenance. In the United Kingdom, there is a general move away from working on transfer and generalization of skills as a separate phase of therapy. Currently, clients are encouraged to be aware of and collect strategies that will help them when they leave the supportive environment of regular therapy sessions. Stewart & Richardson (2004) suggested that these are more dynamic in nature and may include problem-solving skills, risk taking, personal care programs, and development of support networks.

Although these processes are listed as separate, in practice identification is carried out alongside some nonspeech variation or loosening of behaviors. Desensitization and avoidance reduction are often worked on in parallel, with fluency modification introduced only when clients are sufficiently desensitized to their stuttering and their avoidance behaviors have been markedly reduced at all levels.

Let us now consider the interplay of this therapy element with other dynamics. If we adopt the perspective that the above processes are acceptable good practices in current thinking, then it is interesting to reflect on how these processes interact in the dynamic between clinician and client.

## Therapy and Client

One important function of therapy is to match the therapeutic approach with client need. However, this is not as straightforward as it might first appear. For example, a client may request specific fluency management at the onset of therapy. The client may even have researched the evidence and have an idea of the specific type of fluency control he or she wishes to learn (e.g., easy onset, rate control). The clinician may have alternative ideas, perhaps based on observations and assessment of the client's avoidance behaviors and feelings associated with the occurrence of dysfluencies. The clinician may believe that long-term, positive outcomes require a focus on desensitization and avoidance reduction techniques. Taking a client-led approach, the clinician would present the various options to the client with a rationale and allow the client to dictate the starting point. If the client chooses his or her own way, the clinician may have to support the client through a process of failing to use fluency techniques outside the clinic for fear of stammering. Through experiencing this process, the client may come to realize the need for a different approach. Alternatively, should the clinician take a more directive, behavioral approach, presenting the hypothesis and rationale for work on the client's covert feelings toward the stutter with no other options, the client may feel dragged along and consider that therapy is not addressing his or her specific needs. There are at least two possible outcomes: the client's belief in the clinician as expert could help him or her engage in the therapy process, or the client may see little point to it all and opt out of therapy before realizing some benefits.

In the first scenario described above, the clinician almost suspends his or her expertise and allows the client to make the choice. However, the implications of that choice of therapeutic approach are not lost to the clinician, who is aware of the need to support the client, possibly through a number of painful processes, allowing the client to learn from his or her own experiences rather than the clinician's.

In the alternative scenario, the reverse is exemplified. The client is required to accept the clinician's superior knowledge and follow a process defined by the clinician's experiences with other clients. Of course, even the experienced clinician is unable to predict how this particular client will react to the course of therapy, whereas the client may be more able to pre-empt and accurately predict those responses, being his or her own expert.

## Therapy and Clinician

There are also important dynamics that operate between the clinician and therapy options. As we have seen, relationships between individuals are subject to differences, in that some people respond more successfully than others to the development of cooperative dynamic. A similar principle can be applied to the relationship between clinician and a therapeutic approach. There are experienced clinicians who are fully apprised of the range of alternatives in the management of stuttering, who are aware of the various benefits each approach might yield and determining the clients most suited to the different interventions. However, despite this extensive knowledge, many clinicians choose to use one or two of the options available because these are the types of interventions that best fit their practice and with which they themselves are most comfortable. It may be that some of our EBP is negatively affected by this clinician-centered variable. Clinicians may be reporting positive outcomes from the one type of therapeutic intervention they happen to be using as a matter of their choice only. They may well be more confident with this approach and, because of their consistent use of it, be more competent in its application. There will be a lack of reported results of several interventions across their case load, and as a result, the evidence-based data collected will be skewed toward the intervention of their choice. Obviously, this is rather an extreme example, but there are instances of clinicians making some therapy options (e.g., fluency shaping) less available to clients because as clinicians they did not appreciate its long-term validity and/or disliked working in a purely behavioral way for any length of time.

## EFFECTIVENESS

### Assessment Processes

In this section we consider how our current assessment processes relate to the elements of the triad discussed above of client, clinician, and therapy.

Ideally, assessment is an open, informative, and explorative process, with exchange of information between the client and clinician that will assist both parties in identifying, describing, and delineating the nature of the problem and estimating its severity. In some instances (e.g., in late-onset stuttering or acquired stuttering) causative factors may be an important issue for consideration.

When a client and a clinician meet to assess stuttering, there are several questions being addressed by both parties. Some clinical questions typically include issues about the existence of a problem, its nature, its severity, and how best to describe these features. Others will reflect intense curiosity about the client and the effect of the stutter on his or her day-to-day life. Ultimately, the clinician is hopeful that the process will lead to a good understanding of what the problem is for the client, and begin to formulate hypotheses about its nature, its variability, and how to open up possibilities for managing these issues. Some clients' questions may include the following: "What's the meaning of asking all these questions? I know I have a stutter, and how bad it can be, and can explain this, but will I give the wrong impression if I'm fluent? How badly will I stutter today? Why ask me about attitudes? Do they think I have a psychological problem as well as the stutter? Why am I not better informed about this? When will they start doing something to help?" Others may be less knowing and more curious about the therapist and the process, wanting to know more about the stuttering, its description, and its severity, perhaps waiting for the expert to analyze and report on the nature of the problem.

The process will include the clinician informing the client about objectives of the assessment, addressing issues about stuttering, and listening closely to answers. It will usually include some sampling of the client's speech and non-verbal behaviors (and often videorecording these for analysis, identification, and comparison). As some clients will come to therapy having researched various options and read widely about approaches to therapy, it is wise to provide the opportunity for clients to ask questions and to provide comments or answers to questions that are not asked. The recognition of the client as expert in his or her own life and experience of stuttering moves the clinician away from adopting traditional models of therapy and simultaneously encourages client autonomy.

## What Assessment Procedures Reveal: The Client

The variety of published assessment procedures available for working with adults who stutter suggests that all the questions we may have about this area have already been addressed by many clinician–investigators, in many different ways (Crowe, Di Lollo, & Crowe, 2000). Ideas about quantifying and measuring aspects of stuttering are well documented, and despite the knowledge that stuttering is variable in nature and that sampling data are unlikely to provide truly valid or reliable estimates of severity, the false security presented by measurement means that many clinicians persist in prioritizing this form of assessment. Clinic samples (and occasionally outside-of-clinic samples) of the type and frequency of stuttering are usually recorded during the first two or three sessions, and they do serve a useful function in describing the overt impact of stuttering on the listener and for the speaker. However, these types of data corpora cannot hope to capture all of the relevant information for deciding how to create a well-designed therapy program that fits the individual characteristics of the client. Pretherapy and post-therapy comparisons are often made by collecting samples of stuttering type and frequency, to help evaluate the effects of therapy, and these too may serve a useful function in contrasting how overt symptoms have changed over time.

Complementing a focus on overt features, description and evaluation of the covert (or hidden) features of stuttering have been usual features of assessment since authors (including, for example, Johnson, Woolf, and Erikson) developed procedures that describe and measure feelings, reactions, and attitudes that often accompany stuttering. Procedures such as the Stutterer's Self-Ratings of Reactions to Speech Situations (Johnson, Darley, & Spriestersbach, 1963), the Perceptions of Stuttering Inventory (Woolf, 1967), and communication attitude scales (S24; Erikson, 1969) have been widely exploited to attempt to understand the depth of negativity that persons who stutter experience. However, recent research has questioned the usefulness of a number of these procedures (Franic & Bothe, 2008).

The iceberg model (Sheehan, 1984; Stewart, 2008) uses the analogy of the one tenth visible versus the nine tenths concealed parts of the iceberg to represent what stuttering is. That is, the visible overt features (type and frequency of stutters) are only the tip of the iceberg. Feelings of shame, fear, lack of confidence, avoidance, inferiority, and so forth, have all been documented as common elements of stuttering and exist below the surface of the water.

An additional focus of assessment is the qualitative approach that gives the opportunity for the client's experience of stuttering to be explored and for client priorities to take precedence when therapy decisions are made. Qualitative assessment procedures overlap to a large extent with aspects of covert features, but they also seek to estimate the impact of the problem on the client's level of activities and participation in day-to-day life, and they reflect the influence of practice of the International Classification of Functioning & Disability (WHO, 2001). Useful examples of assessments in this area are the Wright and Ayre Stuttering Self-Rating Profile (Wright & Ayre, 2000) and the Overall Assessment of the Speaker's Experience of Stuttering (Yaruss & Quesal, 2006).

There are a number of other, more minor assessment tools available. One notable example is the locus of control scales (Craig et al., 1984). These are useful to discover beliefs about the relative influence of fate, luck, and personal motivation in determining behaviors and motivation to change.

## GAPS IN MEASUREMENT

### The Client

Relating back to our triad, it is clear that there are major omissions in measurement from the client's perspective. Current assessments fail to reflect the client–therapy dynamic. There are no formal or informal procedures in use to gain information on factors that would have a bearing on this area; for example, client understanding of the current approaches available, client preference of approach, and why such a preference has been decided upon. Such information could be collected as part of the case history, but it is clearly not obtained routinely, nor is it considered by many clinicians as providing relevant information when developing their client's management plan.

In addition, clinicians do not obtain data on issues that relate to the client–therapist dynamic. For example, clients' learning style, clients' preferred interaction style (e.g., use of humor, need for theoretical rationale) are rarely considered. If we agree that the nature of the clinical interaction is a crucial part of determining its effectiveness, then clinicians could usefully examine this area and use the information to modify their interactive style in ways that would enhance the clients' learning.

### Therapy

Choices taken by clinicians regarding the predominant approach to assessment taken reveal their theoretical preferences. Where openness, flexibility, and resources are available for clinicians and for clients, assessment and therapy options may be molded to accommodate client preferences. In practical terms, however, we offer what we have to offer. Factors such as service pressures, prioritization of certain clients over others, and resource issues all play a part in determining what is offered to particular clients at particular times. In addition, clinicians negotiate client preferences (i.e., their search for fluency balanced against the search for successful management of stuttering) with their own personal and professional evidence of what works. In terms of effectiveness, however, there is little evidence that these various factors are measured as part of the assessment process. Again, if we agree that they are important in determining the effectiveness of any management program, then questions are raised about the need to reconsider the tools at our disposal.

## Clinician

Finally, how and when do we assess the role we play in the management of individuals who stammer? There is certainly no published protocol available to specialist clinicians that would enable them or their managers to evaluate their effectiveness. However, there are mechanisms that can assist individuals to consider their skill and competencies in general and in relation to specific clients. These include accessing clinical supervision within their workplace or through a specialist network. Such a system, although often optional in the United Kingdom, provides a means of clinical reflection in a safe and constructive environment and within the bounds of a structured process and is to be recommended. Other opportunities for evaluation are often part of an appraisal system carried out by a superior and/or line manager. In the United Kingdom, this would take place at least annually and include a clinical audit and discussion of caseload management issues.

It is incumbent on clinicians at all levels to evaluate and reflect on individual cases as part of their professional development. It is not always easy to acknowledge when particular cases have gone less well but openness to reflection in these situations can be the catalyst to making important changes. As clinicians, we learn a great deal from our clients if we take the time to reflect on and incorporate our learning into future management.

## CONCLUSION

This chapter has considered the unique nature of therapy for adults who stutter. It has argued that the individual experiences in each therapeutic encounter are based on the interaction of a triad of variables: the client, the clinician, and the type of therapy. Each of these variables brings with it a range of characteristics and features intrinsically important in shaping the experience for the participants. In addition, the way in which the elements of the triad fit together can have a fundamental impact on the outcome of therapy. We have considered the individual features brought by each aspect of the triad and have discussed what we consider important dynamics between the components of that triad. In looking at our current understanding of effectiveness in the management of stuttering in adults, it is clear thus far that outcomes have been largely based on the client element of the triad. Little attention has been paid to other elements, such as the role of the therapy itself or the vital role of the clinician. Among the challenges for the clinician is to be aware of the uniqueness she brings to the therapy setting. This means that the clinician must consider how he or she expresses uniqueness, or in referring to O'Donoghue's terms (2007), how the clinician inhabits his or her individuality. We believe that reflection on these individual differences and on the way the elements of the triad interact with them may be a fruitful avenue to improving effectiveness in this field.

## REFERENCES

Bernstein Ratner, N. (2006). Evidence based practice: An examination of its ramifications for the practice of speech & language pathology. *Language, Speech, and Hearing Services in Schools, 37*, 257–267.

Canadian Cochrane Network and Centre. (2003). *A primer on evidence based practice.* Retrieved August 22, 2008, from http://www.cochrane.uottawa.ca/pdf/presentations/EBCPPrimer_July_2003.pdf

Crowe, T. A., Di Lollo, A., & Crowe, B. T. (2000). *Crowe's protocols: A comprehensive guide to stuttering assessment.* San Antonio, TX: The Psychological Corporation.

Craig, A., Franklin, J., & Andrews, G. (1984). A scale to measure locus of control of behaviour. *British Journal of Medical Psychology, 57*, 173–180.

Duchan, J. F., & Leahy, M. M. (Eds.) (2008). Hearing the voices of people with communication disabilities. *International Journal of Language & Communication Disorders, 43*, 1–4.

Erikson, R. L. (1969). Assessing communication attitudes among stutterers. *Journal of Speech and Hearing Research, 12*, 711–724.

Franic, D. M., & Bothe, A. K. (2008). Psychometric evaluation of condition-specific instruments used to assess health-related quality of life, attitudes, and related constructs in stuttering. *American Journal of Speech-Language Pathology, 17*, 60–81.

Fransella, F. (1972). *Personal change and reconstruction.* London: Academic Press.

Johnson, W., Darley, F., Spriestersbach, D. (1963). *Diagnostic methods in speech pathology.* New York: Harper & Row, Publishers.

Kelly, G. A. (1991). *The psychology of personal constructs.* New York: Routledge.

Leahy, M. M. (2002). *Real change can be constructed: Personal construct therapy in stuttering therapy.* Fifth Annual ISAD Conference. Retrieved August 22, 2008, from http://www.mnsu.edu/comdis/isad5/papers/leahy.html

Leahy, M. M. (2008). Multiple voices in Charles Van Riper's desensitization therapy. *International Journal of Language & Communication Disorders, 43*, 69–80.

O'Donoghue, J. (2007). *Benedictus: A book of blessings.* London: Transworld Publishers.

Prochaska, J. O., & DiClemente., C. C. (1982). Transtheoretical therapy: Toward a more integrative model of change. *Psychotherapy: Theory, Research & Practice, 19*, 276–288.

Rolfe, G. (2006). Technical rationality and the theory—Practice gap. *Nursing Sciences Quarterly 19*, 39–43.

Sheehan, J. G. (1975). Conflict theory and avoidance reduction therapy. In J. Eisenson (Ed.), *Stuttering: A second symposium* (pp. 97–198). New York: Harper and Row.

Sheehan, J. G. (1979). Stuttering and recovery. In H. H. Gregory (Ed.), *Controversies about stuttering therapy* (pp. 175–207). Baltimore: University Park Press.

Sheehan, J. G. (1984). Problems in the evaluation of progress and outcome. In W. Perkins (Ed.), *Current therapy of communication disorders: Stuttering disorders* (pp. 223–239). New York: Thieme-Stratton.

Simmons-Mackie, N., & Schultz, M. (2003). The role of humour in therapy for aphasia. *Aphasiology, 17*, 751–766.

Stewart, T. (2008, July). Avoidance reduction in adults who stammer: A clinical discussion. A paper presented at the Oxford Dysfluency Conference, Oxford University, United Kingdom.

Stewart, T., & Birdsall, M. (2001). A review of the contribution of Personal Construct Psychology to stammering therapy. *Journal of Constructivist Psychology, 14*, 215–225.

Stewart, T., & Richardson, G. (2004). A qualitative study of therapeutic effect from a user's perspective. *Journal of Fluency Disorders, 29*, 95–108.

Turnbull, J., & Stewart, T. (1999). *The dysfluency resource book*. London: Speechmark Publishing.

Van Riper, C. (1971). *The nature of stuttering*. Englewood Cliffs, NJ: Prentice-Hall.

Van Riper, C. (1973). *The treatment of stuttering*. Englewood Cliffs, NJ: Prentice Hall.

Van Riper, C. (1977). *Action therapy* (videotapes). Memphis, TN: Speech Foundation of America.

Woolf, G., (1967). The assessment of stuttering as struggle, avoidance, and expectancy. *British Journal of Disorders of Communication, 2*, 158–171.

World Health Organisation (WHO). (2001). *The international classification of functioning, disability and health*. Geneva, Switzerland: WHO.

Wright, L., & Ayre, A. (2000). *WASSP: Stuttering self-rating profile*. Bicester, United Kingdom: Winslow Press.

Yaruss, J. S., & Quesal, R. (2006). Overall assessment of the speaking experiences of stuttering (OASES): Documenting multiple outcomes in stuttering treatment. *Journal of Fluency Disorders, 31*, 90–115.

# 11 Individual Differences That Influence Responsiveness to the Lidcombe Program

*Rosemarie Hayhow and Rosalee C. Shenker*

## INTRODUCTION

The Lidcombe Program (LP) is a behavioral treatment developed for preschool-age children who stutter (Onslow, Packman & Harrison, 2003). In this therapy, the parent is trained to present verbal contingencies (feedback) for stutter-free speech and for stuttering in everyday speaking situations. The treatment begins with parents providing feedback initially for stutter-free speech and then adding less frequent feedback for their child's stuttering in more structured conversations. More structured conversations usually take place in a relatively quiet context, and visual stimuli or specific activities are used so that length and complexity of utterances can be reduced as necessary to obtain plenty of stutter-free speaking. Within a conversation, the structure can be loosened as children become more fluent and then tightened again if more stuttering occurs. As children's stuttering reduces, the treatment gradually changes so that the feedback is given in unstructured or naturally arising conversations throughout the day.

The LP was developed as a two-stage treatment. During Stage 1, the parent and child who stutters visit the clinic once a week. At each visit, the goal of the speech-language pathologist (SLP) is to train parents to deliver the treatment at home. The parent demonstrates how treatment has been conducted at home during the previous week; the SLP provides feedback to ensure that treatment has been appropriately administered. The SLP then demonstrates any adjustments or changes that need to be made in the coming week to promote effectiveness, taking into account how the child is responding to treatment. Fluency and stuttering are both monitored by measuring the percentage of unambiguous stutters (%SS) at the start of each weekly clinic visit and by collecting the parent's daily severity ratings (SRs) made during the previous week. The parent is trained to use a 10-point scale for these ratings, where 1 = no stuttering, 2 = extremely mild stuttering, and 10 = extremely severe stuttering. Continued weekly clinic visits ensure correct implementation of procedures once parents have learned to use the parental verbal contingencies (PVCs) safely, appropriately, and in a ratio of five PVCs for stutter-free speech to every PVC for stuttering. Difficulties that may arise during administration of the home program are discussed; parents and clinicians work together to jointly solve emerging problems so that parents can effectively treat their children's stuttering on a daily basis. Stage 1 is nearing completion when there is less than 1%SS in the weekly clinic sample and SRs for the previous week are 1 or 2, with at least four of these ratings being 1. These criteria must be met for three consecutive weeks (Webber & Onslow, 2003) before starting Stage 2, which aims to maintain program speech criteria and prevent relapse. When the speech criteria are met during Stage 2's clinic visits, PVCs are gradually withdrawn, and the frequency of clinic visits systematically decreases.

There is an extensive and robust evidence base for the LP, showing it to be an efficacious treatment for children who are under 6 years of age at the start of treatment. Evidence is available for the social validity of the treatment (Lincoln, Onslow, & Reed, 1997), and there is evidence that this treatment causes no negative changes to the child's developing expressive language (Bonelli, Dixon, Bernstein Ratner, & Onslow, 2000; Lattermann, Shenker, & Thoradoridottir, 2005; Rousseau, Packman, Onslow, Harrison, & Jones, 2007). A randomized controlled trial (RCT) was conducted comparing the effectiveness of the LP with a control group of preschool-age children who received no treatment for 9 months (Jones et al., 2005). In this study, the effect size of the RCT was large enough to justify the conclusion that "the reduction in stuttering in the LP group was significantly and clinically greater than natural recovery" (Jones et al., 2005, p. 3). Phase I and II trials have shown that low levels of stuttering are maintained 2–7 years after treatment (Lincoln & Onslow, 1997; Miller & Guitar, 2009; Onslow, Andrews, & Lincoln, 1994; Onslow, Costa, & Rue, 1990).

Two retrospective studies (Jones, Onslow, Harrison, & Packman, 2000; Kingston, Huber, Onslow, Jones, & Packman, 2003) presented recovery plot data for 316 children and showed that a median of 11 clinic visits were required to complete Stage 1, and 95% achieved this point of treatment by 21 weeks. The few remaining children took longer, and 22 children who were unable to complete treatment were excluded from the analysis. In some cases, the excluded children had significant language or behavioral problems, and so stuttering was not the primary concern, and in others there were domestic or family issues that impacted on the parents' commitment to stuttering treatment. These data provide benchmarks for expected time in Stage 1; however, it is now recommended (Webber & Onslow, 2003) that these criteria should be maintained for 3 weeks before moving on to Stage 2. When this new criterion is adopted, the median becomes 13 weeks before progressing to Stage 2. The retrospective studies indicate that children will vary in how quickly they respond to the LP; however, the aim of the LP is for children to achieve less than 1% SS in the clinic and SRs of 1 with only occasional 2s, so it is treatment length that varies rather than outcome. Onslow and Yaruss (2007) summarized the available outcome studies and concluded that none have identified a cohort of children who failed to respond to the treatment. Onslow and Yaruss further stated that SRs are expected to reduce by 30% within the first 5 weeks of treatment, and when this benchmark is not met, clinicians should seek assistance in reevaluating their specific approach unless there is evidence suggesting that the child is merely progressing more slowly.

The LP uses behavioral techniques and is supported by empirical research; it is not based on a belief about underlying causal mechanisms of stuttering (Packman & Attanasio, 2004). We could argue that early stuttering is an operant-like behavior and that that is why operant procedures can eliminate it, but many would feel this is an incomplete explanation. In the last 10 years, more information has been published about possible subtle neuroanatomical differences between children who stutter and those who do not (see review by Packman, Code, & Onslow, 2007); it is possible that the LP procedures help children learn a "work-around" (Onslow & Yaruss, 2007, p. 67) for this underlying cause. If this is the correct explanation for an underlying therapeutic mechanism in the LP, it still leaves questions about whether all the components of the treatment are indeed necessary for each client.

For example, Harrison, Onslow, and Menzies (2004) made a preliminary investigation of the importance of PVCs for stutter-free speech and stuttering, as well as the SRs, in the first 4 weeks of treatment. Stuttering reduced with just PVCs for stutter-free speech, but the reduction was more successfully maintained during the nontreatment phase of the study when PVCs for stuttering had also been used. Early in treatment, the SRs did not have an appreciable effect in increasing fluent speech, but this does not rule out the value they may have later in treatment, when clinical decisions are more clearly related to changes in SRs and when parents begin to use them to make ongoing judgments about how to administer home treatment. The possible importance of PVCs for stuttered speech, which encourages self-correction, relates well to Onslow's suggestion noted earlier that children are actively learning how to work around the interruptions they experience to the forward flow of speaking (Onslow & Yaruss, 2007).

The introduction to the LP presented in this chapter does not fully convey the real-life experience of using the LP as a clinician, a parent, or a child. Bernstein Ratner and Guitar (2006) noted that "some observers of ongoing parent–child sessions have commented on their almost Rogerian nature of quiet, cooperative and reflective interaction" (p. 117). LP training emphasizes that the child must enjoy both clinic and home treatment sessions; the PVCs need to occur in a supportive manner and the child's best interests always come first. The PVCs for stutter-free speech are attempts to draw children's attention to their smooth speaking, and the requests for self-correction are made in a neutral manner to reduce the likelihood that the child internalizes a sense of failure but rather perceives an invitation to smooth a bumpy word. For some children, this request may be received like a revelation, because it is interpreted as assurance that they *can* smooth the bumps. They may become further empowered when they find through their experiences with speaking that they do not have to struggle or force the words out. In early treatment, clinicians and parents carefully structure speaking situations to ensure that children speak with little stuttering and can be successful when asked to self-correct. To maximize success, parents also must provide feedback acknowledging a child's response to the PVC in a helpful, positive manner, for example, "that was great; you did a bump and fixed it." Parents often refer to these structured conversations as *talk-times*.

In a qualitative study of parents' experiences of the LP (Hayhow, 2008), a profile of straightforward implementation of the treatment emerged. The key features these parents identified were as follows:

1.  Parents were either enthusiastic when the LP was introduced to them or able to *give it a try* even though it may not fit with their personal view of stuttering or a child's learning processes.
2.  The following experiences were evident in their accounts:
    *   Their children's stuttering had reduced quickly and consistently.
    *   Parents found their own styles of implementing the procedures so that the contingencies became a natural part of treatment conversations.
    *   Overall, parents and children enjoyed the LP, and they had "special times" working together with their children's talking.
    *   The appearance of stuttering gradually became more predictable.
    *   Parents integrated the LP procedures into their everyday lives. They did not find their role as deliverers of the treatment overly demanding
    *   In some cases, there was a gradual shift from parents taking responsibility for their children's talking to the children taking on this responsibility themselves.
    *   Problems that arose with the implementation of the LP were resolved by parents in consultation with their clinician or by the parents' experimentation in adjusting the treatment.
3.  The parents experienced the LP as an evolving process, starting with the rather self-conscious application of contingencies in somewhat contrived conversations and moving to a more natural responsiveness to children's speaking. The responsiveness took account of the children's current need for contingencies and their need for more or less conversational structure. When it worked in this way, parents seemed confident that they had the skills and understanding to help their children, and the children were able to constructively respond to parental help. For these parent–child dyads, the LP was not an overly complex or demanding treatment, and the children's responsiveness validated the view that early stuttering can be a relatively simple problem to address.

In earlier studies, parents and clinicians were reported to have commented favorably on the structure and measurement that are an integral part of the LP (Hayhow, 2005; Shenker, Hayhow, Kingston, & Lawlor, 2005), and some expressed appreciation for the flexibility that is possible within this framework. When discussing this straightforward implementation of the LP, both clinicians and parents have commented that their behavior is also reinforced. The choice of the LP as an appropriate treatment is further supported when children enjoy treatment sessions and their stuttering is reduced in their everyday talking. Parents are reassured that what they are doing at home is right for their children, and their clinicians are reassured that they can use the LP effectively. These successful cases have met the benchmarks identified earlier, which offers further encouragement.

## WHAT IS A TYPICAL CASE FOR THE LP?

Routine case studies showing the progress of preschool children through the LP have been described by Rousseau & O'Brian (2003) and show similarities to the straightforward progression described by some parents in Hayhow's (2008) study. Benchmarks of a median of 13 clinic visits for completion of Stage 1, with 95% completing Stage 1 by 21 visits, were established in the retrospective studies conducted in Australia (Jones et al., 2000) and in the United Kingdom (Kingston et al., 2003). However, Rousseau et al. (2007) reported a mean of 16 clinic visits for the completion of Stage 1 by their participants, which indicates that some variation in median treatment time is to be expected, although the reasons for this are not clear. In Rousseau et al.'s (2007) study, the children all came from a small area within Sydney and were treated by one SLP, whereas the others came from various locations with a variety of clinicians. This suggested that there may be demographic and clinician variables that operate, but further research would be needed to clarify this.

A significant finding from the retrospective studies was that children who had been stuttering for more than 1 year took less time to reach Stage 1 than those stuttering for less than a year. Although age and gender are not significant predictors of treatment time, the trends suggested that girls and older children progress more quickly. Stuttering severity as measured by %SS at assessment was a predictor, with the more severe taking longer. The research conducted by Onslow and colleagues at the Australian Stuttering Research Centre has been primarily concerned with establishing whether or not the LP works as expected, whether there are unwanted side effects, whether it is more successful than awaiting a natural recovery, and whether the treatment results obtained in relatively small samples are more widely achievable. In order to answer these questions, quantitative methods have been used with increasingly large samples of children and using primarily descriptive data that is available in routine assessment and treatment. The investigation of how more subtle individual differences may impact on progress with the LP awaits research. However, SLPs using the LP work with a wide range of children and their problem solving during treatment often needs to take account of these differences. There are subtle differences in the timing, frequency, wording, and general presentation of contingencies that arise in routine cases when parents and clinicians discuss children's progress, their responses to contingencies, and the contexts when treatment occurs outside the clinic. These occur naturally when the procedures are implemented with sensitivity to the needs of individual parent–child dyads.

In this chapter, we approach the issue of individual differences by considering some clinical adjustments that have been made to the routine delivery of the LP in response to clients' individual needs. We will consider these adjustments in relation to (a) speech and language concerns, (b) parent responses to the LP, (c) cultural/linguistic issues, and (d) temperament. These are the differences that we have found require more carefully considered adaptations to the basic structure of the LP and that speech-language clinicians trained in provision of the LP also report to be challenging.

These cases provide examples of how treatment procedures can be adapted for individual child/parent dyads while adhering to the basic LP treatment protocol, for which there is an evidence base. We are not recommending deviation from the manualized (Australian Stuttering Research Centre, 2008) format for clinic sessions or the treatment overall but rather hope to illustrate how responsiveness to individual characteristics and circumstances can optimize progress. We also indicate how we may alter the criteria for Stage 2 in cases where clients present with a cognitive deficit.

## STUTTERING IN THE PRESENCE OF OTHER
## SPEECH AND LANGUAGE CONCERNS

Since stuttering often emerges at the same time as rapid phonological and language development (Bernstein Ratner, 1997; Yairi & Ambrose, 1999), it is not surprising that children who stutter frequently present with concomitant speech and language disorders. However, the extent to which this occurs is presently unknown (Bernstein Ratner, 2005; Hall, Wagovich, & Bernstein Ratner, 2007; Nippold, 1990, 2002, 2004; Thompson Byrd, Wolk, & Davis, 2007). Arndt and Healey (2001) and Blood, Ridenour, Qualls, and Hammer (2003) have noted that a significant number of children who stutter exhibit co-occurring language impairment. Yaruss, LaSalle, and Conture (1998), in a retrospective audit of 100 files, found that 15% of children who stuttered performed below average in receptive vocabulary testing and that 29% performed below average when expressive language was evaluated. Arndt and Healey and Blood et al. found that 56–62% of children who stutter had concomitant language, speech, or phonological disorders. In the Blood et al. findings, 33.5% presented with an articulation disorders and 12.7% with a phonological disorder. Taken together, these studies indicate that children who stutter are variable with regard to their general communication development, and they seem more likely than children who do not stutter to demonstrate disordered language.

Although more global measures of language ability have suggested few differences between children whose stuttering persists, in contrast with those who recover, other, more specific measures have shown some differences between these groups (see Watkins & Johnson, 2004, for spontaneous language; Hakim & Bernstein Ratner, 2004, for poorer nonword repetition characterized by increased numbers of phoneme errors and more errors on words with non-English stress patterns). The work of Watkins, Yairi, and Ambrose (1999) suggested that persistence of stuttering does not appear to be related to language functioning as revealed in standardized testing. Although longer and developmentally more complex utterances are more likely to include stuttering (Logan & Conture, 1995, 1997; Weiss & Zebrowski, 1992; Yaruss, 1999), language profiles of children who recovered from stuttering tended to move from an above age level profile for spontaneous language measures to a more age-appropriate pattern (Watkins & Johnson, 2004). Although, we know little about the interaction between speech and language development and responsiveness to the LP, a few small-$n$ studies have investigated language skills pre- and post-Lidcombe treatment. These investigations have arisen because of anecdotal concern that fluency may be achieved in the LP as a product of curtailed language use, either by producing fewer utterances or by producing utterances with less complex syntactic structure.

Bonelli et al. (2000) reported that the children in their study appeared to use more age-appropriate, less ambitious expressive language at the end of Stage 1, suggesting that the LP may have slowed the rate of language development. Bernstein Ratner and Guitar (2006) discuss these findings and stress that this is not evidence of any loss of language skills but rather "a more adaptive mix of expressive language gambits and sentence production skills on the child's part" (p. 116). This was not the case in a study by Lattermann et al. (2005), who compared pretreatment standardized language tests with spontaneous language samples collected 2 weeks prior to treatment and at weeks 1, 4, 8, and 12 during Stage 1 of the LP, as well as 6 months after the onset of treatment, in four preschool-age boys. Analysis of mean length of utterance (MLU), percentage of simple and complex sentences, number of different words, and percentage of stuttered syllables for the participants of the Lattermann et al. study revealed that all participants presented with language skills in the average or above average range. In fact, the children achieved an increase in stutter-free speech accompanied by increases in MLU, percentage of complex sentences, and number of different words. The authors concluded that for some preschool children who stutter, improved stutter-free speech during treatment with the LP is not achieved at the cost of a decrease in linguistic complexity. This finding was replicated with another group of children who were also bilingual (Guttmann & Shenker, 2006).

The relationship between speech and language skills and treatment time in the LP has recently been investigated. Rousseau et al. (2007) found that children who presented with delays in phonological development did not systematically take more (or less) time to complete Stage 1 of the program. However, MLU correlated significantly with treatment time in Stage 1; children with higher MLUs at the beginning of therapy exhibited shorter treatment times. Although this preliminary study raises further questions about the possible interface between patterns of speech and language development and responsiveness to the Lidcombe treatment, it should be noted that none of the children in the study had significant speech and/or language impairments.

Since there is evidence that a subgroup of children who stutter also present with other speech and language concerns (Hall et al., 2007; Nippold, 1990, 2002), it is important to show how the LP may be adjusted to be successful with these children. That is, if a child has a concomitant language disorder, the treatment plan should be able to accommodate for that. The following case descriptions demonstrate how treatment can be adjusted to suit individual needs stemming from differences in language competencies while retaining the integrity of the treatment.

## CASE 1: ADAPTING THE LP FOR A CHILD WITH SEVERE STUTTERING AND COGNITIVE AND LANGUAGE IMPAIRMENT

In the case of Sara, a 9-year-old with Down syndrome, the parents were not overly concerned about her stuttering. However, they requested treatment for her stuttering after they noted that Sara was becoming reluctant to speak in public, a change from previous sociable behavior. Pretreatment %SS ranged from 16% to 35% for in-clinic and beyond-clinic samples, with parents' SRs at 9 (where 1 = no stuttering, 2 = very mild stuttering, and 10 = extremely severe stuttering). In addition, Sara's language ability, both expressive and receptive, was more than 2 years below age level, although her use of pragmatic/social language was a relative strength. Language comprehension was higher for single-word vocabulary, and she demonstrated understanding of simple sentence structures and grammar but was challenged in understanding and following directions involving multiple pieces of information or abstract concepts. In the area of expressive language, relative strengths were noted in relation to expressive vocabulary, use of grammatical markers, and simple sentence structure. Formulated sentences, as opposed to imitated sentences, were significantly more likely to be ungrammatical. As noted, pragmatic language use was a relative strength, with appropriate nonverbal and interactional skills observed in conversation contexts. Sara responded well to prompts to repair grammatical and syntactic errors, expand simple sentences, and clarify meaning when asked. She was also responsive to requests for correction of stuttering, repeating the word in a more fluent manner.

The reasons for selecting the LP as the treatment of choice for this child were that (a) it was believed that Sara would not be able to learn to use an alternative method of speaking (i.e., fluency shaping technique) in order to be more fluent, (b) there was a positive response to a treatment trial, and (c) the parents were very consistent in providing verbal contingencies beyond the clinic. Treatment adaptations made for this particular child included the decision to initiate therapy in an intensive format for increased carryover to beyond clinic settings and to collaborate with the school SLP for the purpose of integrating simultaneous and continued development of language goals. Contingencies were provided in both structured and unstructured speaking conversations in a variety of settings throughout the day to facilitate effective carryover. Linguistic complexity was restricted to the level that Sara needed in order to be fluent enough to allow for verbal contingencies in the recommended ratio of 5 for stutter-free speaking to 1 for stuttered speech, clearly an accommodation to the LP. This goal was adjusted in consultation with the school-based SLP. A tangible reward system was introduced to increase compliance, assist Sara's comprehension, and ensure that she enjoyed treatment. Use of the tangible reward system was reevaluated, faded, changed, and reintroduced as needed throughout the course of treatment to maintain Sara's motivation and success with the LP.

During the course of treatment, the SRs went from 9 to 3–4, and %SS decreased to a stable 4%. Fluency increased to near normal rates in simple sentences, and instances of sociability increased as well. The latter was assessed through anecdotal parent and classroom teacher reports, supplemented by analysis of videotapes of conversational speech in beyond-clinic settings. Thus, Stage 2 criteria (normally <1%SS and SRs mostly 1 with an occasional 2 noted for 3 consecutive weeks) were adjusted to reflect Sara's cognitive and linguistic limitations. Post-Stage 1 measurement included a videotape made in a beyond-clinic situation that confirmed Sara's increased fluency and willingness to communicate in a social situation. This was compared with parent reports of positive experiences in beyond-clinic settings. In this case, language goals were provided by the school-based SLP, with fluency goals and activities provided by the parent during the structured speaking conversations. These conversations were sometimes restricted to short, complete sentences that were always within the range of Sara's linguistic capability. In unstructured speaking situations, parents were trained to provide feedback using verbal reinforcement or nonverbal signals that were initially paired with verbal feedback and then used as signals or prompts to Sara to "use her smooth speech." This combination of types of feedback typically helped Sara to increase fluency while increasing the length of utterance and communicative interaction.

The reader should remember here that it has been demonstrated that children with more severe stuttering took longer to complete Stage 1 of the LP (Jones et al., 2000; Kingston et al., 2003). In cases of children with severe stuttering and a concomitant cognitive component such as the one described above, established predictors of treatment times may have to be adjusted, as slower progress is to be expected. In addition, the criteria for maintaining fluency during the Stage 2 phase may require adjustment to allow for the possibility that these children may not achieve the same stutter free level that children without these factors are capable of achieving. However, the daily SRs should show the reductions in variability in stuttering and then a steady decrease in stuttering overall.

## CASE 2: TREATING STUTTERING AND PHONOLOGY WITH THE LP

The presence of additional phonology difficulties may influence the clinical decisions made while using the LP. Conture, Louko, & Edwards (1993) raised some questions and concerns regarding this issue. If SLPs focus on treatment of phonology first, would the attention to precision of speech production required in treatment and the corrective feedback that is often related to treatment of phonological processes increase stuttering by drawing the child's attention to his or her speech? On the other hand, leaving phonology untreated might create further problems in intelligibility for the young client. However, leaving stuttering untreated may pose ethical dilemmas, as the window of opportunity for effective early treatment may close in the interim.

Although about one third of children with fluency disorders also have a concomitant phonological problem, there are limited data on treatment outcome with children when these coexisting conditions are identified (Thompson Byrd, Wolk, & Davis, 2007). Several treatment models have been suggested by Conture et al. (1993) as choices for SLPs treating stuttering in children for whom phonological delays are also observed. These have included use of an indirect approach, a direct fluency modification approach, and a concurrent model, and one or another may be best suited to a particular child's learning style or temperament. Two possible scenarios would include sequential or simultaneous treatment. A second question would be to decide which of the coexisting conditions to treat first. Conture et al. (1993) used a simultaneous model to treat four children with stuttering and disordered phonology in a stuttering-phonology group. Stuttering changed considerably in two of the children, and additionally, three of the children in the stuttering-phonology group made significant improvements in their phonology. Although there are no empirical data for a sequential treatment model, the literature is clear that the most important consideration is that phonological goals have to be targeted in a manner that does not exacerbate the child's stuttering (Thompson Byrd et al., 2007, p. 177).

In the case of David, a sequential model, with stuttering treated initially, was used to adjust the LP to allow for the introduction of phonology treatment. David was 5 years 6 months at treatment onset, had been stuttering for more than 2 years, and was in kindergarten when first assessed for stuttering. There was no family history of stuttering; however, David had a history of late talking and was highly unintelligible. Specifically, intelligibility was negatively affected by the following patterns: /s/ and /z/ produced as stops in all positions, s- blends deleted in all positions, l-blends inconsistently deleted, /sh/ became /t/ in all positions, /tsh/ and /dg/ became /t/ and /d/ in all positions, /f/ was inconsistently produced as a stop, and /v/ was inconsistently produced as a /w/. In addition, David presented with a sensitive introverted temperament and became frustrated and reluctant to speak when asked to repeat something when he was misunderstood. Previous treatment received by this child for stuttering had been unsuccessful, and at the time of assessment David produced 16.6%SS with an SR of 8. The LP was the treatment of choice because David was under 6 years of age, his mother was easily able to provide appropriate feedback to her son's speaking, and the treatment trial had been successful in reducing stuttering. The mother's skill with verbal contingencies was established by watching her provide consistent and specific feedback in both structured and less structured speaking conversations from treatment session 1 of the LP, as well as from her detailed diary notes collected during home treatment sessions.

During the early treatment with the LP, David and his mother attended and participated consistently in all aspects of the treatment. After seven sessions, SRs of 3–4 in structured conversations were reported by the mother, but there was still variability in unstructured conversations. David was noted to be poor at monitoring his stuttering, and so little spontaneous self-correction was displayed. At this time, a decision was made to stall the progression of the Lidcombe therapy to introduce the phonology goals. The rationale for this decision was based on the observations that (a) stuttering levels had reduced to a point where communication was functional; (b) severity of stuttering had reduced with no more blocks, and so David was able to continue speaking without stutters of long duration; and c) David's peers continued to abandon conversations with him because of their difficulties in understanding his speech. A further consideration for introducing treatment for phonology took into account David's sensitive temperament. Although little is known about the clinical relationship between temperament and treatment outcome for early stuttering, his clinician believed that the observation that David abandoned speaking when misunderstood might indicate a high degree of reactivity. For further discussion of the relationship between stuttering and temperament, please refer to Guitar (1997) and Anderson, Pellowski, Conture, and Kelly (2003).

In summary, treatment adaptations to the LP for David included the following: (a) a slowing of the progression of the LP when SRs were 4 or lower; (b) introduction of a block of 10 weekly sessions for David's phonology goals; (c) the mother's continued collection of daily SR data for the SLP, as well as a continuation of praise for stutter-free speech in beyond-clinic settings; (d) the mother's introduction of a structured speaking session to increase stutter-free speech on any day when David's SR was above 4; (e) in any clinic session where the stuttering SR had increased over 4, the session in the clinic on that day was dedicated to the LP, not phonology goals; and (f) mother's continuation to praise David's stutter-free speech in beyond-clinic sessions without requesting self-corrections because it was believed that these requests might be confusing for the child when he was receiving verbal feedback for phonology goals.

Although there is no evidence to support this type of sequential treatment model in the literature for children exhibiting both stuttering and speech sound errors, David's stuttering severity did not increase as a result of the introduction of a block of phonology therapy following the initial treatment for dysfluency. This case supports Thompson Byrd et al.'s (2007) statement that "clinical intuitions suggest that it may be most beneficial to first target the disfluency and once fluency begins to improve, attention could be given to the phonological impairment" (p. 177). This is one example of a treatment plan that was adjusted to allow for direct, sequential behavioral intervention for what were perceived by the SLP to be two motor speech issues.

## CASE 3: SEVERE STUTTERING AND LANGUAGE CONCERNS

Sometimes severe stuttering masks the extent of children's language difficulties such that these become apparent only as fluency increases and the children want to say more but have difficulties with vocabulary or sentences structure. This happened in the case of Joe, who was referred when nearly 5 years old with an 8-month history of consistent stuttering preceded by a year of increasingly severe episodes of stuttering. A clinic sample showed 30%SS, with some relaxed syllable repetitions and many tense prolongations with associated pitch rise and volume increase. These prolongations were distressing for both mother and child and had elicited some negative reactions from Joe's peers. Although phonological errors were apparent, Joe's intelligibility was not impaired. Joe showed some avoidance or coping behaviors, in particular by limiting the length of his utterances. The relatively late onset and the increasing severity of Joe's stuttering over the course of 18 months indicated that he had a high risk of persistent stuttering (Yairi & Ambrose, 2005). Initially, stutter-free speaking was achieved in very short utterances, and Joe's attempts at self-correction were only successful when presented with a model, such as, "say *car*." The SLP did not reach the benchmark of 30% reduction in SRs by week 5, but Joe's progress was apparent within structured conversations. By week 8, SRs had reduced from consistent 8s to 5 on four days of the week and a rating of 4 on the other three days. Joe's progress leveled out for another 3 weeks, with some tense prolongations still appearing at the beginnings of some sentences. At this point, the child's classroom teacher commented, "Because of [his] fantastic improvement I have seen a knock on effect with his behaviour and learning. His phonics has really come on and he seems a lot more focused in the classroom environment."

However, Joe's progress stalled, and a language assessment was completed because there were indications of some discrepancy between his receptive and expressive skills, and at the same time, Joe's level of stuttering had reduced sufficiently so that it was now less likely to depress his expressive language scores. The Clinical Evaluation of Language Fundamentals—Pre-school UK (Wiig, Secord, & Semel, 2000) revealed both age-appropriate and above-age expectations in receptive skills and a mixed picture in terms of Joe's expressive language performance. Specifically, the word structure subtest yielded an age-appropriate score, but Joe's performance on the recalling sentences subtest was below age expectations, and the formulation of labels subtest score was even lower. Joe's clinician hypothesized that problems with vocabulary storage and retrieval were affecting the child's speech fluency and that possible difficulties with short-term memory could also be a factor in delaying his progress. Joe's teacher and his mother addressed vocabulary development and use in order to enhance word retrieval. They worked specifically on revising new words that arose in the school curriculum and ensuring that Joe was able to use these words appropriately. In addition, Joe's mother worked imaginatively on vocabulary and memory whenever difficulties arose in their everyday conversations. Throughout this time, verbal contingencies were used to address the sentence initial prolongations that continued to occur. It was a full year before Joe was consistently experiencing stutter-free days, even though it took only 11 sessions for stuttering to dramatically reduce from 30 to 4% SS. However, in hindsight, it seems we were correct in thinking that for Joe there was a relationship between his expressive language skills and stuttering. We could speculate that to effect sustained reduction of stuttering, progress was needed with the child's expressive language competencies, as well as with fluency skills and so this child's treatment took longer.

In conversation, clinicians often report that parents are reluctant to continue with clinic and home treatment when children's progress slows after rapid and significant progress. Some argue that this is a satisfactory outcome, and certainly, Joe's quality of life improved dramatically during those early weeks of therapy. Onslow et al. (2003) have proposed that any residual stuttering places the child at risk of relapse. Fortunately, Joe's mother persisted with the program, although at times she became weary of the need for continued vigilance and was unable to maintain her schedule of weekly clinic visits. Joe showed a remarkable willingness to participate in the LP and never responded negatively to the contingencies provided in response to his speech by either his mother or the clinician. Clinic sessions were supplemented by phone calls when needed. Clinicians unfamiliar with the LP have questioned the feasibility of placing so much responsibility for providing treatment on parents or other caregivers. In this case, Joe's mother was neither highly educated nor financially advantaged, but she had an accepting and patient approach to her son's stuttering, and she expressed genuine delight with Joe's progress and persistence. She showed considerable skill in working with him. It was fortuitous that during this time, Joe's mother was training to be a classroom assistant. She was able to apply what she was learning in the context of her child's stuttering to her college work and school placement, and vice versa.

Currently, it is unclear what the specific relationship between the development of speech and language skills, severity of stuttering, and progress with the LP may be. Given the substantive number of children who present with both stuttering and speech and language delays, additional studies of the patterns of therapeutic change for these children when the LP is used are badly needed to enhance the body of empirical evidence available and to help clinicians make appropriate treatment adaptations.

Thus far we have focused on differences that children who stutter bring to therapy and how these might influence their responses to the LP. Now we consider the broader context in which treatment occurs and how individual differences in parents, parenting, and cultural and multicultural backgrounds may affect progress.

## PARENTS AND STUTTERING THERAPY

Parents' experiences of therapy for different developmental communication problems have not been widely explored, and yet frequently parents play an important role in the treatment of their preschool children. Interview studies have provided some insights into parents' views of therapy for speech and language problems. For example, Glogowska (2002) identified problems around the clarity of parents' perception of their roles in therapy and understanding of the nature of their children's communication problems, as well as the rationale and likely outcomes of their children's treatment. Some parents had experienced what they interpreted as negative attitudes from others toward their children's speech and language difficulties and therapy, and they reported feeling isolated from other parents because of their child's difficulties.

Parents have an important role in treatment approaches for preschool children who stutter. In PCI therapy (Rustin, Botterill, & Kellman, 1996), both parents in two-parent families are required to attend therapy where they learn to modify specific communication targets. In the demands capacities model (Starkweather & Gottwald, 1990; Stewart & Turnbull, 2007), parents are taught to adjust demands for their children's speaking and fluency in line with their capacity to reach these levels of performance. Stewart & Turnbull included working in partnership, empathetic listening, fundamental respect, and a willingness to understand the parents' view in their discussion of "empowering parents" (p. 89) of preschool children. Yaruss, Coleman, and Hammer (2006) reported that they spend two to four sessions of their parent–child training program on education and counseling aimed at preparing parents to become active participants in their children's therapy. It would seem that the parental role is more clearly defined in stuttering therapies than in the therapy Glogowska's (2002) parents and children received.

## PARENTS AND THE LP

The main treatment components of the LP and the process of implementation in structured conversations, and then in increasingly unstructured conversations, have been relatively easy to describe to parents. The clinician always demonstrates the portion of treatment to be carried out at home, which is then tried out by the parent in the clinic, providing an opportunity for the SLP to give feedback, so there is clarity around the weekly aims of the LP and how to achieve them.

The Australian-based LP research program has established benchmarks regarding likely length of treatment and outcome. Interested parents can use the Internet to access the LP manual from the Australian Stuttering Research Centre, copies of the Lidcombe News from the Montreal Fluency Centre, and some articles on the LP from the British Stammering Association. The way the LP is structured, the methods used in parent training and the resources available for parents should help to address the concerns raised by the parents in Glogowska's (2002) study. However, this does not mean that all parents will respond similarly to using the LP; a study of parents' experiences (Hayhow, 2008) provides some insight into different parental perceptions of this treatment in the United Kingdom.

Parents' initial responses to the LP certainly differed (Hayhow, 2008). Some parents did not verbalize any strong feelings about the program, as they were happy to proceed as their clinician advised. Others had definite positive feelings, as the program matched their parenting style, and some expressed more skepticism but were happy to give the treatment a try. One couple said they viewed the PVCs as condescending and so they relied more heavily on nonverbal contingencies, although this interpretation of the LP carries some risk, as nonverbal contingencies provide less information and are less specific. However, many of the children whose parents expressed a range of attitudes and beliefs made demonstrable progress, and the treatment process was relatively trouble free. This suggests that this range can be accommodated without necessarily being detrimental to the treatment process.

Some parents reported feeling daunted by the centrality of their role in the LP, particularly when they had assumed the therapist would do all the work and fix their child. Others were pleased to play such an important role. One made a favorable contrast with professionals who induce feelings of helplessness in parents. That is, the LP is based on the premise that parents play an integral role; they are viewed as the antithesis of helpless in the therapeutic process. In some cases, parents reported that their children's progress was relatively slow or erratic, and so they found the responsibilities weighed more heavily. These parents voiced a need for extra support from their own family or from other parents who had used the LP with their children. Some parents described a reciprocal relationship between the nature of the child's difficulties and responsiveness to treatment and their feelings of competence. Slower progress raised problems for some parents, as the contingencies appeared to become less effective over time, parents' energy and commitment flagged, and weekly clinic visits reportedly became arduous. When this occurs, clinicians may be inclined to introduce other therapies, as documented by Shenker et al. (2005) and Hayhow (2005). However, this is unlikely to be in the children's best interests, as there is no evidence base for the efficacy of "pick and mix" treatments, and the possibility of confusion and inappropriate use of PVCs increases. Of course, clinicians and parents may both need extra support when progress is slower. One parent found that a problem-solving session with her husband, but without the child, provided a much-needed opportunity to reflect on the progress made so far, to explore the problems and their resources, and to then establish their next steps. When progress is slower, children are also getting older, and for this reason treatment may require subtle changes that reflect older children's ongoing development.

Another parent difference that emerged in Hayhow's (2008) interview study related to parents' confidence in their parenting skills and the impact this had on their ability to use contingencies for stuttering. This was an issue for only two parents and so was not a general concern, but in both cases, their comfort with their role in therapy increased after they had, independently, each attended a parenting course. In one case, the mother felt more confident that she was a good enough parent, and in the other case, the mother reappraised her views on boundary setting and discipline. Prior to the parenting course, both mothers had found the use of contingencies for stuttering difficult because they viewed any comments on problematic behavior as potentially harmful and so were tentative or apologetic in their manner of delivery of these PVCs. Subsequently they were more able to view these contingencies as helpful information rather than as criticism, which influenced how they requested self-corrections and, in turn, their children's responses to these.

A family history of stuttering may also influence children's responsiveness to treatment, depending upon the strength of the underlying vulnerability. In addition, when the parent implementing the LP is the one who stutters, this may have a special influence on treatment. There is no evidence to suggest that children respond differently to contingencies provided by parents who stutter compared with those who do not. However, parents who stutter may need to be open to requests from their children that they also correct their stutters. The mothers who stuttered in Hayhow's (2008) study were generally enthusiastic about the LP, and there was nothing in their accounts to suggest that their stuttering had any negative impact on treatment. One mother was an exception to this pattern; she clearly remembered the embarrassment that her stuttering caused her as a young child and the speaking event that made her avoid subsequent speaking in situations that might elicit stuttering. By the skillful use of avoidance strategies, she successfully passed as fluent throughout childhood, even though she experienced many of the internal aspects of stuttering. In her teens she became rebellious and decided to speak regardless of the risks, and so discovered she no longer stuttered. Although able to talk openly about this and able to manage the occasional stutter, she found being open about her son's stuttering extremely stressful and providing contingencies for stuttering almost impossible. Her child made initial progress when she introduced contingencies for stutter-free speaking, but, perhaps predictably, progress stopped when contingencies for stuttering were required. At the time, neither the mother nor the clinician appreciated the extent to which childhood experiences of stuttering as an internal problem might impact on this mother's ability to view stuttering as behavior.

All the parents who contributed to Hayhow's study appeared to enjoy the opportunity to discuss their children and their experiences with implementing the LP. Some also seemed to benefit from the opportunity to discuss different aspects of the treatment, and by talking in this way, they gained a new perspective even though the interviewer was careful to maintain a research rather than clinical role. These observations, along with the analysis and interpretation of the interviews, led Hayhow to suggest that when progress is inexplicably slow, or when parents struggle with parts of the LP, then an interview without the child may provide a context to explore factors that are getting in the way of the family's successful implementation of the program. This step toward clarifying the therapeutic process is probably critical for ensuring a positive therapeutic outcome, a better strategy than immediately introducing another treatment that might also fail if underlying beliefs or inconsistencies are not explored.

## CULTURAL/LINGUISTIC ISSUES

The importance of listening to mothers' beliefs about therapy and communication problems was emphasized by Peacey (2005) in her study of mothers of children with primary language impairment. She suggested that once mothers' beliefs become more explicit, it is then possible to negotiate around them for the benefit of parent and child. She suggested that openness and sharing of beliefs around communication disability and its remediation will facilitate mothers' participation in interventions. This view is shared by Marshall, Goldbart, and Phillips (2007), who argued that ethnographic interviewing during the assessment process could lead to better tailoring of treatment to individual families and hence greater compliance among parents of children with language delay. By ethnographic interviewing, we refer to an approach that is open-ended, thus encouraging families to discuss their individual perspectives and not making assumptions about how families live their lives.

Differences in cultural beliefs were explored by Hettiarachchi (2007) in her study of Tamil-speaking mothers' responses to parent–child interaction (PCI) therapy for language delay. The mothers' beliefs that children learn to talk through being asked questions and being given information were at odds with the child-centered approach of PCI, the treatment selected for them and their children. Hettiarachchi pointed out that most of the information underpinning PCI is based on Caucasian, middle-class, two-parent families in North America. However, there is no cross-cultural evidence to show that learning through incorporation into conversation is superior to learning by exposure to directive language, or that following children's lead is preferable to adult direction. This study questioned the assumption that there is one best way to learn language and identified the need to be respectful of people's cultural origins and beliefs. That is, different perspectives on language learning exist, and in the absence of any proof that one perspective is inherently better than another, it is important for SLPs to make sure that their recommendations for therapy fit a family's point of view (van Kleeck, 1994).

The cornerstone of the LP is perhaps best seen in the observations, made over and over again, that both parents and children participate enthusiastically in the treatment. This is underscored by the findings that the program can be used successfully with families from nonmajority cultures and where families speak a language other than English. Some of the challenges in providing the program in other languages to parents with different belief systems include finding the equivalent terminology and providing verbal contingencies in a manner that is appropriate for the culture. Cultural factors can influence the success of clinical work; differences in cultural aspects of communication may affect treatment outcomes. Verbal and nonverbal communication media are both culturally influenced, and misunderstandings between client and clinician might result if the differences are not factored into the treatment model (Leith, 1986). These factors can extend to whether or not (and how) children should be praised, ways to use verbal contingencies, and how each family's cultural beliefs may influence verbal feedback. Other individual differences, such as use of eye contact, the identification of the parent who takes responsibility for the child's therapy, and how the verbal contingencies will be used, may need to be discussed with family members before starting treatment; the clinician should not assume that these factors will be uniform in nature.

## WHEN CHILDREN ARE BILINGUAL OR MULTILINGUAL

Perhaps a greater challenge in working with children who speak more than one language is the issue of choosing which language to work in and then ensuring that fluency developed in the therapy language transfers to the other languages that the child speaks. With millions of people speaking more than one language, we cannot assume that families are monolingual. In fact, we often find ourselves treating preschool children who speak two or more languages (Shenker & Wilding, 2003). In the LP, parents provide the treatment, and therefore it would seem to be an approach that is easy to use with families when the clinician does not speak the language spoken by the family at home. In studies to date, when preschool children were treated in one language in the clinic, all have transferred treatment gains to the untreated, home language (Rousseau, Packman, & Onslow, 2004; Shenker, Conte, Gingras, Courcy, & Polomeno, 1998). There are currently no studies of children who received verbal feedback simultaneously in two languages with the LP.

## A MULTILINGUAL PRESCHOOL CHILD TREATED FOR STUTTERING

In the case of a multilingual child, Ian, treatment was provided in two languages. Ian began treatment with the LP at age 5, 2 years after the reported onset of stuttering. From birth, Ian had been exposed to French and English at home and was introduced to a third language in school at age 4. Although Ian was more proficient in English, his mother continued to speak only in French and his father in English. There was a family history of recovered stuttering in both Ian's older sister and his mother. At the time of treatment, Ian was aware yet unconcerned about his stuttering. Recently, however, his parents had observed Ian abandon some utterances (e.g., "I just can't say it"), and during these times they saw an increase in frustration and a reduction in their child's eye contact. In pretreatment assessment, stuttering ranged from 3 to 12%SS in English and in French for both within- and beyond-clinic measures, with SRs ranging from 3 to 7. Stuttering was characterized by a high frequency of audible sound prolongations, blocks, and repetitions of sounds and syllables. Some secondary characteristics were noted in the form of pitch and volume increases, loss of eye contact, turning of the head and neck to release a word, and changes in respiration pattern. Both parents attended therapy and provided verbal contingencies (mother in French; father in English). After three sessions, Ian was noted to be initiating spontaneous self-corrections with stuttering characterized by less effort, more whole-word and phrase repetitions, and fewer prolongations noted in both languages. Parents provided SRs in both French and English. Structured speaking sessions were provided in both languages, with Ian's parents splitting the responsibility for contingencies, so that each parent provided a structured speaking session every other day in his or her own language. Verbal contingencies in unstructured conversations that arose naturally in daily living were provided by both parents. Ian met the criteria for Stage 2 in eight clinic visits over 12 weeks; however, he did not meet the criteria at the first Stage 2 session and for the subsequent 3 visits, suggesting that Stage 2 had been initiated too quickly for this child. The parents resumed daily structured treatment conversations and increased verbal feedback in the unstructured conversations, reinstating the criteria on the fourth Stage 2 visit. Ian was discharged from Stage 2 after 12 months at 0%SS and SR of 1. This criterion has been maintained for the past 3 years. Ian's parents noted that they had enjoyed being part of the solution to their son's stuttering and welcomed the opportunity to participate in treatment, giving high priority to attending the sessions and providing the prescribed therapy at home. In this case, verbal contingencies were conveyed in two of the languages that the child spoke, with positive outcomes.

## WHEN THE HOME LANGUAGE IS ONE
## NOT SPOKEN BY THE CLINICIAN

In another situation, a family spoke Arabic at home, and although the father was able to communicate in French, the mother was not; the child, however, had been introduced to French in day care 1 year prior to initiating treatment with the LP. Both parents accompanied the child to treatment sessions, and the clinician trained the father to provide verbal contingencies in French. Once the father was observed to provide the verbal feedback accurately, he translated this information to Arabic for the mother. The mother then provided the feedback to the child in Arabic, while both the father and the therapist collaborated on the appropriateness of the treatment. The father relayed this feedback to mother, who then became the primary person responsible for providing treatment in beyond-clinic settings. The nonverbal feedback from the child (e.g., appropriate smiles upon receipt of verbal contingencies for fluency in both French and Arabic) was one of the confirmations for the therapist that this verbal feedback was both appropriate and well received.

In a study that considered the impact of cultural factors on treatment outcomes, Waheed-Kahn (1998) found that 20% of the school age children who were recent immigrants to Canada reached target fluency levels, compared with 85% of children in native English speaking group. Subsequently, she required parental attendance during therapy, observed the parents practicing with their child, and supported beyond-clinic practice in the child's home language using culturally relevant stimuli. Results showed that 75% of the children achieved fluency criteria, and attendance improved from 73% to 97%. This study provides data to support the use of culturally relevant stimulus applied in beyond clinic contexts identified as appropriate for individual client's culture. Although empirical data elucidating the effect of linguistic and cultural diversity on outcome of the LP are not currently available (Shenker, 2004), there is interest in these issues, given the makeup of our clinical population and the use of the program around the world in a variety of languages.

As the case studies have indicated, cognitive ability, speech and language skills, and cultural and linguistic backgrounds can all potentially interact with the standard, prescribed LP procedures. The final areas of individual difference that we consider in more detail are temperament and the related area of attitude.

## CHILDREN'S TEMPERAMENT AND RESPONSES

There has been an interest in the relationship between children's temperamental characteristics and early stuttering for some years. Riley and Riley (1979) identified distractibility, hyperactivity, poor attention, and low frustration tolerance in approximately a third of their stuttering sample. Guitar (1998) hypothesized that a predisposition to stuttering could include a neurodevelopmental component, along with a sensitive temperament and a reactive limbic system. Temperamental characteristics are evident early in life and are relatively stable across situations and over time. In young children, these characteristics are typically measured by parental rating scales and thus may be telling us something about the parents as well as about their children. Furthermore, studies using these rating scales have often compared children who stutter with those who do not, so this may tell us something about this particular aspect of individual variation.

In a study by Karrass et al. (2006), parents completed the Behaviour Style Questionnaire (McDevitt & Carey, 1978). The authors concluded that children who stuttered were more reactive, were less able to regulate their emotions, and had poorer attention regulation than their nonstuttering peers. They suggested that increased emotional reactivity has the potential to exacerbate or maintain stuttering. Embrechts, Ebben, Franke, and Van de Poel (2000) found that parents rated their children who stutter as more active and impulsive and lower on ratings of attentional focusing, inhibitory control, and perceptual sensitivity than the nonstuttering controls. Their children were not judged to be more fearful or shy, suggesting that when fear and shyness characterize children who stutter, this may be a by-product of stuttering rather than an initial triggering factor.

Conture et al. (2007) have developed a communication-emotional model of stuttering that is based upon their own and others' research. These investigators have argued that both dispositional and situational aspects of temperament have a role to play in both the development and maintenance of stuttering. The model predicts that children who have a predisposition to stronger emotional reactions and difficulties with emotional regulation will be potentially more vulnerable to stuttering when other language or motor vulnerabilities coexist. The inclusion of situational sensitivity relates well to considerations of how children might respond to specific elements in any direct treatment approach, including the LP.

When considering the LP, we could speculate that the recommended openness about stuttering, the development of parent skills specific to managing stuttering, and the opportunities for the children to learn how to manage moments of stuttering target both the possible underlying temperamental predisposition and children's emotional responses. It is possible that "easy" children, whom Williams (2006) categorized as more regular, positive in approach, highly adaptable, and with a typically positive mild to moderate intense mood, may be more amenable to parental contingencies than their peers who have a different constellation of temperamental characteristics.

Parents in Hayhow's (2008) study talked about their children's responses to verbal contingencies and to structured treatment sessions at home, and their accounts may give some insight into this area. Some parents commented that the words *bumpy* and *smooth*, used to describe unambiguous stuttering and stutter-free speech, respectively, were particularly helpful to their children because they are descriptive and nonjudgmental. They expressed their comfort in talking to their children about their speaking in these terms because they made it clear that the labels were referring to behavior and not to the children's more global abilities or value as a person. The higher frequency of contingencies for stutter-free speaking, contrasted with those for stuttering, helped some parents switch from a preoccupation with their children's speaking problems to their children's developing fluency. The parents reported that they benefited from the openness, directness, and positive orientation of the LP and that in turn this helped their children engage in the treatment.

The guidelines for implementation of the LP were derived from learning theory and were refined during the initial development of the approach (Onslow, 2003). The prescribed way in which the contingencies are used by parents conveys information, as well as parental attitudes, to the child. This influences the meanings that the contingencies might have for children. Molden and Dweck (2000) considered the importance of the meanings that praise might have and how this affects children's intrinsic motivation. Their cognitive evaluation theory predicts that when praise passes judgment on a person's enduring characteristics (e.g., such as worth as a person) it may backfire if the person does less well than expected. That is, in a clinical context, the client may feel he or she has failed as a person. However, if clients understand that feedback refers to their current level of ability in relation to a particular behavior or skill, their sense of self-worth is not activated. When the information aspect of praise is salient, there is less risk that it feels judgmental to a client, and so it is less likely to undermine the recipients' sense of autonomy and self-worth. This type of praise is also potentially more useful to children learning how to manage their stuttering than praise or rewards alone that carry little information. An extension of this framework would suggest that contingencies for the speech behavior warranting change would work in a similar way. When a word is identified as "bumpy," this tells children about the manner in which it is problematic, and the request to "smooth" or "fix the bumpy word" implies that the adults believe the children can do something about changing their production. When this information is given in a supportive context and embedded within comments on "smooth talking," it is potentially empowering for children and so may increase their sense of autonomy. In both these respects, providing feedback in the prescribed manner can be more helpful than procedures such as time-out that, when used alone, may seem concerned only with achieving stutter-free performance and adult control.

Occasionally, parents noted that their children did not like any attention drawn to their speaking. Sometimes this related to a specific communication situation. For example, the mother of a child with delayed speech and language development, dyspraxia, and a family history of stuttering discussed how careful she needed to be in requesting self-correction. Not unexpectedly, situations that challenged this child's language skills tended to elicit more stuttering; in addition, he became frustrated by any comments that evaluated his speaking. This mother felt that her child had to work so hard to get his message across that any evaluative comment from her overloaded his system. At other times, when the communication task was easier for him, the child referred to "throwing his bumps out of the window" as he self-corrected, a much more relaxed response.

When discussing the use of verbal contingencies with their children, parents did not present pictures of different temperamental profiles. Instead, they identified a need for parents to modify how they implemented these contingencies in response to daily variations in their children's attitudes toward speaking and in response to the particular communication situations that arose. They described a sensitive interplay between all these elements. The parents and children who seemed most comfortable with the contingencies were those who were able to respond in a natural and genuine manner. Most parents stressed the important role that their clinician played in helping them work out how to achieve this. They valued the support that regular clinic sessions provided, and seeing the contingencies being used successfully with their children by their clinician was an essential part of their learning. The parents' comments raised a question about the possible importance of temperamental compatibility between parents and children rather than their being a particular child profile that might facilitate favorable responses to contingencies. For example, some parents may be relatively sensitive to their child's changing communicative efforts, whereas others may not. There may also be an interplay between temperament and the extent to which stuttering upsets individual children. Parents described a range of responses to stuttering, with generally greater distress occurring when children became stuck with their speaking (i.e., experienced blocks). In contrast, those producing repetitions seemed less upset by their stuttering and in some cases appeared to have little motivation to change their speaking to reduce the frequency of repetitions. We do not yet know whether the type of stuttering a child produces is influenced by temperament, but this may be another interesting focus of future research.

An alternate way of looking at children's responses to contingencies is to consider their self-evaluations rather than their temperaments, bearing in mind there may be a relationship between these. Stipek, Recchia, McClintic, and Lewis (1992) suggested that young children develop through three stages of self-evaluation. The first stage lasts up to around 21 months, when children enjoy experiences of causality, so they enjoy making things happen or watching other people make things happen without self-evaluation. Next, children begin to seek adult approval for successes and avoid negative reactions to failure. Gradually, children internalize these external reactions, so that by 5 years the third stage is reached, and children will react emotionally to success or failure independently of adult reactions. The nature of the emotional reaction may vary according to the difficulty of the task. Lewis, Alessandri, and Sullivan (1992) found that preschool children are more likely to experience pride when succeeding in a task perceived as difficult and more likely to experience shame when they fail an easy task. They summarized:

> It would appear, therefore, that by the age of 3, children are able to discern task difficulty, at some level, and are able to evaluate their behaviour in terms of this factor.... These findings support our hypothesis that children's evaluative processes influence their emotional response. (p. 636)

Whether children perceive speaking as easy or difficult may depend upon their individual experiences of learning to talk, on parental responses, and on the children's age. Self-evaluation, on some level, is assumed to play a major role in speech and language acquisition. This area is an important one for helping us understand some of the individual differences observed in children's responses to the contingencies that parents described, and it may also partly explain why children's responses change with age. A parent described her young child as being "all puffed up" (that is, really pleased with himself) when she first started using contingencies for stutter-free speaking but that with time they became "just a background noise." We can speculate that this initial positive emotional response can only last for a limited time, partly because the novelty wears off and partly because children's self-evaluations may involve some sense of progression. That is, they expect to make progress.

Older preschool-age children may already know that most children talk smoothly; thus, being praised for smooth talking may not always be encouraging but rather remind them that they are failing to do something their peers do naturally. If children think talking is easy, then they may experience shame when they stutter, not necessarily resulting from parental responses but from their own evaluations. Lewis and Ramsay (2002) reported that children as young as 4 have been found to experience two different types of embarrassment: one resulting from negative self-evaluation and the other from a sense of exposure when they are the object of the attention of others. Children may feel both these types of embarrassment when others notice or comment on their stuttering, and even comments about their smooth speaking could lead to a sense of exposure. It seems inevitable that feelings of embarrassment and shame could make contingencies uncomfortable for some children and make self-correction more difficult. There may be a relationship between temperament and susceptibility to feelings of embarrassment, which in turn could influence how easily children are able to self-correct their stuttering.

Furthermore, there is a possibility with any treatment implemented by parents that children will resent their parents' taking on a clinician role. The following two examples show how some children responded to this apparent perception. The first child attends school, which may have influenced how he perceived the LP. His parents reported that he seemed to understand his therapy as an activity in itself, with its own set of rules and structures, a bit like having to go to school, something he needed to do. They thought that the explanations given to their child in the clinic and at home helped him accept the procedures and that he felt he was an active participant in the therapy. Weiss (2004) discussed children as agents for change in phonology therapy, but this concept has not been widely explored in early stuttering treatments.

The second child, Jamie, was younger and attended preschool. He had delayed speech and language development and some behavioral problems. Jamie's stuttering was severe at the beginning of therapy and interfered with his intelligibility, which led to considerable frustration for him and his mother. Jamie's mother described how on difficult days he would stutter more and his behavior would become more challenging (e.g., less compliant). This meant that just when Jamie needed structured therapy the most, he was least receptive. However, by trial and error, his mother learned that if she relaxed with him, chatting and cuddling, he would then suggest that they "play at therapy." Jamie directed his mother to be the therapist and then he cooperated, as he nearly always did in the clinic. From experience, this mother knew that if she suggested a talk-time when Jamie was stuttering and frustrated he would refuse. At these more difficult times, the request for therapy had to come from the child for the therapy to be successful.

The idea that a mother should role-play the therapist did not occur with any other children, but it served an important function with this child. He had a range of problems that could have had an impact on his stuttering, yet he responded very well to treatment. For Jamie, being able to separate the role his mother played from that of his therapist and then bring these roles back together when he was ready seemed to make a big difference on those difficult days. It seems that when Jamie was feeling frustrated by his talking, he needed his mother for her nurturing qualities. As he became more settled and could focus, he could then engage with her to work on his speaking. It is possible that a similar process operated with other parent–child dyads, based on the fact that parents often talked about the importance of timing their contingencies to suit their children. Jamie, who was generally a more difficult child to manage, highlighted the process of tailoring the manner of contingency delivery to the individual child.

Parents had a lot to say about their children's responses to verbal contingencies and talk-times (Hayhow, 2008). They had clearly thought about how to use them effectively and how to be responsive to their children's needs as little people as well as little talkers. There are different ways of accounting for the individual variations, and we have touched on some of these above. Further research into the variations in responsiveness to these key components of the LP has the potential to help clinicians and parents use them more effectively in more challenging cases.

## CONCLUSIONS

In this chapter, we have not attempted to provide a complete account of the differences that make a difference to outcome; as Zebrowski (2007) pointed out, there are other "elements, aside from those specific to a particular treatment approach, that might influence a child's responsiveness to stuttering therapy" (p. 23). These can include variables embedded in the treatment process, including, for example, temperament and personality, locus of control, family perception of improvement or change in treatment, and the client/clinician's expectation for success. The challenge for future research is to account for these variables in the evaluation of treatment outcome so that clinicians and parents have resources to help them achieve good results whatever the compounding factors. We have considered some of the differences that are found in many young children who stutter, their parents, and their broader circumstances. We have also attempted to describe some of these and have referred to the literature, where available, for possible explanations. Many more of our suggestions are based on our speculations as clinicians with many years of experience as SLPs and practitioners of the LP. We hope that we have stimulated the readers' thinking about how a treatment can be used in a manner that is sensitive to clients' individual differences while retaining the integrity of the basic approach.

# REFERENCES

Arndt, J., & Healey, E. C. (2001). Concomitant disorders in school-age children who stutter. *Language, Speech and Hearing Services in Schools, 32*, 68–78.

Anderson, J. D., Pellowski, M. W., Conture, E. G., & Kelly, E. M. (2003). Temperamental characteristics of young children who stutter. *Journal of Speech, Language, and Hearing Research, 46*, 1221–1233.

Australian Stuttering Research Centre. (2008). Manual for the Lidcombe Program for early stuttering intervention. Retrieved July 29, 2009 from http://www.fhs.usyd.edu.au/asrc/health_professionals/asrc_download.shtml

Bernstein Ratner, N. (1997). Stuttering: A psycholinguistic perspective In R. Curlee & G. Seigel, (Eds.), *Nature and treatment of stuttering: New directions* (2nd ed., pp. 99–127). Boston: Allyn & Bacon.

Bernstein Ratner, N. (2005). Evidence-based practice in stuttering: Some questions to consider. *Journal of Fluency Disorders, 30*, 163–188.

Bernstein Ratner, N., & Guitar, B. (2006). Treatment of very early stuttering and parent-administered therapy: the state of the art. In N. Bernstein Ratner & J. Tetnowski (Eds.), *Current issues in stuttering research and practice* (pp. 99–124). Mahwah, NJ: Lawrence Erlbaum Associates.

Blood, G. W., Ridenour, V. J., Jr., Qualls, C. D., & Hammer, C. S. (2003). Co-occurring disorders in children who stutter. *Journal of Communication Disorders, 36*, 427–448.

Bonelli, P., Dixon, M., Bernstein Ratner, N., & Onslow, M. (2000). Child and parent speech and language following the Lidcombe Program of early stuttering intervention. *Clinical Linguistics and Phonetics, 14*, 427–446.

Conture, E., Walden, T., Arnold, H., Graham, C., Hartfield, K., & Karrass, J. (2007). A communication-emotional model of stuttering. In N. Bernstein Ratner & J. Tetnowski (Eds.), *Current issues in stuttering research and practice* (pp. 124–146). Mahwah, NJ: Lawrence Erlbaum Associates.

Conture, E. G., Louko, L., & Edwards, M. L. (1993). Simultaneously treating stuttering and disordered phonology in children. *American Journal of Speech-Language Pathology, 2*, 72–81.

Embrechts, M., Ebben, H., Franke, P., & Van de Poel, C. (2000). Temperament: A comparison between children who do and children who do not stutter. In H.-G. Bosshardt, J. S. Yaruss, & H. Peters (Eds.), *Fluency Disorders: Theory, research, treatment and self-help. Proceedings of the 3rd World Congress on Fluency Disorders* (pp. 557–562). Nyborg, Denmark. Netherlands: Nijmegen University Press.

Glogowska, M. (2002). *Time to talk: Parents' accounts of children's speech difficulties.* London: Whurr Publishers.

Guttmann, V., & Shenker, R. C. (2006, November). *Bilingual preschoolers' linguistic proficiency during treatment with the Lidcombe Program.* Poster presented at the meeting of the American Speech Language and Hearing Association, Miami, FL.

Guitar, B. (1997). Therapy for children's stuttering and emotions. In R. F. Curlee and G. M. Siegel (Eds.), *Nature and treatment of stuttering: New Directions* (2nd ed., pp. 280–291). Boston: Allyn & Bacon.

Guitar, B. (1998). *Stuttering: An integrated approach to its nature and treatment.* Baltimore: Williams & Wilkins.

Hakim, H. B., & Bernstein Ratner, N. (2004). Nonword repetition abilities of children who stutter: An exploratory study. *Journal of Fluency Disorders, 29*, 179–199.

Hall, N. E., Wagovich, S. A., & Bernstein Ratner, N. (2007). Language considerations in childhood stuttering. In E. G. Conture & R. F. Curlee (Eds.), *Stuttering and related disorders of fluency* (3rd ed., pp. 153–167). New York: Thieme Medical Publishers.

Harrison, E., Onslow, M., & Menzies, R. (2004). Dismantling the Lidcombe Program of early stuttering intervention: Verbal contingencies for stuttering and clinical measurement. *International Journal of Language & Communication Disorders, 39*, 257–267.

Hayhow, R. (2005, June). *An exploration of speech & language therapists' experience of using the Lidcombe Program.* Paper presented at the 7th Oxford Dysfluency Conference, Oxford, UK.

Hayhow, R. (2008). *Parents' experiences of the Lidcombe Program.* Unpublished doctoral thesis, University of the West of England.

Hettiarachchi, S. (2007, March). *Speech impairments amongst children from different cultural backgrounds.* Paper presented at the Primary Care Refresh Conference, National Exhibition Centre, Birmingham, United Kingdom.

Jones, M., Onslow, M., Harrison, E., & Packman, A. (2000). Treating stuttering in young children: Predicting treatment time in the Lidcombe Program, *Journal of Speech, Language, and Hearing Research, 43*, 1440–1450.

Jones, M., Onslow, M., Packman, A., Williams, S., Ormand, T., Schwarz, I., et al. (2005). Randomised controlled trial of the Lidcombe program of early stuttering intervention. *British Medical Journal, 331*, 659–661.

Karrass, J., Walden, T., Conture, E., Graham, C., Hayley, S., Arnold, H., et al. (2006). Relation of emotional reactivity and regulation to childhood stuttering. *Journal of Communication Disorders, 39*, 402–423.

Kingston, M., Huber, A., Onslow, M., Jones, M., & Packman, A. (2003). Predicting treatment time in the Lidcombe Program: replication and meta-analysis. *International Journal of Language and Communication Disorders, 38*, 165–177.

Lattermann, C. Shenker, R. C., & Thoradoridottir, E. (2005). Progression of language complexity with the Lidcombe Program for early stuttering intervention. *American Journal of Speech-Language Pathology, 14*, 242–253.

Leith, W. R. (1986). Treating the stutterer with atypical cultural influences. In K. O. St. Louis (Ed.), *The atypical stutterer* (pp. 9–34). London: Academic Press.

Lewis, M., & Ramsay, D. (2002). Cortisol response to embarrassment and shame. *Child Development, 73*, 1034–1045.

Lewis, M., Alessandri, S. M., & Sullivan, M. W. (1992). Differences in shame and pride as a function of children's gender and task difficulty. *Child Development, 63*, 630–638.

Lincoln, M., & Onslow, M. (1997). Long-term outcome of an early intervention for stuttering. *American Journal of Speech-Language Pathology, 6*, 51–58.

Lincoln, M., Onslow, M., & Reed, V. (1997). Social validity of an early intervention for stuttering: The Lidcombe Program. *American Journal of Speech-Language Pathology, 6*, 77–84.

Logan, K. J., & Conture, E. G. (1995). Length, grammatical complexity and rate differences in stuttering and fluent conversational utterances of children who stutter. *Journal of Fluency Disorders, 20*, 35–61.

Logan, K. J. & Conture, E. G. (1997) Selected temporal, grammatical, and phonological characteristics of conversational utterances produced by children who stutter. *Journal of Speech, Language, and Hearing Research, 40*, 107–120.

Marshall, J., Goldbart, J., and Phillips, J. A. (2007). Parents' and speech and language therapists' explanatory models of language development, language delay and intervention. *International Journal of Language & Communication Disorders, 42*, 533–555.

McDevitt, S. C., & Carey, W. B. (1978). A measure of temperament in 3–7 year old children. *Journal of Child psychology and Psychiatry and Allied Disciplines, 19*, 245–253.

Miller, B., & Guitar, B. (2009). Long-term outcome of the Lidcombe Program for early intervention. *American Journal of Speech-Language Pathology, 18*, 42–49.

Molden, D., & Dweck, C. (2000). Meaning and motivation. In C. Sansone & J. Harakiewicz (Eds.), *Intrinsic and extrinsic motivation: The search for optimal motivation and performance* (pp. 131–159). San Diego, CA: Academic Press.

Nippold, M. (1990). Concomitant speech and language disorders in stuttering children: A critique of the literature. *Journal of Speech Hearing Disorders, 55*, 51–60.

Nippold, M. (2002). Stuttering and phonology: Is there an interaction? *American Journal of Speech-Language Pathology, 11*, 99–110.

Nippold, M. (2004). Phonological and language disorders in children who stutter: Impact on treatment recommendations. *Clinical Linguistics and Phonetics, 18*, 145–159.

Onslow, M. (2003). From laboratory to living room: The origins and development of the Lidcombe Program. In M. Onslow, A. Packman & E. Harrison, (Eds.), *The Lidcombe Program of early stuttering intervention: A clinician's guide* (pp. 21–25). Austin, TX: Pro-Ed.

Onslow, M., Andrews, C., & Lincoln, M. (1994). A control/experimental trial of an operant treatment for early stuttering. *Journal of Speech, Language, and Hearing Research, 37*, 1244–1259.

Onslow, M., Costa, L., & Rue, S. (1990). Direct early intervention with stuttering: some preliminary data. *Journal of Speech and Hearing Disorders, 55*, 405–416.

Onslow, M., Packman, A., & Harrison, E. (Eds.) (2003). *The Lidcombe Program of early stuttering intervention: A clinician's guide.* Austin, TX: Pro-Ed.

Onslow, M., & Yaruss, J. S. (2007). Differing perspectives on what to do with a stuttering preschooler and why. *American Journal of Speech-Language Pathology, 16*, 65–68.

Packman, A., & Attanasio, J. (2004). *Theoretical issues in stuttering.* Hove, United Kingdom: Psychology Press.

Packman, A., Code, C., & Onslow, M. (2007). On the cause of stuttering: Integrating theory with brain and behavioural research. *Journal of Neurolinguistics, 20*, 253–362.

Peacey, L. (2005). *Mothers' beliefs about their children with primary language impairments*, Unpublished doctoral thesis, City University, London.

Riley, G., & Riley, G. (1979). A component model for diagnosing and treating children who stutter. *Journal of Fluency Disorders, 4*, 279–293.

Rousseau, I., & O'Brian, S. (2003). Routine case studies. In M. Onslow, A. Packman, & E. Harrison (Eds.), *The Lidcombe Program of early stuttering intervention: A clinician's guide* (pp. 103–118). Austin, TX: Pro-Ed.

Rousseau, I., Packman, A., & Onslow, M. (2004, September). *Treatment of early stuttering in a bilingual child.* Conference Program and Abstracts of the 26th World Congress of the International Association of Logopedics and Phoniatrics, Brisbane, Australia.

Rousseau, I., Packman, A., Onslow, M., Harrison, E., & Jones, M. (2007). An investigation of language and phonological development and the responsiveness of preschool age children to the Lidcombe Program. *Journal of Communication Disorders, 40*, 382–397.

Rustin, L., Botterill, W., & Kelman, E. (1996). *Assessment and therapy for young dysfluent children: Family interaction.* London: Whurr Publishers.

Shenker, R. (2004). Bilingualism in early stuttering. In A. K. Bothe (Ed.) *Evidence-based treatment of stuttering, empirical bases and clinical applications* (pp. 81–96). Mahwah, NJ: Lawrence Erlbaum Associates.

Shenker, R. C., Conte, A., Gingras, A., Courcy, A., & Polomeno, L. (1998). The impact of bilingualism on developing fluency in a pre-school child. In E. C. Healey & H. F. Peters (Eds.), *Second world congress on fluency disorders proceedings* (pp. 200–204). Nijmegen, The Netherlands: Nijmegen University Press.

Shenker, R., Hayhow, R., Kingston, M., & Lawlor, D. (2005, June). *Evaluation of clinician's attitudes regarding treatment of stuttering following participation in the Lidcombe Program Training Workshop.* Paper presented at 7th Oxford Dysfluency Conference, Oxford, United Kingdom.

Shenker, R. C., & Wilding, J. (2003). Canada. In M. Onslow, A. Packman, & E. Harrison (Eds.), *The Lidcombe Program of early stuttering intervention: A clinician's guide* (pp. 161–172). Austin, TX: Pro-Ed.

Starkweather, C. W., & Gottwald, S. R. (1990). The demands and capacities model II: Clinical implications. *Journal of Fluency Disorders, 15,* 143–157.

Stewart, T., & Turnbull, J. (2007). Working *with dysfluent children* (Revised edition). Brackley, United Kingdom: Speechmark Publishing.

Stipek, D., Recchia, S., McClintic, S., & Lewis, M. (1992). Self-evaluation in young children. *Monographs of the Society for Research in Child Development, 57,* 1–95.

Thompson Byrd, C., Wolk, L., & Davis, B. L. (2007). Role of phonology in childhood stuttering and its treatment. In E. Conture & R. Curlee (Eds.), *Stuttering and related disorders of fluency* (3rd ed., pp. 168–182). New York: Thieme Medical Publishers.

van Kleeck, A. (1994). Potential cultural bias in training parents as conversational partners with their children who have delays in language development. *American Journal of Speech-Language Pathology, 3,* 67–78.

Waheed-Kahn, N. (1998). Fluency therapy with multilingual clients. In E. C. Healey, & F. M. Peters (Eds.), *Second world congress on fluency disorders proceedings* (pp. 195–199). San Francisco. Nijmegen, The Netherlands: Nijmegen University Press.

Watkins, R., V. Yairi, E., & Ambrose, N. G. (1999). Early childhood stuttering III: Initial status of expressive language abilities. *Journal of Speech, Language, and Hearing Research, 42,* 1125–1135.

Watkins, R., & Johnson, B. (2004). Language abilities in children who stutter: Towards improved research and clinical applications. *Language, Speech, and Hearing Services in Schools, 35,* 82–89.

Webber, M., & Onslow, M. (2003). Maintenance of treatment effects. In M. Onslow, A. Packman, & E. Harrison (Eds.), *The Lidcombe Program of early stuttering intervention: A clinician's guide* (pp. 195–199). Austin, TX: Pro-Ed.

Weiss, A. (2004). The child as agent for change in therapy for phonological disorders. *Child Language Teaching and Therapy, 20,* 221–244.

Weiss, A. L., & Zebrowski, P. (1992). Disfluencies in the conversations of young children who stutter: Some answers about questions. *Journal of Speech and Hearing Research, 35,* 1230–1238.

Wiig, E. H., Secord, W., & Semel, E. (2000). *Clinical evaluation of language fundamentals— Pre-school UK edition.* London: Psychological Corporation, Harcourt Education.

Williams, M. (2006, November). *Children who stutter: Easy, difficult or slow to warm up?* Paper presented at the Annual Convention of the American Speech-Language and Hearing Association, Miami, FL.

Yairi, E., & Ambrose, N. G. (1999). A longitudinal study of stuttering in children: A preliminary report. *Journal of Speech and Hearing Research, 35,* 775–760.

Yairi, E., & Ambrose, N. G. (2005). *Early childhood stuttering: For clinicians by clinicians.* Austin, TX: Pro-Ed.

Yaruss, J. S. (1999). Utterance length, syntactic complexity, and childhood stuttering. *Journal of Speech, Language, and Hearing Research, 42,* 329–344.

Yaruss, J. S., LaSalle, L. R., & Conture, E. G. (1998). Evaluating stuttering in young children: Diagnostic data. *American Journal of Speech-Language Pathology, 7,* 62–76.

Yaruss, S., Coleman, C., & Hammer, D. (2006). Treating preschool children who stutter: Description and preliminary evaluation of a family-focused treatment approach. *Language, Speech, and Hearing Services in Schools, 37*, 118–136.

Zebrowski, P. (2007). Treatment factors that influence therapy outcomes of children who stutter. In Conture, E. G., & Curlee, R. F. (Eds.), *Stuttering and related disorders of fluency* (3rd ed., pp. 23–38). New York: Thieme Medical Publishers.

# 12 Predictors of Success for Children With Cochlear Implants
## *The Impact of Individual Differences*

*Holly F. B. Teagle and Hannah Eskridge*

Difference is of the essence of humanity.

**John Hume**

Cochlear implantation is an intervention for deafness that has exceeded the expectations held by those instrumental in its early, controversial development. The initial goal of sound awareness seems a meager benefit compared with the phenomenal results afforded by the state-of-the-art technology and the habilitation tools and strategies available today for persons with severe to profound hearing loss. Cochlear implantation has proven to be effective to restore auditory function and to develop audition skills necessary for normal spoken communication. In the scheme of medical interventions, it ranks high in a model of cost efficiency, with both short- and long-term financial impact (Cheng et al., 2000; Francis, Koch, Wyatt, & Niparko, 1999; Johnson & Stewart, 2004; Koch, Wyatt, Francis, & Niparko, 1997; Palmer, Niparko, Wyatt, Rothman, & de Lissovoy, 1999). The development of this medical invention coincided with an evolution in therapeutic approaches to achieve the outcomes appreciated today by both the recipients and the providers of service delivery. The combination of cochlear implantation and effective habilitation for children who are deaf has resulted in a resounding triumph for the fields of audiology, speech-language pathology, and deaf education.

In this chapter, we will review the collective knowledge gathered from 20 years of clinical experience in the use of multichannel cochlear implants for children, with emphasis on understanding the variables that lend themselves to infinite combinations of individual outcomes. We may arrive at the recommendation to pursue cochlear implantation for a child after a standardized protocol to screen, identify, diagnose, and initiate early intervention services. A standardized protocol does not imply a homogeneous implementation of the diagnostic process and subsequent intervention, however. Children present for cochlear implantation with distinctive audiological profiles, medical conditions, and developmental characteristics. Unique composites of individual differences of each child must be recognized at every stage of therapeutic intervention, from the earliest parent session to the fitting and use of technology and the ongoing focus on developmental or remedial therapy. At every stage, children should be considered in the context of their families and their social, economic, cultural, and educational environments. This is pivotal to understanding how individual differences interface with clinical success in cochlear implantation.

For the purposes of understanding the characteristics of a client that may make him or her more amenable to therapeutic change, we will identify some of the potential sources of variability. Among them are (a) the child's hearing history, including age at onset and age at diagnosis of hearing loss; (b) the fitting and management of assistive technology; (c) the child's medical status and general development and personality; (d) the family's acceptance, vigilance, and rigor in their ability to navigate and participate in the medical and educational web of services; and (e) the implementation of educational and therapeutic resources. See Figure 12.1 for a schematic perspective on the influence of various factors for success of cochlear implementation.

What does it take for a child with severe to profound hearing loss to overcome the barriers imposed by sensory deprivation and loss of access to spoken language? The combined knowledge and experience of clinicians, researchers, educators, therapists, and parents have led us to our current level of knowledge and understanding. Indeed, the 2007 Joint Committee on Infant Hearing (JCIH) Position Statement (2007) is a complete guide to the fundamentals of early management of children with hearing loss. This work is the culmination of years of effort to gain recognition for the need for a universal neonatal hearing screening, rather than screening based on selected risk factors. The principles and guidelines of this statement outline each step in the process of identifying hearing loss and implementing habilitation. Table 12.1 summarizes the key points of this statement.

One aspect of service delivery described in this document is the level of competence and commitment each professional involved in the process must possess to achieve a successful outcome for any individual child. Inherently implied, but certainly beyond the control of professionals, is a level of commitment and understanding that the family must have to seek out the professionals, embrace trust and acceptance, and then glean the benefits of their combined knowledge. And finally, implicit in this position statement is recognition by interventionists of the unique abilities and needs of the individual child and his or her family. We must acknowledge, accept, and understand the differences of each set of circumstances and characteristics of the individuals involved. However, we must also strive for the ideal if we are to be successful. When the process of identification, diagnosis and intervention varies from these guidelines that reflect the ideal management, the potential benefits of systematic, timely, accurate and effective management are lost, and variability in outcome becomes more likely.

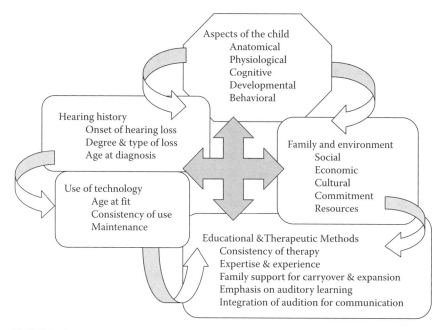

**FIGURE 12.1**    Hellman et al. (1991) and later Fee (2004) developed a clinical index of factors affecting the outcome of cochlear implantation that considered various aspects of the child, the family, and the educational environment. These tools, entitled the Children's Implant Profile (CHiP) and the CHiP-modified, have been used in clinical settings to assist in parent counseling. These predictors of success can be viewed as sources of variability in outcome and are included in this model.

## HEARING HISTORY AND DIAGNOSIS

To begin with, each child possesses a unique hearing history: the status of the cochlea, the presence of residual hearing, and the integrity of the auditory system are distinctive features of the individual child. Consider the deaf infant who was a "preemie," a neonatal intensive care unit (NICU) survivor, a victim of infectious disease, or a host for a combination of disorders expressed as a syndrome or a genetic condition. The anatomical and physiologic characteristics of the infant that cause deafness may also result in other developmental, cognitive, and sensory concerns. The features of an infant's short but often complex medical history are considered to determine which protocol for hearing screening applies, as separate protocols are recommended for NICU babies versus those in the well-baby nursery. Some children have significant health concerns that make the presence of a hearing loss less of a priority for assessment. With that said, timeliness of diagnosis is a cornerstone of the 2007 JCIH Position Statement, since early diagnosis enables planning for early intervention. For either protocol, if the screening for the presence of hearing loss is positive, it is critical to maintain momentum for pursuing a full diagnosis. Although the recognized goal is diagnosis by 3 months

**TABLE 12.1**

**Key Points of the Year 2007 Position Statement: Principles
and Guidelines for Early Hearing Detection and Intervention (EHDI)
Programs**

### Hearing screening and rescreening protocols

- Universal hearing screening should occur through an integrated and interdisciplinary system of EHDI programs.
- All infants should be screened by 1 month of age.
- Those who do not pass screening should have a comprehensive audiological evaluation at no later than 3 months of age.
- Babies admitted to the neonatal intensive care unit for more than 5 days should have an auditory brainstem response (ABR) screening.
- Children who fail screening should be referred to an audiologist for rescreening and the comprehensive evaluation.
- Rescreening should be done on both ears.
- Children readmitted in the first month of life who are at risk for hearing loss should have a repeat screening.

### Diagnostic audiology evaluation

- Experienced pediatric audiologists should complete the evaluation.
- At least 1 ABR should be completed for referred children less than 3 years of age.
- Children who pass screening but have risk factors for hearing loss should be reevaluated.
- Amplification should be fit within 1 month of diagnosis for families who choose it.

### Medical evaluation

- Genetic evaluation should be offered to parents of children with hearing loss.
- An ear, nose, and throat doctor and an ophthalmologist with pediatric experience should examine children with hearing loss.
- All infants with or without risk factors should receive ongoing surveillance of communicative development, beginning at 2 months of age during well-child visits.

### Early intervention

- Infants with confirmed hearing loss should receive appropriate intervention at no later than 6 months of age from expert care.
- Central specialized referral sites should be available.
- Both home-based and center-based intervention options should be offered.
- Families should have access to all technologies.
- Families should have access to all options for treatment and intervention.
- Interdisciplinary intervention should be provided from experienced professionals; programs should be family oriented and culturally sensitive.

### Communication

- The birth hospital and EDHI program should ensure parental and medical home receipt of results.
- Parents should be provided with appropriate resource and referral information.

**TABLE 12.1** (*Continued*)

- Information to parents should be presented in a culturally sensitive and understandable way.
- Individual diagnostic and habilitation information should be conveyed to the medical home and EDHI program coordinator.
- Families should be made aware of all communication options and technologies so they can make informed decisions.

The goal of early hearing detection and intervention is to maximize linguistic competence and literacy development for children who are deaf or hard of hearing. The definition of hearing loss includes congenital, permanent, bilateral or unilateral, sensory, neural, and permanent conductive hearing loss.

*Source:* Adapted from Busa, J., Harrison, J., Chappell, J., Yoshinaga-Itano, C., Grimes, A., Brookhouser, P. E., et al. (2007). Year 2007 position statement: Principles and guidelines for early hearing detection and intervention programs. *Pediatrics, 120*(4): 898–921.

of age, the infant's parents' ability to understand and act on the recommendations of the screening is a source of considerable variability. Bonding with a new baby, not to mention one with potentially life-altering medical conditions, may be challenging for some parents, and that acceptance, or lack thereof, affects the efficiency and immediacy of intervention service delivery. Additional time delays may occur as the baby is rescreened before undergoing a full diagnostic battery, which requires further time and expertise.

Before we can pull something from our bag of technological wonders to begin remediation, we must define the hearing loss for each ear by frequency to the best of our ability. A combination of electrophysiological (auditory brain stem response, auditory steady state response, otoacoustic emissions, acoustic immittance[1]) and behavioral (behavioral observation audiometry, visual response audiometry, conditional play audiometry[2]) audiological measures must be used to corroborate the degree and configuration of hearing loss. Typically, diagnosis is a process,

---

[1] Auditory brain stem response and auditory steady state response are noninvasive objective tests in the battery used by pediatric audiologists to diagnose degree and type of hearing loss. They are accomplished by recording the electrical far-field response to stimulation of the auditory system using electrodes attached at designated positions on the child's head while the child is asleep or inactive. Otoacoustic emissions are measured by placing a probe in the child's ear canal to measure elicited or naturally occurring acoustic emissions from the cochlea. Immittance audiometry is use of a tool that infers middle ear function. All of these procedures provide indices of residual hearing and require no voluntary response or participation by the child.

[2] Behavioral observation audiometry, visual response audiometry, and conditional play audiometry are techniques used by pediatric audiologists that involve observing a child's response to sound, or conditioning or teaching a child to respond to sound, in a controlled manner. These types of measures require the child to be awake, alert, and (depending on the task) involved in the testing. They are voluntary, behavioral responses to sound that are used to determine degree and configuration of hearing loss.

not an event. For many infants with a conductive hearing loss overlying the sensorineural loss and/or progressive hearing loss, the definitive diagnosis may be a moving target. Other comorbid conditions may also deter acquiring a complete audiological profile. For example, the incidence of auditory neuropathy, which has been linked to neonatal concerns such as prematurity, hyperbilirubinemia, and respiratory distress resulting in the need for ventilation, will limit the audiologist's ability to rely on electrophysiological measures to determine the degree of hearing loss. Hearing levels may fluctuate, and the child may not be developmentally able to provide reliable behavioral information to document the hearing loss. This is a prime example of the challenges an audiologist encounters in trying to produce an infant's first audiogram. Expertise and patience, combined with support from parents and insight from early interventionists, contribute to the diagnostic process. Once hearing loss is defined, hearing levels should be monitored for stability, and appropriate amplification should be pursued. Deviation from the recognized ideal timeline to diagnose hearing loss and pursue amplification can result in less than optimal results. This is a significant source of variability in outcomes for children with cochlear implants.

Children who have progressive hearing loss may not be identified by newborn hearing screening. Astute parents and pediatricians who recognize the characteristic behaviors associated with hearing loss must follow up their concerns with a hearing screening, and then a full diagnostic assessment if indicated. The sooner hearing loss is identified, the sooner intervention in the form of amplification and therapy can begin. Late identification of hearing loss results in a greater need for remedial services to bridge the gap in communication development as the child ages (Yoshinaga-Itano, 2003; Yoshinaga-Itano, Sedey, Coulter, & Mehl, 1998).

## USE OF ASSISTIVE TECHNOLOGY

The recognized best practice for fitting amplification in infants with hearing loss is to collect the audiological data as soon as possible and then use prescriptive targets when setting hearing aids to achieve audibility within the child's residual dynamic range (Pediatric Working Group, 1996; Seewald, Moodie, Sinclair, & Scollie, 1999; Westwood & Bamford, 1995). This should be done in a timely manner, with the goal of fitting amplification within a month of diagnosis. A significant source of variability in outcomes begins to take root at this stage of intervention. When actual practice deviates from this best-practice model, the deaf infant, already deprived of audition for the first few months of life, and possibly before birth, continues to develop without the necessary input to develop the auditory areas of the brain.

The longer a child functions with limited or no auditory information, the greater the delay in spoken language acquisition becomes. Deaf children who use visual communication, including American Sign Language, Signed English, or Cued Speech, may develop language constructs that enable communication, but they do not develop audition skills, which are the basis of spoken language. The goal of fitting amplification is to deliver sound that is meaningful to the developing infant. The child's degree of hearing loss dictates the effectiveness of amplifica-tion. Distortion and noise often accompany the signal from high-gain hearing aids. Deaf children may obtain sound awareness and the ability to detect their parents' and their own voices, but sound may not be sufficiently clear to convey the acoustic features of connected speech in a manner that they can meaningfully process. If this is the case, then timely discovery of this situation is essential. On the contrary, if children have residual hearing and have been diagnosed early and well fit with amplification, and have had abundant and purposeful auditory stimu-lation in a controlled environment, they may develop the foundation skills upon which to build a spoken language system. This is the crucial decision point when determining a baby's candidacy for cochlear implantation. Children with some auditory experience, even if it has not afforded spoken language acquisition, are likely to recognize the presence and potential meaning of sound. Children who have no previous experience with sound will have to acclimate to its presence and then learn to attend before they begin to associate it with meaningful information. Thus, the reasons to pursue conventional amplification prior to cochlear implan-tation are twofold: first, to determine whether conventional amplification will enable access to spoken language acquisition, and second, to stimulate remaining hearing, and thus the auditory brain, to the fullest extent possible. If the child is a candidate for cochlear implantation, even limited auditory experience via conventional amplification could expedite the continued development of auditory skills. On occasion, a hearing aid trial will be deferred, but this should be the case only when it has been established that the child's residual hearing is insufficient for noninvasive measures to be of benefit.

Per U.S. Food and Drug Administration guidelines, cochlear implantation is limited to children who fail to make progress in auditory skills development using conventional hearing aid technology. The lower age boundary for a child to undergo cochlear implant surgery has changed over the years. In 1986, when multichannel cochlear implants were first used in a clinical trial to evaluate safety and efficacy, the lower age limit was 2 years. In 1998, this changed to 18 months, and by 2000 it was lowered to 12 months of age. The limiting factors in provid-ing a cochlear implant at an even younger age include confidence that the child is indeed a candidate by audiological and surgical criteria.

The theories propelling earlier implantation are based in developmental research (see Harrison, 2002, for review). They speak to the importance of providing meaningful auditory stimulation before critical periods of normal development are missed, causing delays in language development, which in turn leads to barriers in cognitive and social-emotional development. In the auditory system, areas of the cortex will reorganize following a period of sound deprivation (Kral, Hartmann, Heid, Tillein, & Klinke, 2001; Sharma, Gilley, Dorman, & Baldwin, 2007). If cortical reorganization is arrested, ensuing auditory development will follow a more normal course. Clinical research investigating the effect of age at implantation has supported the notion that earlier implantation impacts speech perception performance. Fryauf-Bertschy, Tyler, Kelsay, Gantz, and Woodworth (1997) found that speech perception outcomes for prelingually deaf children implanted prior to age 5 were significantly better than outcomes for children implanted after age 5. Kirk et al. (2002) studied differences between prelingually deaf children implanted before and after 3 years of age and, again, found significant differences in group performance, with early implanted children demonstrating faster rates of growth in performance on speech perception tasks. Recent studies have explored the risks versus the benefits of implantation under 12 months of age. Dettman, Pinder, Briggs, Dowell, and Leigh (2007) demonstrated that in the hands of experienced pediatric cochlear implant centers, cochlear implantation may be performed safely in very young children. In this study, progress was measured using an infant language scale; language growth rates for children receiving implants before the age of 12 months were significantly greater than rates achieved by children receiving implants between 12 and 24 months, and they matched growth rates achieved by normally hearing peers.

In addition to age at implant, the audiological criteria for pediatric cochlear implantation have changed over the years as the benefits of this technology have become more widely recognized. The candidates for the first multichannel cochlear implants were children with essentially no measurable hearing; today, we provide cochlear implants to children who can be reliably tested and are able to recognize up to 30% of words presented in isolation. Studies of adults comparing residual hearing and postimplant performance suggest that some correlations exist, but outcomes are confounded by other factors, such as duration of deafness (Cullen et al., 2004; Friedland, Venick, & Niparko, 2003; Gomaa, Rubinstein, Lowder, Tyler, & Gantz, 2003). However, there is evidence that this comparison is more compelling and multifaceted in pediatric studies. Children with more residual hearing often make greater progress with cochlear implants and progress at a faster rate than children with little or no residual hearing (Cowan et al., 1997; Gantz et al., 2000, Zwolan et al., 1997). This may be due to development of the central auditory pathway, afforded by better peripheral stimulation and greater plasticity in early development.

Previous experience with sound is another source of variability among children who use cochlear implants. Children with sudden onset of hearing loss or a progressive loss with onset of deafness after language acquisition have historically demonstrated speech perception benefits more quickly than children who are congenitally deaf (Fryauf-Bertschy, Tyler, Kelsay, & Gantz, 1992; Miyamoto, Osberger, Robbins, Myres, & Kessler, 1993; Nicholas & Geers, 2006). The benefits of an established language base and previous auditory experience provide the child with reference points when hearing with an electrical signal. That is, children learn to map the new signal to their memory of sound and spoken language.

The postimplant audiological care and management is of great importance when considering differences among deaf children with cochlear implants. This is a significant source of diversity in outcomes, and one that can be impacted if the parent and child are motivated and resourceful. This includes the consistency of device use, regularity in monitoring hearing and optimizing the programming of the speech processor, and consistent maintenance and upgrading of the hardware

(Geers, Brenner, & Davidson, 2003). Selective use or nonuse translates to a delay in the development of auditory skills. Use of well-maintained equipment and frequent checks of hearing levels and speech perception performance are critical to ensure that a child is realizing the full benefit of the technology. Children who receive cochlear implants at older ages often have more difficulty in maintaining the motivation to use a device that may not provide immediate benefit. Support from family and an educator is essential and is another source of the variability in a child's acceptance of and benefit from a cochlear implant.

## ANATOMICAL, MEDICAL, AND DEVELOPMENTAL FACTORS

The audiological aspects of a child's development are only one facet of the whole child that will affect the outcome of therapeutic interventions. A critical medical consideration is the anatomical status of the cochlea and the integrity of the auditory nerve and the higher auditory pathways. In addition, the presence of cognitive delays and developmental conditions may impact a child's ability to use the technology and benefit from therapy.

Advancements in the medical science of anatomical imaging have provided the cochlear implant surgeon with the tools needed to clearly visualize the cochlea and its nerve supply (Buchman et al., 2006; Gleeson et al., 2003; Kerr & Backous, 2005). The computed tomography scan and magnetic resonance imaging are clinical tools that are used to determine cochlear patency and the presence of the auditory nerve. More recent research has led to means of imaging the electrode array in vivo (Skinner et al., 2007), which illuminates the interface between the implant array and cochlear structures. It must be recognized that cochlear implant technology has limitations when applied to grossly abnormal anatomy. Some children with cochlear malformations have received implants and attained good detection and reasonable speech perception abilities, but for many, the devices serve mostly to supplement visual information (Buchman, Copeland, Brown, Carrasco, & Pillsbury, 2004). Expectations for outcome and the goals of therapy may need to be adjusted for a child if, despite aggressive programming of the device and consistent auditory intervention, there is insufficient stimulability resulting in reduced clarity of sound.

The cochlear implant delivers stimulation at the peripheral end-organ of hearing: the cochlea. We can engineer the way sound is detected and changed from an acoustic signal to electrical impulses and then amplified, filtered, and coded before it is delivered to the cochlea. However, the way the auditory nervous system analyzes the information and processes it in the higher regions of the auditory brain stem and cortex is beyond our control. Herein lies a major source of variability among children. Although an individual child's brain may be able to recognize patterns of stimulation that are perceived as words or phrases, that child's attention, cognition, and memory abilities affect the overall ability to process language (Fagan, Pisoni, Horn, & Dillon, 2007; Pisoni, 2000). These may be target areas for therapy that require a comprehensive approach.

It has been reported that 30–40% of children with significant hearing loss who may be candidates for cochlear implants also have other development issues (Karchmer & Allen, 1999; Parrish & Roush, 2004; Picard, 2004). These handicaps often affect a child's prognosis for success, when success is defined as age-appropriate spoken language development. Many clinical reports have been published regarding children with blindness, mental retardation, autism, and other sensory and cognitive disorders who have received cochlear implants (Fryauf-Bertschy, Iler Kirk, & Weiss, 1993; Holt & Kirk, 2005; Waltzman, Scalchunes, & Cohen, 2000). In general, these studies support the position that children with multiple handicapping conditions can learn to use audition with varying levels of benefit and, typically, at slower rates of progress compared with their peers with no other diagnoses. For some of these children, cochlear implantation will support communication, and for others, its benefit can better be described as providing a connection to the environment. Especially in these cases, it is critical that family and educators work together to explore and capitalize on each child's potential. The presence of other handicapping conditions certainly increases the need for counseling with the family in regard to appropriate expectations and the need for supplemental resources.

## THE FAMILY AND ITS GOALS, ENVIRONMENT, AND RESOURCES

Cochlear implantation, being an elective procedure, is a choice parents make for a child for the purpose of gaining the sense of hearing. The functional use of hearing may vary depending on a child's general development and parents' goals for the child. Before discussion of the individual differences in families, environments, and therapies that affect outcomes in children who use cochlear implants, it is important to recognize that the conventional way to measure results in the area of communicative disorders is to compare performance with the developmental patterns and timelines of normal speech and language acquisition. However, normal speech and language acquisition is not necessarily commensurate with the definition of success for every child with a cochlear implant. Success is defined as a function of the goal for the individual; that goal may be very conservative, such as sound awareness for safety, or it may be ambitious, such as age-appropriate speech and language acquisition. For the purposes of this discussion, we acknowledge that the long-term goal for each child is to reach his or her potential in communicative competence. However, to quantify outcomes in cochlear implantation, we use measures of speech perception performance and normative indices of speech and language acquisition. Thus, the measurement tool of choice depends on the purpose of assessment.

In counseling parents about what it will take to help their child achieve the goal of effective communication, which is a cornerstone to building a life's achievement academically, socially, and personally, we sometimes refer to the technology as the "tools" and the parents and therapists as the "technicians." Undoubtedly, the tools have improved and will continue to improve over time. Certainly, the hearing aid and cochlear implant technology that is available today is more sophisticated, flexible for individual fitting, durable, and user friendly than the first generations of these devices. Simply said, better tools or technology provides better results. However, to understand the variability of individual outcomes in cochlear implantation, we must also recognize that some technicians have more natural ability, practice, and expertise than others. In addition, some families have more barriers to overcome as they strive to become competent technicians. Much of the variability in therapeutic outcomes for children with cochlear implants correlates with the family's ability to navigate medical and educational needs independently by overcoming potential language, economic, and/or social barriers. Other family variables that influence a child's rate and level of progress with a cochlear implant include acceptance and vigilance, stability of the family's structure, and access to and commitment to therapy.

The family's acceptance of the diagnosis and the family's ability to move forward will likely affect the timeliness and efficacy of intervention. A family with no history or experience with hearing loss may struggle to recognize the long-term impact and permanency of deafness. For example, the family members may perceive cochlear implantation as "the fix" for deafness, with little appreciation for the importance of ongoing therapy. Families must be counseled to understand that the continuous use of well-maintained technology, coupled with consistent and appropriate therapy, is the key to deriving maximum benefits from its use. This requires thorough counseling from clinicians who recognize when a family needs more instruction and support in using and maintaining hardware as well as encouragement to participate in therapy services.

Family structure and support are considerable sources of variability in cochlear implant outcomes. However, it is difficult to objectively measure these because of the number of confounding factors they include and our inability to conduct a causal study. It is typical for children to learn language from parents and other family members. Families whose members participate in regular therapy with their children and learn how to carry over the therapeutic principles and practices to everyday life contexts will provide the optimal environment for a language-developing child. It is important to look at individual differences in families' organization to help determine how provision of therapy will best work for their particular situations and obligations. Some of these potential differences include single-parent families, families where both parents work full time, families that live in rural areas, and families with low socioeconomic status, who often have fewer economic and educational resources. Regularly scheduled intervention, ideally weekly therapy sessions, is essential to support parents as they nurture the language development of the child. Single parents may need help analyzing their schedule to determine when a weekly therapy session can take place. It will be important for them to establish support from family and/or friends in order to meet all of their responsibilities, including therapy with their child. The implant team can provide documentation to employers as needed to allow time off for the session. A letter explaining the importance of therapy and why it is critical for the parent to be consistently involved can often convince an employer to allow a longer lunch hour or for the parent to leave work early once a week. Families with two working parents and a child who spends a great deal of time in daycare or with another primary caregiver may need other types of flexibility. The primary caregiver can attend therapy with the parent or the session can be recorded for parents to view later so that they too can carry over goals while they are with the child.

The economics of acquiring therapy services is a concern for many families. Most families can access resources through insurance, Medicaid, scholarships, and local community organizations or parent support groups. When families do not have access to resources, either because of logistics or the lack of financial means to acquire them, valuable time may be lost in intervention, which impacts overall outcomes (Yoshinaga-Itano, 2003; Moeller, 2000).

Families living in metropolitan areas may find a variety of sources to access appropriate services. Families that do not have appropriate services available in their local area may have to travel long distances for services. One strategy for overcoming this problem may be to find a local therapist who can work with an experienced therapist in a mentoring relationship. Current technology such as videotaping and webcams to provide distance health services can make this process more feasible. This not only allows for access to qualified professionals but also decreases costs for families for both therapy and transportation. Although Medicaid law does not currently recognize this as a distinct service, Medicaid reimbursement can be obtained for practitioners using Telemedicine (http://www.cms.hhs.gov/Telemedicine; U.S. Department of Health and Human Services, 2009).

We cannot presuppose that socioeconomic factors that can be quantified, such as income and number of parents in the household, will always impact outcomes in a predictable way. The University of North Carolina-Chapel Hill's Center for Acquisition of Spoken Language Through Listening Enrichment (CASTLE) provided weekly parent sessions to 20 children in December 2007. The families of these children represent many of the individual differences found in families throughout the country. Three of the families did not speak any English, four of the children were in single-parent homes, six mothers worked full-time jobs, and seven families' annual gross income was less than $30,000. All but 4 of the children were demonstrating average to above average progress, as defined by making a year's progress in a year's time.

## EDUCATIONAL AND THERAPEUTIC METHODS

In addition to the variables previously discussed, successful therapeutic intervention hinges on the ability of intuitive and creative therapists to lead parents in the art of developing the auditory skills of the child. In recent years, there have been a multitude of books, guides, materials, and intervention programs developed to help parents and therapists teach children with cochlear implants to meet their communicative potential. From a therapeutic standpoint, to apply the same theories and practices without regard for the strengths and weaknesses of the individuals involved in the process can result in frustration, disappointment, and ultimately, failure to achieve the personal potential of the child and family. The ideal scenario includes (a) access to experienced therapists, (b) parental involvement in therapy, (c) carryover of concepts from therapy to daily life,

(d) importantly, an emphasis on the development of audition skills, and (e) the integration of and reliance on hearing as the main mode for communication.

## EXPERIENCED THERAPISTS

Although aggressive audiological management is being pursued, parents also need to establish appropriate auditory-based therapy services with a therapist trained in the development of spoken language through audition. It is important for parents to work with their cochlear implant team to discuss the types of services that are available in their area and how to advocate for and establish services. Parents should determine the following (Estabrooks, 1998; Ernst, 2001): Does the therapist (a) expect the child to learn through listening and teach the child how to obtain information through hearing, (b) understand how the environment can interfere with listening, (c) follow the normal patterns of language and speech development, and (d) work with the parents as partners in developing the child's goals as prescribed in family-centered practice? That is, parents must be encouraged to assess the quality of therapy they are receiving. See Table 12.2 for a delineation of features of adequate therapy.

## PARENTAL INVOLVEMENT

It is important for one or both parents or another caregiver who is very knowledgeable about the child to participate in these sessions on a weekly basis. The goal of the therapist in this session is not to directly teach the child but to teach the parent how to, first, stimulate the child to develop the child's auditory and language potential, and then to implement the carryover of goals at home on a daily basis. Parents and caregivers need to be their children's primary language teachers. Therapists can make the greatest impact on a child's development by teaching the parent the skills for developing audition skills and language. Effective therapists must incorporate elements of adult learning into the time spent with the parent and child so that parents develop confidence, competence, a level of energy, and motivation. Parents then incorporate therapy goals into normal caregiver routines, facilitating children's learning of language in their home environment.

## CARRYOVER AT HOME

Once appropriate services are established, parents will need to carry over goals established in therapy at home. Many of the scheduling issues previously discussed can impact parents' consistency in doing this. However, without carryover, the child's progress will be very slow based on the limited amount of time spent with the therapist. The therapist can help parents prioritize their day and determine where daily carryover activities best fit.

Daily activities focusing on carryover need to take place in a quiet environment. Many normal-hearing adults are not aware of the various environmental noises that can negatively impact a child's successful listening, such as the dishwasher,

## TABLE 12.2
## Principles of Listening and Spoken Language Specialist (LSLS) Auditory-Verbal Therapy

Families can consult the document "Principles of LSLS Auditory-Verbal Therapy" as a first step when learning about the components of appropriate therapy.

1  Promote early diagnosis of hearing loss in newborns, infants, toddlers, and young children followed by immediate audiologic management and Auditory-Verbal therapy.

2  Recommend immediate assessment and use of appropriate, state-of-the-art hearing technology to obtain maximum benefits of auditory stimulation.

3  Guide and coach parents[1] to help their child use hearing as the primary sensory modality in developing spoken language without the use of sign language or emphasis on lip-reading.

4  Guide and coach parents[1] to become the primary facilitators of their child's listening and spoken language development through active consistent participation in individualized Auditory-Verbal therapy.

5  Guide and coach parents[1] to create environments that support listening for the acquisition of spoken language throughout the child's daily activities.

6  Guide and coach parents[1] to help their child integrate listening and spoken language into all aspects of the child's life.

7  Guide and coach parents[1] to use natural developmental patterns of audition, speech, language, and cognition and communication.

8  Guide and coach parents[1] to help their child self-monitor spoken language through listening.

9  Administer ongoing formal and informal diagnostic assessments to develop individualized Auditory-Verbal treatment plans to monitor progress and to evaluate the effectiveness of the plans for the child and the family.

10 Promote education in regular schools with peers who have typical hearing and with appropriate services from early childhood onwards.

[1] The term "parents" also includes grandparents, relatives, guardians, and any caregivers who interact with the child.

*Source:* Adapted from Pollack, D. (1970). *Principles of LSLS auditory-verbal therapy.* Adopted by the AG Bell Academy for Listening and Spoken Language. With permission.

ringing phones, and television. These sources of noise need to be minimized or eliminated during time set aside for home carryover activities. Other elements that may enhance the listening environment include parents and/or therapists sitting beside the child's chair on the side of the best ear, speaking to the child close to their cochlear implant microphone, at a normal speaking volume, and using a technique referred to as *acoustic highlighting* (Estabrooks, 1998). One example of acoustic highlighting is to use a sing-song voice, also referred to as *parentese*, to make the phrase more audible and interesting to the child.

### CONSISTENT AUDITORY AND SPOKEN LANGUAGE INPUT

Language and listening should be incorporated into the child's daily routine throughout the day. Isolated drills in "auditory training" once per day for an hour will be insufficient for a child to learn to integrate sound for meaningful, age-appropriate communication. Instead, a child must be immersed in an environment of "auditory learning," where all routines are seen as opportunities for the child to listen and be exposed to language. The child needs to know that he or she is expected to listen. Normal caregiver routines such as feeding and dressing a child are rich in language that is repetitive and includes the vocabulary first learned by children with normal hearing. These care-giving routines should be done within close proximity to the child, which is important for providing an optimal auditory environment. Incorporating phrases from routines that the child participates in every day can help children pick up auditory and language skills in a developmentally appropriate way. Including songs in daily activities that embed age-appropriate language features will gain the child's interest and attention.

## COMMUNICATION MODE

Communication mode is the predominant feature of various theories and methods for educating children with hearing loss that are often described on a continuum ranging from no codependence on auditory information for communication to total and complete integration of audition for communication. Children with cochlear implants use a variety of communication approaches including American Sign Language, Total Communication, Cued Speech, Auditory–Oral, and Auditory-Verbal, as well as forms of augmentative alternative communication. Although the literature does not support a single communication mode as being clearly superior for children with hearing loss as a group because of their heterogeneity (Moeller, 2000; Yoshinaga-Itano, 2003), the preponderance of studies of children with cochlear implants show higher levels of speech perception performance and spoken language acquisition among children utilizing oral communication modes over those using visual or combined communication modes. Research has shown that children educated in a spoken language approach without the use of sign demonstrate more sophisticated narrative skills, greater vocabulary size, greater use of more bound morphemes, and use of longer utterances with more complex syntax in their spontaneous language than children taught a signed communication system (Geers, Nicolas, & Sedey, 2003). In addition children from oral programs have also been shown to demonstrate higher speech perception scores and more age-appropriate speech production, oral language, and total language (Kirk et al., 2002; Moog & Geers, 2003; Osberger, Fisher, Zimmerman-Phillips, Geier, & Barker, 1998). Improved spoken language skills have been shown to result in increases in reading skills. Although a recent study by Geers (2003) demonstrated that speech perception scores did not contribute as an independent variable to reading outcome in children with hearing impairments, speech production and language skills were shown to predict their reading success.

　　Reasons for selecting a particular communication mode should be the prerogative of well-informed parents who recognize their child's potential and limitations. Most parents seeking cochlear implantation for their child have normal hearing themselves; they often express the desire for their deaf child to acquire intelligible speech and achieve speech understanding that will enable the child to participate in a mainstream educational setting. Parents need to be counseled regarding expectations for their child; other medical or developmental characteristics of the child may make mainstream education unrealistic. It may be necessary for a child to rely on a combination of visual and spoken communication. Parents are the most powerful force influencing a child's success with any communication approach. As stated by Luterman (1999), "No educational method is going to work unless parents freely choose it and take responsibility for it" (p. 31). Thus, although choice of communication mode is very important, the family's commitment to following through with supporting the remedial practices for becoming competent teachers of language through that chosen option is even more important. An environment that provides consistent and appropriate language models, whether signed, cued or spoken, is the most desirable. The parents' or primary caregiver's role is pivotal in affecting competent use of that communication mode.

## CASE STUDIES

As noted, a child's success with a cochlear implant is impacted by many variables. The following case studies represent a range of patient characteristics, expectations, and outcomes among children who have received cochlear implants.

### SARAH

Sarah was diagnosed with a severe to profound hearing loss at 6 weeks of age after being referred by an infant newborn hearing screening at her birth hospital. There was no history of hearing loss in her family and no risk factors associated with her mother's pregnancy or the birth. Genetic testing later revealed her cause of deafness was related to a Connexin 26 mutation. She had normal cochlear anatomy and was a healthy baby. She was the second child born to a two-parent home. Both of her parents were college educated, and the family was socially and financially stable. Sarah was fit with hearing aids at 2.5 months of age and began receiving early intervention services with a certified auditory verbal therapist shortly thereafter. Sarah's developmental milestones unrelated to speech and language were typical. Despite consistent hearing aid use and some evidence of sound awareness, Sarah did not make the expected progress in acquiring auditory skills. She received an implant at 12 months of age. The expectations of the cochlear implant team and Sarah's parents were that she would develop age-appropriate spoken language skills and be able to successfully enter a mainstream kindergarten classroom with her peers.

Sarah and her mother attended weekly auditory-verbal therapy consistently, and her family carried over her goals on a daily basis at home. Her audiological management was consistent and aggressive. She began to make progress right away, producing more frequent and varied vocalizations and alerting to voices and sounds in the environment. At the age of 2, she received a second cochlear implant. Her annual speech, language, and hearing assessment at the age of

3 years, 2 years after receiving her first cochlear implant, revealed detection of sound at 20–25 dB HL across audiometric frequencies, excellent speech recognition abilities, and speech production and receptive and expressive language scores within normal limits or above. She continues to demonstrate communication skills comparable to those of normal hearing children of her age.

## Rob

Rob is a child with multiple disabilities, including profound hearing loss. After a normal pregnancy, birth, and early childhood development, Rob contracted meningitis at 9 months of age, which resulted in a total loss of hearing as well as concomitant cognitive and motor delays. He was fit with conventional hearing aids by his first birthday, but he obtained little more than sound awareness. His general development stagnated for months after the meningitis, but he slowly began to recover motor function. However, his cognitive abilities were severely and negatively affected by the insult of meningitis.

Rob is the second child born to college-educated parents who are highly motivated for him to succeed. They are very aware of and have accepted his other disabilities. Rob received a cochlear implant at the age of 4 years. The expectations of the cochlear implant team were for Rob to develop some sound awareness skills to augment communication. Although his responses to sound were slow to emerge after implantation, he eventually became very attached to his cochlear implant, requested it, and wore it consistently. Rob responds alertly to his name and many environmental sounds that are routine in his environment.

Rob attends a special education class in his local school system. He also receives weekly therapy from the cochlear implant center to address his audition goals. Because of the dedication of his mother, he has not only met expectations for sound awareness but has also begun to understand some functional spoken phrases and words. Rob has demonstrated limited use of his voice. He will vocalize for attention or with emotion, but does not vocalize for expressive communication. His receptive language, however, appears to be emerging. His parents have begun to pair signs with speech and very recently, he has begun to use sign expressively in specific situations and in response to information being presented to him through listening. Expectations for his continued growth in communication are unknown but unlimited by his parents' support and this educational and therapeutic environment.

## Jennifer

Jennifer received a cochlear implant at the age of 13. Even though she was diagnosed as profoundly deaf shortly after birth, she did not use assistive technology, as her severe bilateral cochlear malformations led surgeons to believe that neither hearing aids nor cochlear implants would enable auditory stimulation. Her parents approached communication aggressively and began using Cued Speech with her at a very young age. With no residual hearing but with consistent intervention services, Jennifer was able to maintain academic achievement commensurate with her hearing peers through use of Cued Speech and her parents' ongoing support. In a final attempt to obtain sound awareness, her parents elected to pursue an auditory brain stem implant (ABI) in Europe. Although it is not approved for use in nontumor patients in the United States, the ABI has been used with a small number of children in Europe, with reportedly good results for sound awareness. In gathering medical records for the ABI consultation, new imaging was collected that, due to improved resolution, suggested to an experienced surgeon that Jennifer may in fact have a patent internal auditory canal with an intact eighth nerve on one side. She underwent cochlear implantation with guarded expectations that she would hear. The result was a partial insertion of the electrode array with effective stimulation on about one third of the available channels. Although the development of auditory skills has been reliant on intensive therapy and painstaking drill, Jennifer uses her cochlear implant during all waking hours and increasingly relies on sound. She alerts to her name, recognizes the voices of her family, and understands words and phrases in closed-set tasks. Her lip reading has also improved, and her reliance on Cued Speech has declined, which affords her many more communication partners. Jennifer's intelligibility is also improving, as she is finally able to monitor her voice. She is highly motivated and determined to make continued progress.

For these children, expectations for benefit from a cochlear implant were varied. They have all been successful based on their individual differences and goals. Although they differ in many ways, all three case studies include the important variable of supportive parents who are involved in the therapeutic process.

## WHERE DO WE GO FROM HERE?

As a nation, our success in identifying hearing loss at birth and following up with timely fitting of assistive technology is improving. In 1985, when multichannel cochlear implants were first used under investigational trials, hearing screening procedures were insensitive and nonspecific, identifying only a fraction of children in the population with hearing loss. There was no consensus regarding the best way to identify and habilitate children with hearing loss before important milestones in their development had passed. At the time of this writing, our success rate has greatly improved. A survey of state-mandated hearing screening programs by Harrison, Roush, and Wallace (2003) indicated a positive trend toward earlier identification of hearing loss and hearing aid fitting as a direct result of newborn hearing screening. Efforts are now focusing on subsequent intervention and the availability of well-trained professionals to implement early intervention and preschool and elementary school services. Although more parents are choosing cochlear implant technology and spoken language for their children who are deaf, university training programs are not responding quickly to this need. A recent survey indicated that out of the 70 universities in the United States that have deaf education programs, only 8 have a specialization in auditory-based education. Training programs for teachers of the deaf and speech-language pathologists need to prepare future professionals to become competent in teaching children to develop spoken language skills through listening (White, 2006).

Continued development of effective therapeutic methods to use with *all* children with severe to profound hearing loss is critical. We should target special populations of children who require a flexible and thoughtful approach, such as those with multiple handicapping conditions, children from families who are not native speakers of English, and children from families who are socially and economically disadvantaged and may require assistance with general living and parenting skills. The diversity among children with hearing loss and their families is unlimited. Our ability to recognize and appreciate differences among children is the first step in helping them achieve their individual potential after cochlear implantation.

> Diversity is the one true thing we all have in common. Celebrate it every day.
>
> **Anonymous**

## REFERENCES

A. G. Bell Academy for Listening and Spoken Language. (2007). *Principles of LSLS auditory-verbal therapy*. Retrieved July 27, 2009, from http://www.agbellacademy. org/principal-auditory.htm (Adapted from the principles originally developed by Doreen Pollack.)

Buchman, C. A., Copeland, B. J., Brown, C. J., Carrasco, V. N., & Pillsbury, H. C. (2004). Cochlear implantation in children with congenital inner ear malformations. *Laryngoscope, 114*, 309–316.

Buchman, C. A., Roush, P. A., Teagle, H. F. B., Brown, C. J., Zdanski, C. J., & Grose, J. H. (2006). Auditory neuropathy characteristics in children with cochlear nerve deficiency. *Ear and Hearing, 27*(4), 399–408.

Busa, J., Harrison, J., Chappell, J., Yoshinaga-Itano, C., Grimes, A., Brookhouser, P. E., et al. (2007). Year 2007 position statement: Principles and guidelines for early hearing detection and intervention programs. *Pediatrics, 120*(4), 898–921.

Cheng, A. K., Rubin, H. R., Powe, N. R., Mellon, N. K., Francis, H. W., & Niparko, J. K. (2000). Cost-utility analysis of the cochlear implant in children. *Journal of the American Medical Association, 284*(7), 850–856.

Cowan, R. S., DelDot, J., Barker, E. J., Sarant, J. Z., Pegg, P., Dettman, S., et al. (1997). Speech perception results for children with implants with different levels of preoperative residual hearing. *American Journal of Otology, 18*(6 Suppl.), 125–126.

Cullen, R. D., Higgins, C., Buss, E., Clark, M., Pillsbury, H. C., & Buchman, C. A. (2004). Cochlear implantation in patients with substantial residual hearing. *Laryngoscope, 114*(12), 2218–2223.

Dettman, S. J., Pinder, D., Briggs, R. J., Dowell, R. C., & Leigh, J. R. (2007). Communication development in children who receive the cochlear implant younger than 12 months: Risks versus benefits. *Ear and Hearing, 28*(2 Suppl.), 11S–18S.

Estabrooks, W. (1998). Learning to listen with a cochlear implant: A model for children. In W. Estabrooks (Ed.), *Cochlear implants for kids*. Washington, DC: Alexander Graham Bell Association for the Deaf.

Ernst, M. (2001). How to know your child has a qualified auditory based therapist. In W. Estabrooks, (Ed.), *Fifty frequently asked questions about auditory-verbal therapy.* Toronto, Ontario, Canada: Learning to Listen Foundation.

Fagan, M. K., Pisoni, D. B., Horn, D. L., & Dillon, C. M. (2007). Neuropsychological correlates of vocabulary, reading, and working memory in deaf children with cochlear implants. *Journal of Deaf Studies & Deaf Education, 12*(4), 461–471.

Fee, R. (2004). *Children's Implant Profile (ChIP-modified).* Center for Childhood Communication, The Children's Hospital of Philadelphia. Available from http://www.chop.edu/service/cochlear-implant-program/home.html

Francis, H. W., Koch, M. E., Wyatt, J. R., & Niparko, J. K. (1999). Trends in educational placement and cost-benefit considerations in children with cochlear implants. *Archives of Otolaryngology-Head & Neck Surgery, 125*(5), 499–505.

Friedland, D. R., Venick, H., & Niparko, J. (2003). Choice of ear for cochlear implantation: The effect of history and residual hearing on predicted postoperative performance. *Otology & Neurology, 24*(4), 582–589.

Fryauf-Bertschy, H., Iller Kirk, K., & Weiss, A. L. (1993). Cochlear implant use by a child who is deaf and blind: A case study. *American Journal of Audiology, 2,* 37–48.

Fryauf-Bertschy, H., Tyler, R. S., Kelsay, D. M., & Gantz, B. J. (1992). Performance over time of congenitally deaf and postlingually deafened children using a multichannel cochlear implant. *Journal of Speech and Hearing Research, 35,* 913–920.

Fryauf-Bertschy, H., Tyler, R. S., Kelsay, D. M., Gantz, B. J., & Woodworth, G. G. (1997). Cochlear implant use by prelingually deafened children: The influences of age at implant and length of device use. *Journal of Speech, Language, and Hearing Research, 40*(1), 183–199.

Gantz, B. J., Rubenstein, J. T., Tyler, R. S., Teagle, H. F., Cohen, N. L., Waltzman, S. B., et al. (2000). Long-term results of cochlear implants in children with residual hearing. *Annals of Otology, Rhinology & Laryngology, 185*(Suppl.), 33–36.

Geers, A. E. (2003). Predictors of reading skill development in children with early cochlear implantation. *Ear and Hearing, 24*(1 Suppl.), 59S–68S.

Geers, A. E., Brenner, C., & Davidson, L. (2003). Factors associated with development of speech perception skills in children implanted by age five. *Ear and Hearing, 24*(Suppl.), 24S–35S.

Geers, A. E., Nicholas, J. G., & Sedey, A. L. (2003). Language skills of children with early cochlear implantation. *Ear and Hearing, 24*(Suppl.), 46S–58S.

Gleeson, T. G., Lacy, P. D., Bresnihan, M., Gaffney, R., Brennan, P., & Viani, L. (2003). High resolution computed tomography and magnetic resonance imaging in the pre-operative assessment of cochlear implant patients. *Journal of Laryngology & Otology, 117*(9), 692–695.

Gomaa, N. A., Rubinstein, J. T., Lowder, M. W., Tyler, R. S., & Gantz, B. J. (2003). Residual speech perception and cochlear implant performance in postlingually deafened adults. *Ear and Hearing, 24*(6), 539–544.

Harrison, R. V. (2002). Representing the acoustic world within the brain: Normal and abnormal development of frequency maps in the auditory system. In R. C. Seewald & Judith S. Gravel (Eds.), *A sound foundation through early amplification 2001: Proceedings of an International Conference* (pp. 3–24). Great Britain: St. Edmundsbury Press.

Harrison, M., Roush, J., & Wallace, J. (2003). Trends in age of identification and intervention in infants with hearing loss. *Ear and Hearing, 24*(1), 89–95.

Hellman, S. A., Chute, P. M., Kretschmer, R. E., Nevins, M. E., Parisier, S. C., & Thurston, L. C. (1991). The development of a children's implant profile. *American Annals of the Deaf, 136,* 77–81.

Holt, R. F., & Kirk, K. I. (2005). Speech and language development in cognitively delayed children with cochlear implants. *Ear and Hearing, 26*(2), 132–148.

Johnson, R. F., & Stewart, M. G. (2004). Outcomes research in pediatric otolaryngology. *Journal for Oto-Rhino-Laryngology and Its Related Specialties, 66*(4), 221–226.

Karchmer, M. A., & Allen, T. E. (1999). The functional assessment of deaf and hard of hearing students. *American Annals of Deaf, 144*(2), 68–77.

Kerr, J., & Backous, D. D. (2005). Cochlear implantation in the partially ossified cochlea. *Operative Techniques in Otolaryngology-Head & Neck Surgery, 16*(2), 113–116.

Kirk, K. I., Miyamoto, R., Lento, C. L., Ying, E., O'Neill, T., & Fears, B. (2002). Effects of age at implantation in young children. *Annals of Otology Rhinology & Laryngology, 189*(Suppl.), 69–73.

Koch, M. E., Wyatt, J. R., Francis, H. W., & Niparko, J. K. (1997). A model of educational resource use by children with cochlear implants. *Otolaryngology Head & Neck Surgery, 117*, 174–179.

Kral, A., Hartmann, R., Heid, S., Tillein, J., & Klinke, R. (2001). Delayed maturation and sensitive periods in the auditory cortex. *Audiology & Neurootology, 6*, 346–362.

Luterman, D. (1999). *The young deaf child*. Baltimore: York Press Inc.

Miyamoto, R. T., Osberger, M. J., Robbins, A. M., Myres, W. A., & Kessler, K. (1993). Prelingually deafened children's performance with the nucleus multichannel cochlear implant. *American Journal of Otology, 14*(5), 437–445.

Moeller, M. P. (2000). Early intervention and language development in children who are deaf and hard of hearing. *Pediatrics, 106*(3), e43.

Moog, J., & Geers, A. E. (2003). Epilogue: Major findings, conclusions and implications for deaf education. *Ear and Hearing, 24*(1 Suppl), 121S–125S.

Nicholas, J. G., & Geers, A. E. (2006). Effects of early auditory experience on the spoken language of deaf children at 3 years of age. *Ear and Hearing, 27*(3), 286–298.

Osberger, M. J., Fisher, L., Zimmerman-Phillips, S., Geier, L., & Barker, M. J. (1998). Speech recognition performance of older children with cochlear implants. *American Journal of Otology, 19*(2), 152–157.

Palmer, C. S., Niparko, J. K., Wyatt, J. R., Rothman, M., & de Lissovoy, G. (1999). A prospective study of the cost-utility of the multichannel cochlear implant. *Archives of Otolaryngology-Head & Neck Surgery, 125*(11), 1221–1228.

Parrish, R., & Roush, J. (2004). When hearing loss occurs with other disabilities. *Volta Voices, 11*(7), 20–21.

Pediatric Working Group. (1996). Amplification for infants and children with hearing loss. *American Journal of Audiology, 5*, 53–68.

Picard, M. (2004). Children with permanent hearing loss and associated disabilities. Revisiting current epidemiological data and causes of deafness. *The Volta Review, 104*, 221–236.

Pisoni, D. B. (2000). Cognitive factors and cochlear implants: Some thoughts on perception, learning, and memory in speech perception. *Ear and Hearing, 21*(1), 70–78.

Seewald, R. C., Moodie, K. S., Sinclair, S. T., & Scollie, S. D. (1999). Predictive validity of a procedure for pediatric hearing instrument fitting. *American Journal of Audiology, 8*(2), 143–152.

Sharma, A., Gilley, P. M., Dorman, M. F., & Baldwin, R. (2007). Deprivation-induced cortical reorganization in children with cochlear implants. *International Journal of Audiology, 46*, 494–499.

Skinner, M. W., Holden, T. A., Whiting, B. R., Voie, A. H., Brunsden, B., Neely, G., et al. (2007). In vivo estimates of the position of Advanced Bionics electrode arrays in the human cochlea. *Annals of Otology, Rhinology, & Laryngology, 116*(4 Suppl. 197), 1–24.

U.S. Department of Health and Human Services. (2009). *Overview telemedicine*. Retrieved July 27, 2009 from http://www.cms.hhs.gov/Telemedicine

Waltzman, S. B., Scalchunes, V., & Cohen, N. L. (2000). Performance of mutiply handicapped children using cochlear implants. *The American Journal of Otology, 21*, 329–335.

Westwood, G. F., & Bamford, J. M. (1995). Probe-tube microphone measures with very young infants: Real ear to coupler differences and longitudinal changes in real ear unaided response. *Ear and Hearing, 16*(3), 263–273.

White, K. (2006). Early intervention for children with permanent hearing loss: Finishing the EHDI revolution. *The Volta Review, 106*(3), 237–258.

Yoshinaga-Itano, C. (2003). From screening to early identification and intervention: Discovering predictors to successful outcomes for children with significant hearing loss. *Journal of Deaf Studies and Deaf Education, 8*, 11–30.

Yoshinaga-Itano, C., Sedey, A. L., Coulter, D. K., & Mehl, A. L. (1998). Language of early- and later-identified children with hearing loss. *Pediatrics, 102*, 1161–1171.

Zwolan, T. A., Zimmerman Phillips, S., Ashbaugh, C. J., Hieber, S. J., Kileny, P. R., & Telian, S. A. (1997). Cochlear implantation of children with minimal open-set speech recognition skills. *Ear and Hearing, 18*(3), 240–251.

# 13 How Focus on Individual Differences Informs our Clinical Practice for Individuals With Communication Disorders: A Summary and a Look Ahead
## *Epilogue*

*Amy L. Weiss*

Reading through the chapters of this text, it may be obvious that there was general agreement by this collection of authors, all of whom are clinicians as well as researchers, that the individual differences their clients embody are essential to consider when making clinical decisions. Likewise, there is an evident thread running through the chapters supporting the belief that the most effective therapy for a client is one that takes into account a client's individual characteristics. This may have been the result of a nonscientific sampling. That is, the researcher–clinicians who agreed to participate in this writing project may have been attracted to it because the theme resonated with their already-held beliefs. Even if that is the case, it is interesting for me to note how differently the authors approached the task of describing how individual differences played a part in clinical practice with one or another communication disorder diagnosis.

## THE CASE FOR CASE STUDIES

Many of the authors express some frustration at trying to balance adherence to the principles of evidence-based practice (EBP) with the relative lack of empirical information about the impact of individual differences incorporated into available treatment studies. One of the barriers to studying the role of individual differences that is frequently mentioned is the difficulty of carrying out powerful, large-scale population studies of intervention approaches due to the heterogeneity of subject pools for persons with communication disorders, including the age of the subjects and the particular type of communication disorder observed. Without results from sophisticated intervention studies with sizeable populations at their disposal, the question of how to weigh the remaining two aspects of EBP, clinician experience and client preference, becomes even more critical. This is made especially evident by the fact that some of the authors use a case study approach to illustrate how intervention can be adapted to individual clients.

For example, Brinton and Fujiki (Chapter 2) observe that they could easily provide case histories of several children with highly similar language abilities, but when they scratched the surface, it was clear that each child presented with a distinctive social profile (p. 17). Determining the specific makeup of that individual social profile turned out to be critical. As demonstrated in their informative descriptions of the paths taken for successful therapy with each case, each of the children presented with a different set of challenges to social development and ability to use social language (p. 17). The authors are dubious that intervention could have been successful without consideration of these individual challenges. For Brinton and Fujiki, knowledge about the social competencies and social temperament of a child with a language impairment is essential both to ultimately understand a young client's needs and to then factor into clinical decision making and programming.

Similarly, in their discussion in Chapter 9 of the treatment options available for children with cleft lip and palate, Chapman and Hardin-Jones present three case studies illustrating the individuation of therapy programs for children depending on their specific presenting characteristics. The authors demonstrate how general principles of intervention for children with this category of orofacial anomaly and resultant communication disorder could be accommodated to yield a workable program depending on an individual child's specific complex of anatomical, physiological, linguistic, and motivational features.

In Chapter 11, Hayhow and Shenker describe how the Lidcombe Program (LP), a behavioral treatment that was designed to eliminate stuttering in preschool-age children, could be altered to take into consideration a young child's particular circumstances. That is, because the LP places so much emphasis on the ability of the family to shoulder the lion's share of therapy administration, taking into account the individual differences represented by a child's familial milieu takes on added importance. That is not to suggest that a family-centered orientation has not been considered by other authors, but it is inescapable that clinicians do so with the LP.

Note that Hayhow and Shenker have assumed that the LP is a general therapy template that does not need to be administered in one way only. They illustrate this point by describing how a clinician might make accommodations for a child who has a concomitant cognitive and linguistic impairment or for a child in a family whose cultural background dictates a change in the way the program would be delivered by the child's parents. Hayhow and Shenker demonstrate that the LP is a flexible therapy program; to administer it in one standardized way only and not adapt it to the needs of each client and family would invite failure or at least prolonged therapy.

When Stewart and Leahy (Chapter 10) reflect on the clinical decision making of clinicians who treat adults who stutter, they give the consideration of individual differences an even more central role. That is, they suggest that the very nature of the therapeutic enterprise involves the dynamic interaction of at least two people, the client and the clinician, and a third entity, the therapy approach selected. Thus, it is impossible not to tailor-make therapy to fit its individual participants. Stewart and Leahy's careful delineation of how the inherent features of the therapy process intersect provides a framework for all clinicians to rethink their approach to service delivery regardless of the specific communication disorder tackled.

## SELECTING APPROPRIATE INDIVIDUAL CHARACTERISTICS

Another barrier described by many of the authors in service to fully capitalizing on their clients' individual differences involves knowing how to select the individual differences that would be most fruitful to study. To that end, Teagle and Eskridge (Chapter 12) challenge clinicians to delineate all of the relevant personal factors of their clients that influence the success of using a relatively new technology, that of cochlear implantation. Although the degree of the hearing impairment rendering a client eligible for a cochlear implant is probably the most important criterion for choosing this type of intervention, clinicians must also determine how to weigh additional factors, such as the age of the client, ability to use residual hearing (if any), and so forth.

Hewitt's discussion in Chapter 7 of the individual differences in responses to intervention observed in children and adults diagnosed on the autism spectrum reveals that the although there has been an exponential increase in the information now available about autism spectrum disorders (ASDs), treating the problem—even defining the problem—remains highly complex. In particular, the number of varieties of ASD, with their multiple potential concomitant problems, has continued "to pose a challenge to unraveling commonalities and individual differences alike" (p. 134). In addition, Hewitt mentions that when looking at the trajectories of change observed in children with ASD receiving therapy, one has to consider both within-subject and between-subject variables. With so much potential for individual differences, each client with ASD in therapy might be thought of as exemplifying a natural single-subject design. This fits well with a statement I have frequently heard from clinicians who work with individuals on the autism spectrum: When you meet one child with autism, you have met one child with autism. That is, do not make the mistake of thinking you now understand the scope of the disorder from one observation. There is far too much variability for most practitioners to get a handle on all of the varieties this communication disorder can manifest. It remains for future research to delineate the most salient individual differences for study, although in Chapter 7 Hewitt suggests several as a start including neurobiological underpinnings, sensory differences, and relative cognitive-linguistic competencies.

Vander Woude (Chapter 5) was given the difficult task of considering the individual differences most relevant to consider when providing intervention for preschool age children diagnosed with specific language impairment (SLI). Sometimes referred to as a disorder of exclusion (Paul, 2007), most clinicians know what a child diagnosed with SLI cannot show (e.g., hearing loss, significant cognitive deficit), but that does not mean that a homogeneous group of children with SLI results following diagnosis. Vander Woude delineates several inherent problems in deciding the individual differences to pursue, such as the scope of the disorder (i.e., which language components are affected?), the relative strength of the child's expressive and receptive language skills, differences shown in the maturational trajectories of children with SLI, the presence of variability, and the conversation style the child uses that often is impacted by features of the child's home environment (pp. 81–83). Vander Woude concludes that what we know about language impairment, even SLI, does not yet provide us with a blueprint for how to incorporate individual differences between children with this diagnosis into a direct pathway to the most appropriate therapy program.

## WHY BOTHER WITH INDIVIDUAL DIFFERENCES?

Another question that was addressed by some of the authors was, "What drives the pursuit of the role of individual differences?" One common answer to this question from the authors in this text is the hope that doing so would lead to provision of the best-suited intervention for clients with communication disorders. However, Weiss notes in Chapter 8 that "clinical investigators are generally aware that a one-size-fits-all approach to selecting treatment for speech sound disorders, as Powell (2008) noted, ignores the diversity of potential for change represented by the individual children who make up our clinical caseloads" (p. 165). That is, as pleasant as it might be to find a uniform magic bullet for provision of therapy for the large proportion of our clients who present with difficulties learning the speech sound system of their language, this is not very likely to be the case without the consideration of individual differences.

The danger of not considering individual differences is overlooking factors that may make or break therapeutic success. The particular danger involved in not considering individual differences is described by Hammer and Rodríguez in Chapter 4, which deals with bilingual children's language competencies. Of course, one of the first major decisions that clinicians need to be comfortable with, in dealing with clients on our multilingual and multicultural caseloads, is determining with certainty whether the client is presenting with a language difference or a language disorder. In order to accomplish this, clinicians must be aware of typical, normal differences in language acquisition that have been shown to exist when comparing the language development of monolingual and bilingual speakers. Specifically focusing on children who are native Spanish speakers learning English as a second language in the United States, Hammer and Rodríguez point out that a variety of factors (not always considered by clinicians when working with monolingual clients) must be taken into account, including the client's generational status, the length of time living in the United States, parents' and siblings' language use, gender, age of the client and amount of language exposure, and makeup of the child's larger language community. Although these may not be the individual differences delineated by the other authors in this text, clearly they are pertinent to providing the most accurate diagnosis and, if a disorder is found, the most appropriate intervention. Failure to accurately make the distinction between difference and disorder potentially has serious academic, social, and legal ramifications.

In their chapter, Larrivee and Maloney (Chapter 6) tackle a common question dealt with by classroom teachers, speech-language clinicians, special educators, parents, and school administrators alike: Why is it that although most children learn to read with little difficulty, others find reading to be an almost insurmountable task? This is far from a trivial question. Any nation wanting to compete on the world stage needs a literate population. As a result, millions of state, local, and federal dollars are distributed to school districts and researchers each year in the United States to attempt to find workable solutions to this problem. The authors focus on several prerequisite skill sets necessary for successful literacy learning, suggesting that clinicians cannot assume that all children failing to read represent children with the same needs. Among the individual differences discussed by Larrivee and Maloney are children's levels of phonological awareness, semantics and morphosyntactic knowledge, language comprehension, and their underlying oral language competencies. According to the authors, each of these areas of learning, if representing a deficit in a child's skill repertoire, will need to be addressed, with a resulting improvement in word recognition and/or comprehension, the root skills of reading. Again, as noted by other authors in other chapters, a thorough evaluation of a client's entering competency levels (read: individual differences) should dictate the shape of the intervention program for success to follow.

In a somewhat similar vein, Capone and Sheng (Chapter 3) make it clear that the road to vocabulary learning is not uniform for all children, whether we investigate the child considered to be typically developing or the child who has a bona fide language impairment. Again, understanding what may be contributing to a disordered pattern of vocabulary learning is essential to determining the most appropriate programming to resolve the deficit. This chapter certainly provides ample evidence that not only is vocabulary development not a one-size-fits-all process but that clinicians also cannot assume that they have the luxury of providing a one-size-fits-all solution to the problem.

## RECOMMENDATIONS FOR FUTURE STUDY

The study of individual differences and their impact on therapy planning and therapy success in the field of communication disorders is in an interesting phase. Although our research does not always reflect it, there seems to be an overwhelming, if anecdotal, consensus that the individual differences that our clients present with do matter. In fact, as illustrated by many of the authors in this text, speech-language pathologists and audiologists believe that individual differences are critical to providing the most appropriate services for clients. All of the cases presented here have been compelling; the inclusion of individual differences in thinking through assessment, diagnosis, and the design of therapy is nonnegotiable.

Does this mind-set represent a counterpoint to EBP? I do not believe so. I do believe that sometimes we have a tendency to forget about all of the components of EBP. Specifically, we may find it easy to forget, dismiss, or not give full credence to the importance of clinician experience and client preference. As was apparent with all of the authors, a strong case was made for looking beyond group data supporting one or another therapy approach and asking, "Yes, and how does this fit with what I know about this particular client?"

The statements above were not meant to subvert the importance of large, carefully controlled intervention studies. They are difficult to carry out, to be sure, given the heterogeneity of the populations of persons with communication disorders, but they add essential knowledge for clinical decision making. However, regardless of whether we have an exponential increase in the completion of such studies with their resultant data, I believe that it will always be important for clinicians, from clinicians-in-training to seasoned professionals, to be reminded of the importance of considering who we are treating as individuals. When we consider our clients (and their families, of course) as individuals, we are ultimately providing more comprehensive, better suited intervention and fulfilling the true intention of the dictum of EBP.

I look forward to a time when I can be assured that reading intervention research in our most prestigious journals will always include a delineation of the role of the subjects' individual differences in contributing to the reported results.

## REFERENCES

Paul, R. (2007). *Language disorders from infancy through adolescence: Assessment and intervention* (3rd ed.). St. Louis, MO: Mosby Elsevier.

Powell, T. (2008). The use of nonspeech oral motor treatments for developmental speech sound production disorders: Interventions and interactions. *Language, Speech, and Hearing Services in Schools, 39,* 374–379.

# Author Index

# Subject Index